KU-053-662

Lecture Notes
Immunology

IAN TODD

MA, PhD
Reader in Cellular Immunopathology
University of Nottingham
School of Molecular Medical Sciences
Queen's Medical Centre
Nottingham

GAVIN SPICKETT

MA, DPhil, BM BCh, FRCPath, FRCP, FRCPE
Consultant and Senior Lecturer in Clinical Immunology
Royal Victoria Infirmary
Newcastle upon Tyne

Fifth Edition

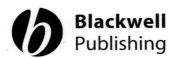

Blackwell
Publishing

© 2005 I. Todd and G. Spickett
© 1987, 1991, 1996, 2000 by Blackwell Science Ltd
Published by Blackwell Publishing Ltd

Blackwell Publishing, Inc., 350 Main Street, Malden, Massachusetts 02148-5020, USA
Blackwell Publishing Ltd, 9600 Garsington Road, Oxford OX4 2DQ, UK
Blackwell Publishing Asia Pty Ltd, 550 Swanston Street, Carlton, Victoria 3053, Australia

The right of the Authors to be identified as the Authors of this Work has been asserted in accordance with the Copyright, Designs and Patents Act 1988.

All rights reserved. No part of this publication may be reproduced, stored in a retrieval system, or transmitted, in any form or by any means, electronic, mechanical, photocopying, recording or otherwise, except as permitted by the UK Copyright, Designs and Patents Act 1988, without the prior permission of the publisher.

First published 1987
Reprinted 1990
Four Dragons edition 1990
Second edition 1991
Four Dragons edition 1991
Third edition 1996
Fourth edition 2000
Reprinted 2002, 2003, 2004
Fifth edition 2005

Library of Congress Cataloging-in-Publication Data
Todd, Ian, Ph. D.
    Lecture notes. Immunology. — 5th ed./Ian Todd, Gavin Spickett.
      p. ; cm.
    Rev. ed. of: Lecture notes on immunology / Gordon Reeves, Ian Todd. 4th ed. 2000.
    Includes bibliographical references and index.
    ISBN-13: 978-1-4051-2662-5 (alk. paper)
    ISBN-10: 1-4051-2662-0 (alk. paper)
    1. Immunology. I. Spickett, Gavin. II. Reeves, W. G. Lecture notes on immunology. III. Title.
    [DNLM: 1. Immune System. 2. Immunity. 3. Immunologic Diseases. QW 504 T634L   2005]
    QR181.R35   2005
    616.07′9—dc22

                                           2004025323

ISBN-13: 978-1-4051-2662-5
ISBN-10: 1-4051-2662-0

A catalogue record for this title is available from the British Library

Set in 8/12 Stone Serif by SNP Best-set Typesetter Ltd., Hong Kong
Printed and bound in India by Replika Press Pvt., Ltd.

Commissioning Editor: Vicki Noyes
Development Editor: Mirjana Misina
Production Controller: Kate Charman
Text and cover designer: Simon Witter

For further information on Blackwell Publishing, visit our website:
http://www.blackwellpublishing.com

The publisher's policy is to use permanent paper from mills that operate a sustainable forestry policy, and which has been manufactured from pulp processed using acid-free and elementary chlorine-free practices. Furthermore, the publisher ensures that the text paper and cover board used have met acceptable environmental accreditation standards.

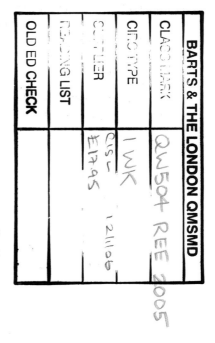

BARTS & THE LONDON QMSMD

CLASS MARK	CIRC TYPE	SUPPLIER	READING LIST	OLD ED CHECK
QW504 REE 2005	1WK	CIG £17.95	12/1/06	

Contents

Preface to the Fifth Edition, vii
From the Preface to the First Edition, viii
Key to Symbols Used in the Figures, ix
An Overview of the Immune System, x

Part 1 Immunity and the Immune System

1   The Nature of Immunity, 3
2   Antigen Recognition, 14
3   Lymphocyte Development and Activation, 28
4   Lymphocyte Interactions, Cytokines and the
    Lymphoid System, 37
5   Immunoglobulins, 50
6   Complement, 64
7   Phagocytes, 71
8   Mast Cells, Basophils and Eosinophils, 77
9   Killer Cells, 84

Part 2 Immunopathology

10   Immunity and Infection, 93
11   HIV Infection and AIDS, 107
12   Immunodeficiency Disorders, 112
13   Inappropriate Responses to Extrinsic and
     Intrinsic Antigens, 128
14   Mechanisms of Immunological Tissue
     Damage, 140
15   Susceptibility to Immunological Disease, 150
16   Lymphoproliferative Disease, 158
17   Transplantation, 170
18   Immunological Therapy, 181

Index, 190

Preface to the Fifth Edition

The first edition of *Lecture Notes on Immunology* that was published in 1987 was conceived and written entirely by Professor Gordon Reeves. The guiding principles, as laid out in the extract from the Preface to the first edition on the following page (p. viii), were to provide an introduction to immunology and its relevance to students of medicine and biology in a straightforward and comprehensible way, avoiding unnecessary detail and jargon. These principles were maintained in successive editions, while updating the text to take account of advances that clarified understanding of the immune system and the application of this knowledge to medicine. The same criteria have been applied in formulating this fifth edition of *Lecture Notes on Immunology*. The topics that have been updated in particular are as follows: innate mechanisms of pathogen recognition; the key role of dendritic cells in the induction of adaptive immunity and the polarization of T cell responses; the nature and function of regulatory T cells; mechanisms of target cell recognition by natural killer cells; HIV infection and AIDS, primary immunodeficiencies, allergies and lymphoproliferative diseases. An entirely new chapter on Immunological Therapy is included that provides an overview of the modern therapeutic applications of immunological understanding. Numerous new diagrams and tables have been added to complement the updated text. Having said this, much of the fabric of the text remains as written by Gordon Reeves in the first to fourth editions of *Lecture Notes on Immunology* and we pay tribute to his talent for distinguishing the essentials of immunology from the 'small print', and presenting these with clarity and literary elegance. We wish him well as he redirects his skills in retirement to the medieval history of Southern France.

Ian Todd
Gavin Spickett

From the Preface to the First Edition

The undergraduate student meeting immunology during a busy medical or biological sciences curriculum or the qualified doctor attempting to get to grips with the subject for specialist training is often daunted by what appears to be an opaque wall of mystifying jargon surrounding a mass of intricate information. The aim of *Lecture Notes on Immunology* is to provide a concise statement covering the basic facts and concepts that are essential for a first understanding of the subject and its relevance to medicine and allied disciplines. Nomenclature has been simplified and appropriately defined and the major principles introduced in a biological setting. Figures and tables are used to summarize or highlight important information and key words are emphasized in the text in bold type.

This text is based on the teaching modules developed in the Nottingham Medical School which have been designed to provide sufficient grounding to enable students to comprehend and utilize developments in immunology in their practice of medicine. Students often feel more comfortable with the detail when they have glimpsed the whole and for this reason the initial chapter outlines the salient features of immunity. These are also summarized in an 'overview of the immune system' presented as the frontispiece. Many of these thoughts have been stimulated by the, often penetrating, questions of first-year students as well as the more clinically informed enquiries of medical graduates and I hope that this text will assist the questioning process.

Gordon Reeves

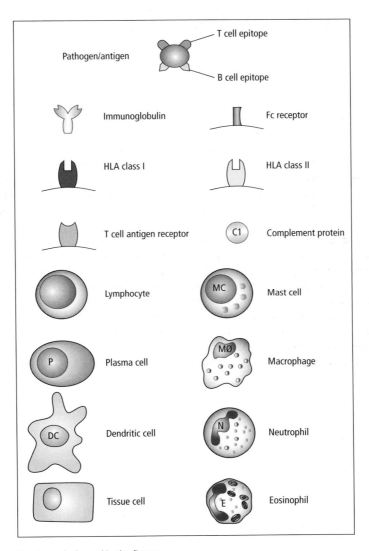

Key to symbols used in the figures.

An overview of the immune system. The upper part concerns the **RECOGNITION** of pathogens and other forms of antigenic material (P/A, pathogen/antigen) that leads to activation of T helper cells (Th0). This process is initiated by signals that induce **innate immunity**. Dendritic cells (DC), which function as the main transducers from innate immunity to **adaptive immunity**, activate Th0 cells by means of antigen presentation and co-stimulation. The innate response also generates polarizing signals (e.g. cytokines such as IL-12 and IL-4), whose nature is determined by the type of infection: intracellular pathogens (e.g. viruses and mycobacteria) induce signals that steer the differentiation of T helper cells into the Th1 subset, whereas extracellular pathogens (e.g. parasitic worms) induce signals that promote Th2 differentiation. These T cells then activate, or promote the differentiation of, other cells of the immune system (e.g. cytotoxic precursor T cells, Tcp) that produce cytotoxins or digestive enzymes and reactive oxygen species (ROS), and release cytokines (cytotoxic T cells, Tc, and macrophages, MØ) or immunoglobulins (plasma cells, PC) mediating **DEFENCE** against the antigen-bearing pathogen (as illustrated in the lower part).

Cytotoxic T cells and macrophages are more effective against intracellular pathogens (e.g. viruses and mycobacteria, respectively) whereas immunoglobulin-mediated activation of complement (C), phagocytes (MØ and neutrophils, N), eosinophils (E) and mast cells (MC) is more effective against extracellular pathogens (e.g. bacteria and parasitic worms). The appearance of macrophages in more than one part of this sequence indicates their ability to respond in different ways depending on the nature of the activating stimulus.

Each component of this overview is described in Chapter 1 and the more detailed chapters that follow.

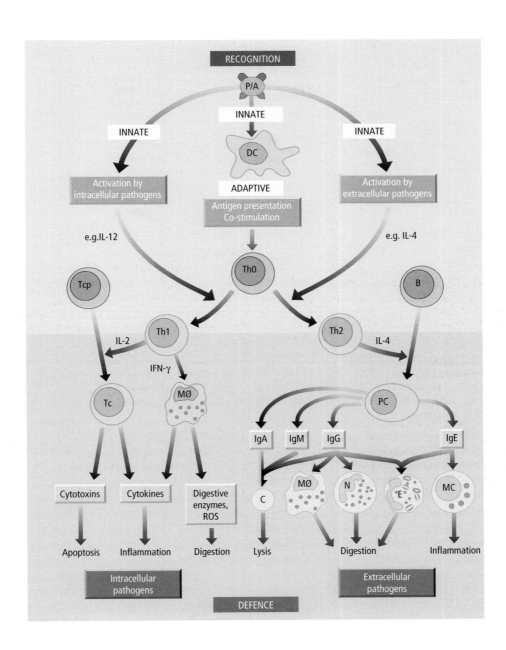

Part 1

Immunity and the Immune System

Chapter 1

The nature of immunity

Infectious diseases, frequently compounded by malnutrition, are still the major cause of illness and death throughout the world. In developed countries, however, the situation has changed dramatically. In Britain, eighteenth-century Bills of Mortality listed cholera, diphtheria, smallpox, tetanus and typhoid as major causes of death whereas today the annual mortality statistics emphasize the importance of cardiovascular disease and cancer. The balance has shifted so much that a series of deaths from a particular infectious disease is likely to precipitate the setting up of a committee of inquiry. These changes have been brought about by the introduction of successful immunization programmes in conjunction with chemotherapy and various public health measures. The key role of the immune system in defence against pathogens of many kinds has recently received dramatic emphasis with the rapid spread of the acquired immunodeficiency syndrome (AIDS). Allergic hypersensitivity and autoimmunity are also disturbances of immunity that cause many other kinds of disease, e.g. asthma and glomerulonephritis. Manipulation of the immune system has become of increasing importance in the treatment of disease and in organ transplantation.

This all began with the centuries-old knowledge that an individual who had recovered from a life-threatening infection, e.g. plague, could subsequently nurse another affected individual without fear of contracting the disease again. He or she had become **immune**. The term **immunity** was originally used to indicate exemption from taxes and this meaning still exists in the term 'diplomatic immunity'.

The sequence of events that led to the global eradication of smallpox in 1980 spans more than two centuries and demonstrates vividly the way in which the immune response can be modified to render a previously life-threatening pathogen ineffective in causing disease.

Variolation and vaccination

It is estimated that over 50 million people died of smallpox in eighteenth-century Europe. In 1712, a duke's daughter from Nottinghamshire, Lady Mary Pierrepont, eloped with a diplomat, Edward Wortley-Montagu, and later travelled with him when he became British Ambassador to Turkey. She wrote from Constantinople in 1717 concerning the local habit of preventing smallpox by inoculating material obtained from smallpox crusts. She introduced it into England with royal patronage following initial experiments on condemned criminals and orphaned children. However, this procedure was not without risk of causing smallpox (variola) itself and the high morbidity and mortality associated with it made others look for less dangerous and more effective ways of controlling the disease.

Edward Jenner—a Gloucestershire family doctor—made the important observation that dairymaids, who frequently contracted cowpox (an infection of the hands acquired during milking), were remarkably resistant to smallpox and did not develop the disfigured pock-marked faces of those who had had smallpox infection. Hence the rhyme:

'Where are you going to, my pretty maid?'
'I'm going a-milking, sir', she said.
'What is your fortune, my pretty maid?'
'My face is my fortune, sir', she said.

Edward Jenner had suffered painfully from variolation performed when he was 8 years old. The increasing spread of smallpox throughout the population led him to develop the alternative technique of vaccination. This was first performed in 1796 when he inoculated material obtained from cowpox pustules into the arm of a healthy boy. He was subsequently able to inoculate him with smallpox more than 20 times without any untoward effect. This courageous experiment aroused much criticism but Jenner offered his new preventive treatment to all who sought it and performed many of his vaccinations in a thatched hut—which became known as the Temple of Vaccinia—in the grounds of his house at Berkeley. Recently, these buildings have been restored and contain a Jenner Museum and Conference Centre.*

Many other forms of immunization have followed from this work and one of the current goals of the World Health Organization's Tropical Disease Programme is to identify immunological ways of controlling and, hopefully, eliminating other major infections, e.g. malaria (against which vector control has largely failed and chemotherapy is becoming less effective).

Several other kinds of immunological manipulation have proved to be of therapeutic benefit, e.g. the administration of specific antibody in the prevention of rhesus haemolytic disease of the newborn. The advent of monoclonal antibodies of many different specificities offers promise for

* Further information can be obtained from the Custodian, The Chantry, Church Lane, High Street, Berkeley, Gloucestershire GL13 9BH, UK.

targeting therapeutic agents to tissues and tumours as well as having many diagnostic applications. Experimental work has shown that the administration of antigen or antibody can be used to turn off specific immune responses—a situation known as immunological tolerance or enhancement. This is of particular relevance to clinical transplantation and the treatment of many immunological and metabolic disorders.

Recognition and defence components

Before considering the complexity of the immune system as it exists, it is useful to consider some of the general design requirements of an immune system in order for it to protect the host organism and display the characteristic features already described. Clearly, the two important biological events are **recognition** of the target pathogen and effective **defence** against it. Using a military analogy, the former is equivalent to reconnaissance and the latter might include artillery support invoked by those in the front line. A major consideration is how many recognition specificities are required and how many kinds of defence, i.e. methods of pathogen destruction, are necessary. The next question to be decided is whether the units that recognize and the units that defend should be combined together or whether a division of labour is preferable in which recognition units and defence units operate as separate entities. These possibilities are illustrated in Figs 1.1 and 1.2, and examples are given in the captions of components of the immune response that use these different strategies.

There exists an enormous variety of infectious pathogens, including many types of viruses, bacteria, fungi, protozoa and multicellular parasites, each with its own mechanisms of transmission, infection and reproduction. This means that no single recognition or defensive strategy is effective against all pathogens and therefore a wide variety of cellular and secreted components are present within the body that collectively constitute the immune system. Examples of the main cells and molecules of the immune system are given in Tables

1.1 and 1.2, respectively. These components vary in terms of whether their main role is recognition or defence, although many possess a combination of these properties.

Innate and adaptive immunity

The cellular components that mediate recognition and defence can be categorized by various criteria, including their developmental lineage from stem cells in the bone marrow (**myeloid** or **lymphoid**), and their morphology as mature blood leucocytes (Table 1.1). **Polymorphonuclear leucocytes** (PMNs) are distinguished from **mononuclear cells** by their lobulated nuclei and they largely coincide with the **granulocytes**

Table 1.1 Cells of the immune system.

Cell type	Developmental lineage	Morphological definition	Type of immunity
Neutrophils	Myeloid	Polymorphonuclear leucocytes or granulocytes	Innate
Eosinophils	"		"
Basophils	"	"	"
Mast cells	"	"	"
Monocytes/macrophages	"	Mononuclear leucocytes	"
Dendritic cells	"	"	"
Natural killer cells	Lymphoid	"	"
Cytotoxic T lymphocytes	"	"	Adaptive
Helper T lymphocytes	"	"	"
B lymphocytes	"	"	"

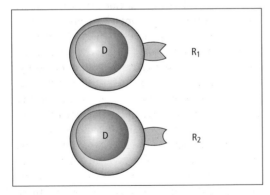

Figure 1.1 Combined recognition (R) and defence (D) units to deal with a pathogenic invader: R and D units with single recognition specificities (exemplified by cytotoxic T cells).

Table 1.2 Secreted mediators of immunity.

Antimicrobial
Antibodies/immunoglobulins (IgM, IgG, IgA, IgE, IgD)
Pentraxins (e.g. C-reactive protein)
Collectins (e.g. mannan-binding lectin)
Complement proteins
Defensins
Lytic enzymes
Interferons
Cytotoxins (perforins, granzymes)

Regulatory/inflammatory
Cytokines (e.g. interleukins, interferons, tumour necrosis factors)
Chemokines (and other chemoattractants)
Eicosanoids (e.g. prostaglandins, leucotrienes)
Histamine

Figure 1.2 Separate recognition (R) and defence (D) units to deal with a pathogenic invader: R units can have different specificities (R₁, R₂, etc.), and interact with different D units (e.g. IgG binding to Fc receptors on neutrophils and IgE binding to Fc receptors on mast cells).

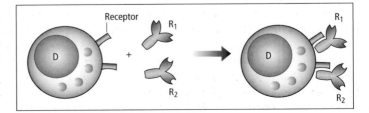

defined by distinctive cytoplasmic granules. The immune system's cellular components can also be considered as mediators of either **innate** or **adaptive immunity** (Table 1.1).

The recognition properties associated with innate immunity may have evolved to recognize chemical structures that are characteristic of infectious pathogens and differ from constituents of host organisms. These include various microbial lipids, carbohydrates, proteins and even nucleic acids that are collectively termed **pathogen-associated molecular patterns (PAMPs)**. They are bound by secreted proteins (e.g. mannose-binding lectin and C-reactive protein) and by cell surface proteins (e.g. macrophage mannose receptor and Toll-like receptors) called **pattern recognition receptors (PRRs)** that are inflexible in their specificities and identical between cells. Innate immunity is rapidly activated in the early stages of an infection and its defensive properties can limit the proliferation and spread of a pathogen within the body. However, it is only moderately efficient in clearing infection, and its capabilities remain the same on repeated exposure to the same microbe.

The resolution of an infection usually requires an additional adaptive immune response by **T lymphocytes** and **B lymphocytes** (often referred to simply as T cells and B cells). Each lymphocyte specifically recognizes an individual **antigen** (usually a protein, but also other types of chemical for B lymphocytes), and there are mechanisms for enhancing the specificity of recognition. Thus, the antigen receptor expressed by a particular lymphocyte is different from that of virtually all other lymphocytes in the body. In addition, the B lymphocytes produce and secrete a soluble form of their antigen receptors called **antibodies** or **immunoglobulins**. An adaptive immune response takes longer to activate than innate immunity but generates more effective defence which improves upon repeated exposure to the same microbe. The details of antigen recognition are considered in Chapter 2, and the development, activation and functions of lymphocytes are described in Chapters 3 and 4; immunoglobulins are considered in Chapter 5.

Cardinal features of adaptive immune responses

It is the cardinal features of adaptive immunity mediated by lymphocytes that Edward Jenner recognized in immunity to smallpox and utilized in the development of vaccination. Furthermore, an individual who is immune to smallpox will not be protected against diphtheria unless he has also met the *Corynebacterium diphtheriae* on a previous occasion. This illustrates the **specificity** of the adaptive immune response. Lymphocytes can detect remarkably small chemical differences between antigens, e.g. subtly differing strains of influenza virus, minor substitutions of a benzene ring, or the difference between dextro and laevo isomers. Were it not for the fact that cowpox and smallpox viruses share important antigens, the experiments of Jenner would have been a dismal failure (although he would not have attempted them without the evidence of the milkmaids).

Another feature of adaptive immune responses is the **memory** that develops from previous experiences of foreign material—a characteristic that enables immunization to be of clinical value. This altered reactivity may last for the entire lifespan of the individual. The ability of an organism to respond more rapidly and to a greater degree when confronted with the same antigen on a second occasion is illustrated in Fig. 1.3. This compares the speed and magnitude of the human response to an antigen that the subjects had not previously encountered (bacteriophage ϕX174). In the first or **primary** response there is a delay of at least 10 days before the antibody level in the circulation reaches its maximum and this level shows considerable variation between individuals, rarely exceeding a titre* of 1000. In the **secondary** response, all individuals respond maximally within 10 days and in all cases the levels attained are of a titre of 10 000 or more. The outcome of an acute infection is often a close race between the activities of the replicating pathogen and the adaptive

---

*The titre is the reciprocal of the weakest dilution of serum at which antibody can still be detected.

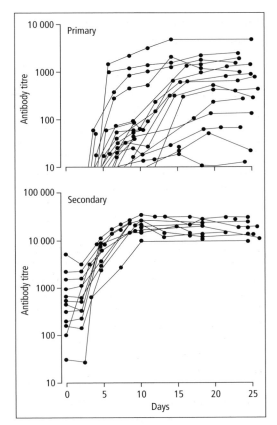

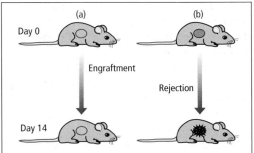

Figure 1.4 Discrimination between self and non-self illustrated by skin grafting in a rodent. (a) The graft was of 'self' type; (b) the graft was from an unrelated animal.

and demonstrate not only the recognition ability of lymphocytes, but also the efficient way in which they fail to react against tissue of 'self' origin. Previously, it was thought that components of the immune system failed to recognize self at all but it is now clear that self-recognition does occur in a controlled and regulated manner such that—except in the special circumstance of autoimmune disease—tissue damage does not take place.

Biological recognition systems

Chemical specificity is a feature of various other biological recognition systems, e.g. enzyme–substrate and nucleotide interactions, although these lack features that characterize immunological responses. It is likely that the recognition component of immune responses has developed from a more basic cellular attribute by which cells are able to recognize each other. Evidence for complementary cell surface interactions has come from several different areas of biological research, e.g. the cellular reaggregation of multicellular invertebrate organisms, such as sponges and slime moulds; the processes whereby cells differentially associate during embryogenesis; the way in which synaptic connections are established in the nervous system; and the recognition events involved in pollination and fertilization. Analogy with these other systems suggests that recognition of self is a primary requirement in phylogeny which, in complex organisms, has developed into a more sophisticated

Figure 1.3 Primary and secondary antibody responses following intravenous injection of bacteriophage φX174 used as a test antigen in humans. (Data kindly provided by Drs Peacock and Verrier Jones.)

immune response and it is for this reason that prior exposure, e.g. to a vaccine, can give the host a considerable advantage.

A third important feature of adaptive immune responses is **self-discrimination**, which is illustrated in Fig. 1.4. If split-skin grafts are placed on the flanks of rodents, it is possible to observe within 2 weeks whether they have healed well and been accepted (Fig. 1.4a) or whether they have been rejected (Fig. 1.4b). In this experiment, the successful graft was obtained from another animal of identical genetic composition (i.e. another member of the same inbred strain). The rejected graft came from an unrelated member of the same species. These chemical differences are relatively minor arrangement whereby reactions to self and non-self have been separately harnessed. Antigens and their recognition are discussed in more detail in Chapter 2.

Stages of an immune response

The different properties of innate and adaptive immunity mean that they are complementary, and they cooperate with each other in order to give the best possible defence. This can be exemplified by considering the stages of a generalized response to a bacterial skin infection (Fig. 1.5). The skin itself constitutes an effective barrier to infection because most microbes cannot penetrate the hard, kera-tinized surface of the epidermis (Fig. 1.5a), but if

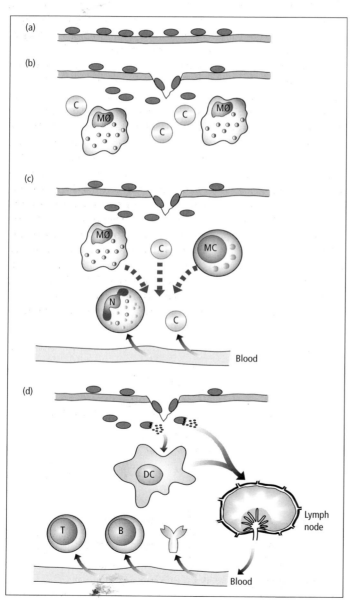

Figure 1.5 Stages of an immune response to bacterial skin infection. (a) Bacteria are unable to penetrate the intact keratinized epithelial barrier; (b) bacterial entry (e.g. via a cut) stimulates an immediate local innate response by tissue macrophages and complement proteins; (c) an early induced inflammatory response is stimulated by inflammatory mediators produced by macrophages, complement proteins and mast cells leading to infiltration by neutrophils from the blood and plasma containing more complement; (d) bacterial antigens are carried in the lymph, and associated with dendritic cells (DC), to draining lymph nodes where specific T and B lymphocytes are activated. These lymphocytes, and antibodies produced by the B cells, return to the infected tissues via the blood circulation.

this is breached (e.g. by a cut), then microbes may infiltrate and start to replicate in the softer underlying dermal tissues. If this is a primary response to infection (because it is the first time this particular microbe has infected the body), then there will be no immunological memory to generate an early adaptive response, but components of the innate immune system that are resident in the infected tissues can be rapidly activated, including **complement proteins** in the tissue fluid and **macrophages** (Fig. 1.5b). The activation of a range of complement proteins triggered by interactions with bacterial surface molecules may result in bacterial **lysis** by the **membrane attack complex** of complement and/or **opsonization** (i.e. coating) of the bacteria by complement proteins that help to adhere the bacteria to the macrophages, which express **complement receptors** as well as the pattern recognition receptors mentioned above. Macrophages are **phagocytes** that can engulf microbes and bring about their **digestion**.

The activation of complement proteins and macrophages not only results in microbial destruction directly, but also induces amplifying events (i.e. **inflammation**). In addition, tissue resident **mast cells**, which are a major source of inflammatory mediators, are activated by complement-derived peptides. These amplifying events can be divided into several categories: local **vasodilatation** and increase in **vascular permeability**; **adhesion** of inflammatory cells to the blood vessel wall; their chemical attraction, i.e. **chemotaxis**; **immobilization** of cells at the site of infection; and **activation** of the relevant cells and molecules to liberate their lytic products (Fig. 1.6). In the present example, the inflammatory mediators induce the influx of leucocytes (particularly **neutrophils** that, like macrophages, are phagocytes) and plasma containing further supplies of complement proteins (Fig. 1.5c).

While the innate response is being established during the first few hours and days of the infection, the processes are being set in train to generate the adaptive response. This involves the transport of microbial components (i.e. antigens) from the site of infection to neighbouring lymphoid tissues, which is where the majority of lymphocytes reside transiently during their circulation around the body. Lymphocytes develop in **primary lymphoid organs**, consisting of **bone marrow** and **thymus**, in the adult. Lymphocytes circulate through **lymph nodes**, the white pulp of the **spleen**, and **mucosa-associated lymphoid tissue** (**MALT**): these locations are referred to as **secondary lymphoid organs** (Fig. 1.7). The total weight of these various lymphoid components can exceed that of the liver. It is at these sites that large

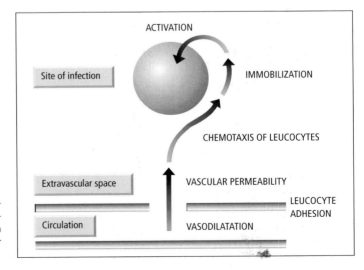

Figure 1.6 Amplifying events involved in the local recruitment of inflammatory cells and molecules from the circulation into an extravascular site of infection.

ACTIVATION

Site of infection

IMMOBILIZATION

CHEMOTAXIS OF LEUCOCYTES

Extravascular space

VASCULAR PERMEABILITY

LEUCOCYTE ADHESION

Circulation

VASODILATATION

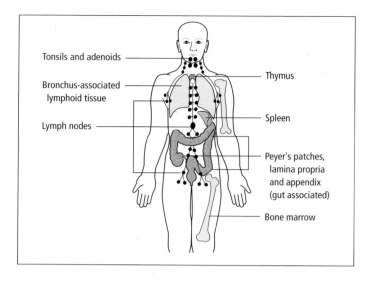

Tonsils and adenoids

Bronchus-associated
lymphoid tissue

Lymph nodes

Thymus

Spleen

Peyer's patches,
lamina propria
and appendix
(gut associated)

Bone marrow

Figure 1.7 The lymphoid system in humans, showing the distribution of primary and secondary lymphoid organs and tissues.

numbers (i.e. hundreds of millions) of the different varieties of lymphocyte come into intimate contact with each other and with specialized **antigen-presenting cells** so as to provide an optimal environment for the activation of the small proportion of the body's lymphocytes that specifically recognize the antigens of a particular microbe. This is why antigens are carried to lymphoid tissues to induce lymphocyte activation rather than these interactions occurring initially within the site of infection. For example, tissue fluid that drains from infected tissues into the lymphatic system may carry microbial antigens to draining lymph nodes where they can be recognized by specific B cells. In addition, microbial antigens are captured and processed by antigen-presenting cells, called **dendritic cells**, which are present in most tissues. The dendritic cells then migrate to the draining lymph nodes where they present the antigens to T cells (Fig. 1.5d). The activated T and B cells return to the blood circulation whence they enter the inflamed, infected tissues, together with antibodies secreted by terminally differentiated B cells called **plasma cells**, in a similar manner to the earlier influx of other leucocytes and complement proteins (Fig. 1.5d). The efficiency of bacterial elimination will then be enhanced by antibodies that opsonize the bacteria, thereby augmenting complement ac-

tivation and phagocytosis, and regulatory proteins called **cytokines** produced by the T cells that increase the antimicrobial activity of the phagocytes.

Some of the T and B cells activated by antigens of the infecting microbe revert to a resting state and constitute the body's population of **memory lymphocytes** specific for that microbe. A subsequent infection with the same, or a closely related (i.e. antigenically similar), microbe would induce a faster and bigger secondary response by these lymphocytes, as described earlier in this chapter.

Immunological defence strategies

The nature of the defensive strategy that the immune system employs in order to eliminate a microbe is determined not only by the biological nature of the microbe, but also by the tissue compartment in which the infection is concentrated. In particular, it is critical whether the microbe remains **extracellular** (i.e. in fluids or at the surfaces of cells of the tissues it infects), or enters the cytoplasm of cells to become **intracellular**. Extracellular pathogens (including many types of bacteria and parasitic worms), which do not cross the plasma membrane of cells, are vulnerable to opsonization by antibodies and complement proteins; bacteria can then be phagocytosed by

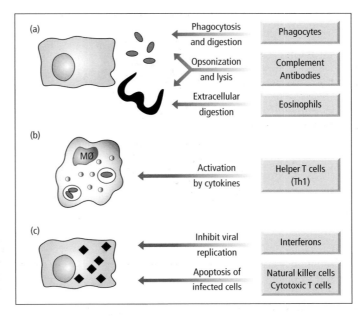

Figure 1.8 Immunological defence strategies. (a) Extracellular pathogens (e.g. bacteria and parasitic worms) are directly exposed to antibodies, complement, phagocytes (macrophages and neutrophils) and eosinophils; (b) microbes that are resistant to digestion (e.g. mycobacteria) can survive intracellularly in macrophage vesicles, but Th1-derived cytokines (e.g. γ-interferon) can enhance the digestive activity of the macrophages; (c) intracellular pathogens, like viruses that generate cytosolic antigens, are targeted by interferons that block their replication, and killer cells (NK and Tc cells) that induce apoptosis of the infected cells.

macrophages and neutrophils and parasitic worms are attacked by eosinophils (Fig. 1.8a). Antibodies and complement proteins are considered in Chapters 5 and 6, respectively, phagocytes in Chapter 7 and eosinophils in Chapter 8. However, some phagocytosed microbes are resistant to intracellular digestion and can survive and replicate in cytoplasmic vesicles of macrophages where they are no longer exposed to antibodies and complement: mycobacteria that cause tuberculosis and leprosy are important examples of this. The macrophages must then be stimulated into a heightened state of activation by cytokines derived from **helper T lymphocytes (Th cells)** in order to overcome the microbes' resistance to digestion (Fig. 1.8b). Some microbes deliberately invade cells: this applies to all viruses, which hijack the metabolic machinery of the cells they parasitize in order to replicate. In order to combat intracellular viruses, **interferons** induce an **antiviral state** in cells, which inhibits viral replication. In addition, **natural killer** (NK) **cells** and **cytotoxic T lymphocytes (Tc cells)**, which are described in Chapter 9, deliberately kill infected cells, thus inhibiting viral replication (Fig. 1.8c).

An overview

The complexities of the immune system often seem rather daunting to the novice, although students usually find the necessary detail more manageable when they can see how the individual parts fit together into a coherent whole. The frontispiece gives a diagrammatic overview of the immune system incorporating the individual components to which reference has already been made and emphasizes the important distinction between those parts of the immune system that specifically recognize the chemical nature of the pathogen and those components that are triggered to act non-specifically and effect its inflammatory destruction. The upper part of the frontispiece concerns the recognition of antigenic material that leads to the activation of helper T cells. These T cells then activate, or promote the differentiation of, other cells of the immune system that mediate defence against the antigen-bearing pathogen (illustrated in the lower part of the frontispiece).

The recognition and defence processes that are effective against intracellular pathogens (e.g. viruses and mycobacteria, as discussed in the preceding section) are shown on the left of the frontispiece. These differ from those, shown on the right, that are involved in immunity to extracellular pathogens (e.g. parasitic worms). The activation of naïve helper T cells (**Th0**) involves both antigen-specific and non-specific elements, and the most important antigen-presenting cells in this context are the dendritic cells. Initially, dendritic cells are activated by PAMPs, and by tissue factors (in the form of cytokines and other inflammatory mediators) derived from both immunological cells (e.g. macrophages, NK cells, mast cells) and other tissue cells (e.g. epithelial cells and fibroblasts). Another view of the signals required for immune response is provided by the 'danger hypothesis'. This states that the antigen recognition that generates an immune response must be accompanied by 'danger signals' released from damaged tissue cells. These signals could include, for example, damaged mitochondria, immature glycosylated proteins or heat shock proteins that bind to innate receptors and provide signals to facilitate an adaptive lymphocyte response to antigen.

The dendritic cells present antigens to the helper T cells and provide co-stimulatory signals that are also necessary for T cell activation. The dendritic cells and other cell types also provide polarizing signals that promote the Th0 cells to differentiate into either **Th1** or **Th2** cells. This is dependent on the nature of the PAMPs and tissue factors that initially activated the innate response: in general, many cell-associated microbes have Th1 polarizing effects, whereas Th2 polarizing signals may predominate during extracellular infections. Cell-mediated immunity against intracellular pathogens is then stimulated by the production of cytokines (e.g. interleukin-2 and γ-interferon) by Th1 cells that promote the activity of cytotoxic T cells and macrophages. The cytokines produced by Th2 cells (e.g. interleukin-4 and interleukin-10) stimulate B cells to make antibodies, which mediate the activation of complement proteins, phago-cytes (e.g. macrophages and neutrophils), eosinophils and mast cells against extracellular pathogens.

The abundance of means by which recognition and defence can be achieved is surprising and begs the question of why so many alternative pathways have developed during evolution. However, there are similarities as well as differences, and the various forms of recognition units, effector systems and lytic processes show considerable homology and may have developed as genetic variants of common ancestral systems. The stimulus for such diversification arises from the enormous task that confronts the immune system, i.e. the constant threat to the survival of the host from a universe of pathogenic organisms ranging from the smallest viruses, through bacteria, protozoa and fungi, to metazoan parasites with their often complex life cycles. The remarkable ability of successful pathogens to evolve mechanisms by which they can evade the immune response adds a further dimension, which is considered in detail in Chapter 10.

Immunopathology

The outcome for the host is often 'survival at a price' and damage to host tissues by the immune system is a common finding during the course of most infectious diseases—a situation referred to as **hypersensitivity** or **allergy**. Furthermore, the development of **autoimmunity** (i.e. immune recognition of self components) is not uncommon during infection and the chronicity of these reactions may be related to the difficulties involved in eliminating certain pathogens from host cells. Some pathogens are also able to initiate various forms of **lymphoproliferative disease** and can cause **immunodeficiency**. **Immunopathology** is comprised of these various deviations from the ideal, many examples of which are found in human disease. These are described in Part 2.

Key points

1 Immunity provides protection against pathogenic organisms, and the functions of the immune system are recognition of these foreign pathogens and defence of the body against them.

2 A wide variety of cells and secreted molecules necessarily constitute the immune system in order to deal with the vast array of pathogenic organisms that can infect the body.

3 Innate and adaptive immunity constitute the two main arms of the immune system which differ in their recognition and activation properties. Adaptive immunity improves upon repeated exposure to the same antigens.

4 Lymphocytes are responsible for the specificity, memory and self-discrimination of adaptive immune responses, as exemplified in vaccination.

5 The early innate response to infection stimulates an inflammatory response and initiates the processes that result in the adaptive lymphocyte response.

6 Defence is mediated by a range of innate and adaptive cells and molecules that stimulate inflammation and cause digestion or lysis of foreign pathogens or infected cells. Different defence mechanisms are required to deal with extracellular pathogens, and with intracellular pathogens either in macrophage vesicles or in the cytosol.

7 Pathogens whose infectious cycles are intracellular usually induce Th1 cells and cell-mediated immunity. Extracellular pathogens usually induce Th2 cells and antibody-mediated immunity.

8 Activation of the immune system can also lead to damage to host tissues and some pathogens can induce abnormal proliferation of the lymphoid system or cause it to become deficient. These together constitute the various forms of immunopathology.

Chapter 2

Antigen recognition

Lymphocytes, as the immunocompetent cells of the immune system, are collectively endowed with the ability to recognize and respond to a wide variety of **antigens**. Most biological materials can serve as antigens, which function either as **immunogens** or **tolerogens** depending on the effect they have on lymphocytes. The recognition and binding of an immunogen by lymphocytes results in the induction of an immune response against the antigenic substance. However, tolerogens induce a specific immunological response of a negative kind, known as **immunological tolerance**, in which an individual becomes specifically unresponsive to subsequent challenge with a normally immunogenic form of the same material.

Factors governing immunogenicity

Whether an antigen induces an immune response or not (i.e. has **immunogenicity**) is dependent on a variety of factors.

Nature of the antigen

1 Macromolecular proteins are the most potent immunogens, but polysaccharides, glycoproteins, synthetic polypeptides and synthetic polymers can also be immunogenic. Lipids and nucleic acids are not usually immunogenic unless conjugated to a protein moiety. Nucleoproteins readily induce antibodies reactive with nucleic acids. The more structurally complex a molecule is, the greater is the likelihood of it being immunogenic in most individuals.

2 Smaller molecules are less immunogenic and the smaller the molecule the greater is the variation in response between individuals. The threshold for immunogenicity varies but is of the order of 1500 daltons (Da) molecular weight.

3 Charged residues tend to contribute to the specificity of immunogens as they are usually expressed on the hydrophilic surface of the molecule but uncharged molecules such as dextrans can be immunogenic.

4 The degree of foreignness of a molecule is an important factor. Thus, molecules exhibiting the greatest differences from constituents of the responding animal are usually the most immunogenic, and molecules that do not elicit an immune response in their normal state may do so when denatured. Aggregated molecules tend to be immunogenic, whereas aggregate-free proteins administered in soluble form can induce tolerance.

Exposure to the antigen

1 Every antigen has an optimum dose for immunogenicity and in experimental systems doses substantially lower or higher than the optimum can induce 'low zone' tolerance (principally in T cells) or 'high zone' tolerance (in both T and B cells), respectively.

2 Intermittent immunization usually produces a greater response than a period of continuous administration of antigen.

3 The route of immunization is also of importance: oral administration of antigen can induce tolerance to subsequent challenge via the usually immunogenic parenteral route (the Schulzberger–Chase phenomenon).

4 Experimentally, the immune response is usually increased by mixing the antigen with a powerful adjuvant, e.g. a mycobacterial extract, which intensifies the inflammatory response non-specifically.

Nature of the recipient

1 Exposure of very young animals (and of immature lymphocytes generally) to an antigen will often induce tolerance rather than immunity. The immune system also becomes less efficient in the elderly.

2 Significant genetic effects can be observed when relatively 'simple' antigens of modest size are used (e.g. insulin). Thus, animals of a single species, but possessing different relevant genes, may differ in their ability to respond to such antigens. This variation has been shown to associate with particular phenotypes of both the human leucocyte antigen (HLA) and immunoglobulin allotype systems (see pp. 25 and 53).

3 Malnutrition or metabolic disturbances (as in uncontrolled diabetes) impair immune responsiveness.

Receptor–antigen interactions

B and T lymphocytes possess different surface receptors for antigens, and immunoglobulins or antibodies are a secreted form of the receptors expressed by B cells. The part of an antigen recognized by the **antigen combining sites** of these receptors is called an **antigenic determinant** or **epitope**, and usually consists of a small portion of the foreign material (Fig. 2.1). Studies using defined antigens have indicated that the size of an antigenic determinant recognized by an antibody's combining site is roughly equivalent to a tetrapeptide or hexasaccharide. Thus, even some of the

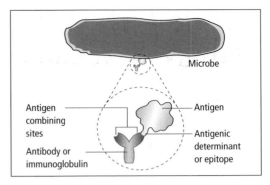

Figure 2.1 The interaction between an antibody and an antigen.

simplest viruses or bacterial toxins possess numerous potential determinants.

The binding of an antigenic determinant to a receptor combining site is analogous to hormone–receptor or substrate–enzyme interactions in being dependent on non-covalent intermolecular attractive forces. Both electrostatic interactions (ionic, hydrogen bonding and van der Waals forces) and hydrophobic interactions contribute to this binding. These can only occur if the epitope and combining site come into very close contact. Strong association is therefore dependent on a close fit between the determinant and combining site to maximize the opportunities for attractive interactions between complementary chemical groups in appropriate positions. Thus, an antibody, for example, shows **specificity** for an epitope whose shape and charge properties are complementary to those of its own combining site, so that they bind together with a high **affinity**. The same antibody lacks specificity for an antigenic determinant with a very different shape and/or charge for which its binding affinity is negligible. If, however, they are sufficiently complementary to show a degree of interaction, then the antibody is said to **cross-react** with this other determinant (Fig. 2.2).

Antigen receptors of B and T lymphocytes

The first antigen-specific recognition units of the immune system to be identified were the immunoglobulins. These are secreted by plasma cells

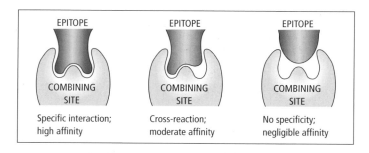

Specific interaction; high affinity

Cross-reaction; moderate affinity

No specificity; negligible affinity

Figure 2.2 The interaction between an antigen combining site and epitopes of different shapes.

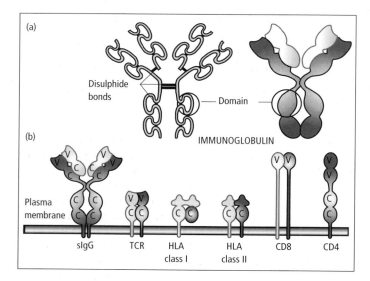

Figure 2.3 Members of the immunoglobulin superfamily. (a) Two representations of the domain structure of an immunoglobulin; (b) some immunoglobulin-related molecules showing the occurrence of C-like and V-like domains (although the V-like domains in CD4 and CD8 are not actually variable). TCR, T cell receptor for antigen.

derived from activated B cells. The polypeptide chains of immunoglobulins are made up of a series of disulphide-bonded peptide loops of β-pleated sheets called **domains**, which are composed of sequences of about 110 amino acids. A number of protein molecules expressed on the surface of lymphocytes and other cells involved in immune responses contain domains that show considerable similarity in amino acid sequence and three-dimensional structure to immunoglobulin domains. These molecules constitute the **immunoglobulin superfamily**, and some of them are illustrated in Fig. 2.3.

B lymphocytes express immunoglobulin molecules in their surface membranes and these can be detected by immunofluorescence (see Chapters 4

and 5). Surface immunoglobulins are the B cell receptors for antigen (Figs 2.3 and 2.4), and differ in structure from secreted immunoglobulins (described in Chapter 5) in having a carboxyterminal amino acid sequence which anchors them in the cell membrane. A receptor is made up of two identical heavy chains (molecular weight between 50 000 and 70 000 Da each) and two identical light chains (molecular weight 25 000 Da). It has a pair of identical binding sites for antigen, each composed of the **variable** (V) domains of one heavy and one light chain (Fig. 2.4), which vary in amino acid sequence among the large variety of receptors with different antigenic specificities. The **constant** (C) domains do not contribute directly to antigen recognition and differ within heavy chains

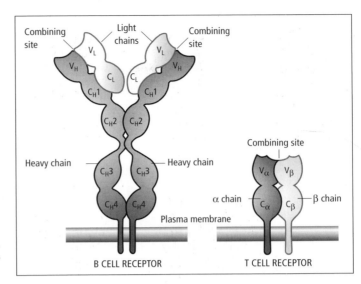

Figure 2.4 The structure of B- and T-cell receptors for antigen (the former exemplified by monomeric IgM).

only between the five **classes** of immunoglobulins (IgM, IgD, IgG, IgA and IgE), and differ within light chains between the two types, κ and λ, both of which can associate with the five types of heavy chains.

The T cell receptor for antigen (often called the **TCR**) is a member of the immunoglobulin superfamily (Fig. 2.3) and consists of two polypeptide chains (α and β), which form a disulphide-linked dimer. The α and β chains each have one constant domain proximal to the cell membrane and one variable domain. The two variable domains form the single combining site of the receptor distal to the cell membrane (Fig. 2.4). A minority of T cells express an alternative form of receptor composed of γ and δ chains instead of α and β chains. The overall structure of the γδ dimer is similar to the αβ receptor, containing two constant and two variable domains. Although the role of γδ-expressing T cells has yet to be clarified, they accumulate in the intestinal epithelium and may be important in the response to infection and in immune regulation.

All the antigen receptors expressed by a single B or T cell have identical combining sites so that each lymphocyte has a particular antigenic specificity. The individual possesses about 10^8 varieties of lymphocyte receptor and it is this diversity of receptors that endows the immune system with the

potential to respond to a vast array of antigens, any of which may gain entry to the body. The genetic mechanisms underlying the generation of this diversity are described in Chapter 5.

The proliferation of a lymphocyte will result in a **clone** of cells with receptors of identical specificity. From the repertoire of specificities available, an antigen will selectively interact with those clones of lymphocytes whose receptors bind it with highest affinity, resulting in their activation and proliferation. It is this **clonal selection** that ensures that an immune response is specific for the immunizing antigen (Fig. 2.5).

Antigen recognition by B and T lymphocytes

The form in which antigen is recognized and bound by receptors on B and T lymphocytes is very different (Fig. 2.6). This reflects the different functions of B and T cells following activation by antigen.

An activated B cell can mature into a plasma cell which secretes large numbers of antibody molecules with the same antigenic specificity as the receptors of the B cell from which it arose (Fig. 2.6). The function of antibody molecules is to bind directly to the stimulating antigen (which may, for

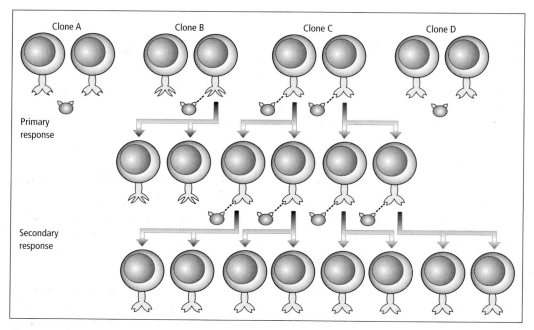

Figure 2.5 Clonal selection of specific lymphocytes by antigen recognition. Clone C interacts with the epitope with high affinity, clone B shows moderate affinity, while the interactions with clones A and D are negligible. Thus, competition between lymphocytes for interaction with the antigen results in clone C being preferentially selected by the antigen for activation and proliferation, with some selection of clone B. Note that this competition leads to increasing specificity of the response upon repeated exposure to the antigen.

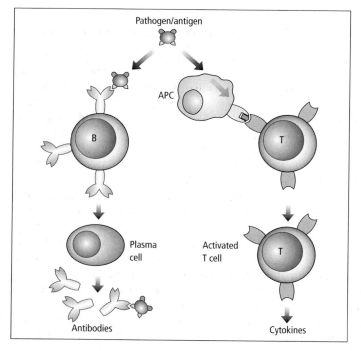

Figure 2.6 A comparison of antigen recognition by B and T lymphocytes. APC, antigen-presenting cell.

example, be a bacterium or a virus) and thereby either neutralize its activity or trigger immune defence mechanisms which bring about its elimination. In practice this means that a B cell antigen receptor or an antibody can interact with an antigen in its native, unmodified state, e.g. on the surface of a bacterium or in free solution (Fig. 2.6). It is thus not surprising that epitopes recognized by B cells and antibodies are often the most accessible regions on the surface of antigen molecules.

T cells have two main functions, both of which involve effects on other cells. **T helper (Th) cells** activate other cells of the immune system, particularly B cells and macrophages. **T cytotoxic (Tc) cells** kill infected cells and, sometimes, cancer cells. Thus, T cells are required to interact with other cell types to achieve their functional effects. This may explain why, in contrast to B cells, T cells can only recognize, and be activated by, antigen bound to specialized cell surface glycoproteins (called **HLA molecules** in humans) encoded by genes of the **major histocompatibility complex (MHC)** (see p. 25). Cells bearing surface antigen bound to HLA molecules are termed **antigen-presenting cells** if their role is to activate T cells (Fig. 2.6), or **target cells** if they are killed by T cells.

T cell receptors do not bind antigen or HLA molecules alone, and only bind effectively to a combination of both. This is called **associative** or **dual recognition**. Most unmodified antigens are unable to associate effectively with HLA molecules, but can do so when they have been processed by the antigen-presenting cell. **Antigen processing** involves partial degradation by enzymes to yield peptides, some of which are of the appropriate length and amino acid sequence to bind to HLA molecules and hence can serve as T cell epitopes (see p. 23). These antigenic determinants can be derived from any part of the original antigen and thus, unlike the B cell epitopes discussed above, may not be exposed on the surface of the antigen in its native configuration. A corollary of this is that B and T cells may interact with totally different epitopes yet still show specificity for the same overall antigen. This is illustrated in Fig. 2.7 using

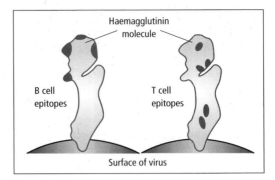

Figure 2.7 Immune recognition of the influenza haemagglutinin molecule. The dark shading indicates the regions of the antigen recognized by B cells (and antibodies) or by T cells.

as an example the haemagglutinin protein expressed on the surface of the influenza virus. The epitopes recognized by antibodies (and B cell receptors) are accessible on the exposed parts of the native molecule. By contrast, as a result of antigen processing, peptides that can associate with HLA molecules and be recognized by specific T cell receptors may originate from internal, as well as external, regions of the haemagglutinin protein.

The HLA system and its proteins

Although the physiological role of cell surface glycoproteins encoded within the **major histocompatibility complex** (MHC) is to present antigenic determinants to T cells, these molecules were initially identified by their role in transplant rejection. Indeed, they were found to play the most significant (*major*) part in determining whether a tissue transplant is recognized as foreign or not (*histocompatibility*).

Considerable interest in the biochemical uniqueness of the individual followed the introduction of organ transplantation in the 1960s. Although blood group antigen systems were already well defined, it soon became clear that the individual tissue type was of paramount importance in determining the rate and severity of graft rejection. Tissue exchanged between genetically identical members of the same species is tolerated indefinitely, whereas the exchange of tissue between genetically different members of the same species, and between members of different species, are both followed by the development of graft-reactive T cells and antibodies, culminating in rejection of the foreign tissue. (The discrimination between self and foreign material is presented as a cardinal feature of the immune system on p. 7, and the details of tissue transplant rejection are considered in Chapter 17.) The MHC genes exist in a large number of alternative (allelic) forms in different individuals (i.e. they exhibit **polymorphism**). This results in significant differences in the amino acid sequences of MHC proteins from one individual to another. It is these differences that permit tissue transplants between individuals to be recognized as foreign by the recipient's lymphocytes.

The structure of HLA molecules

The unravelling of the human MHC has largely been achieved by documenting protein variations on the surfaces of peripheral blood leucocytes; hence the term **human leucocyte antigen** (HLA) system. Multiple pregnancies or blood transfusions often induce antibodies to these HLA proteins because of the allelic differences between mother and fetus or donor and recipient, and sera from such individuals have been used to type for these proteins. This is why HLA proteins are referred to as 'antigens'.

There are two main forms of HLA glycoproteins, called **class I** and **class II**. HLA class I and II molecules are made up of different types of polypeptide chains but they are both members of the immunoglobulin superfamily (Fig. 2.3). Their overall three-dimensional structures are similar and they both bind antigenic peptides for presentation to T cell receptors (Fig. 2.8). HLA class I glycoproteins are expressed on the surface of almost all nucleated cells. They consist of a large α polypeptide chain (molecular weight 45 000 Da) and a smaller polypeptide of 12 000 Da known as β_2-microglobulin (Fig. 2.8). The former contains three domains designated α_1, α_2 and α_3 with the lowermost part of the α chain extending through the cell membrane into the cytoplasm. The single domain of β_2-microglobulin associates non-covalently with the α chain. The α_3 domain and β_2-microglobulin are proximal to the cell membrane and are structurally related to immunoglobulin constant domains (Fig. 2.3). The α_1 and α_2 domains are distal to the cell membrane and together form an antigen-binding groove, the walls of which are two α helices lying across a platform of β-pleated sheet (Fig. 2.9a). The groove can accommodate an antigenic peptide of eight or nine amino acids (Fig. 2.9a) and a T cell receptor can bind simultaneously to the exposed surface of the epitope and the regions of the HLA molecule around the perimeter of the groove (Fig. 2.8).

The expression of HLA class II molecules is mainly confined to cells directly involved in immune responses, i.e. macrophages, other antigen-presenting cells (e.g. dendritic cells and

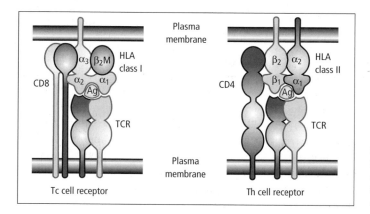

Figure 2.8 The structure of HLA class I and II glycoproteins, and their interactions with antigenic determinants (Ag), T cell receptors (TCR) and CD8 or CD4. β_2M, β_2-microglobulin.

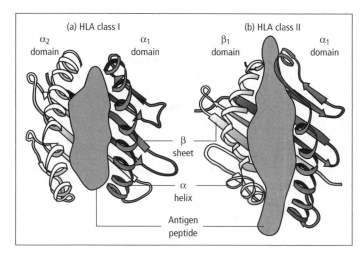

Figure 2.9 The three-dimensional structure of (a) HLA class I and (b) HLA class II antigen peptide-binding grooves which are formed by two α helices lying on a platform of β-pleated sheet. The HLA class II binding groove has open ends and can accommodate longer antigenic peptides than the HLA class I binding groove with closed ends.

Langerhans' cells), B cells and activated T cells. HLA class II molecules are heterodimers of α and β polypeptide chains (33 000 and 28 000 Da, respectively); each chain contains two polypeptide domains and traverses the cell membrane (Fig. 2.8). As with class I proteins, the two domains of HLA class II molecules proximal to the cell membrane (α_2 and β_2) show marked structural homology to other members of the immunoglobulin superfamily (Fig. 2.3). The distal domains (α_1 and β_1) form an antigen-binding groove similar to that of HLA class I molecules, except that the groove of HLA class II molecules has open ends so that longer antigenic peptides of 12–20 amino acids can be accommodated (Fig. 2.9b).

Antigenic peptides bound to HLA class I proteins are recognized by T cells that express, in addition to their antigen receptors, a protein called **CD8**, whereas the T cells that interact with HLA class II-associated peptides express **CD4** protein (see Table 2.1 for the definition of CD molecules). This is because, as illustrated in Fig. 2.8, CD8 molecules interact with the α_3 domain of HLA class I, and CD4 with the β_2 domain of HLA class II (i.e. at sites distinct from the antigen-binding groove engaged by the TCR), thus enhancing the overall interaction between the T cell and the antigen-bearing cell. CD4 and CD8 are also involved, together with CD3 (see p. 31), in triggering T cell activation via cytoplasmic tyrosine kinases. Normally, approximately

Table 2.1 Examples of CD molecules.

CD designation	Function/description
CD2	Receptor for LFA-3 (CD58)
CD3	TCR-associated triggering molecule
CD4	HLA class II binding molecule
CD8	HLA class I binding molecule
CD11/CD18	The two chains of leucocyte integrins: receptors for ICAM-1 (CD54)
CD25	Receptor for interleukin-2
CD28	Co-stimulatory molecule on T cells: receptor for B7.1 (CD80) and B7.2 (CD86)
CD40	Co-stimulatory molecule on B cells: receptor for CD40 ligand
CD45	Protein tyrosine phosphatase which activates tyrosine kinases which interact with CD3 and CD4/CD8
CD49/CD29	The two chains of the VLA integrins: receptors for VCAM-1 (CD106) and connective tissue proteins
CD62	Selectins

The CD nomenclature has been devised to catalogue cell surface molecules as they are identified and characterized. These molecules are often initially defined on certain cell types by producing monoclonal antibodies (see p. 61), which bind to them specifically. CD stands for 'cluster of differentiation', referring to the *cluster* of monoclonal antibodies that define a particular *differentiation* molecule. Over 240 CD molecules have been designated. Some examples referred to in this chapter and in Chapters 3 and 4 are listed here.

BARTS & THE LONDON Queen Mary's School of Medicine & Dentistry

65% of T cells in the blood circulation are CD4+ and 35% are CD8+, although this bias is reversed in some diseases. There are important functional associations of these phenotypes, because most Th cells express CD4, whereas most Tc cells express CD8 (see Table 2.2).

Antigen processing and antigen-presenting cells

An important function of Tc cells is to eliminate other cells that could be detrimental to the body as a whole, e.g. virus-infected cells. Because most cell types can become infected by different types of viruses, it is important that all cells are subject to

surveillance by Tc cells. This is achieved by the expression of CD8 by most Tc cells, which restricts them to the recognition of antigen associated with HLA class I, and the fact that most cell types of the body do express HLA class I molecules (Table 2.2). Figure 2.10 illustrates this recognition of a virus-infected **target cell** by a Tc cell. Viruses do not possess the biological machinery necessary to replicate their own genetic material, and can only proliferate by infecting cells and subverting cellular components for their own ends. Tc cells prevent this replication by specifically recognizing and killing virus-infected cells; this would not be achieved if Tc cells had receptors that could directly recognize free viral particles as antigens.

Table 2.2 Relationship between T cell phenotype, HLA restriction and function.

T cell type	HLA restriction	HLA distribution	Immune function
CD8+ Tc	Class I	Most cells	Surveillance of all cells, e.g. for viral infection
CD4+ Th	Class II	Mainly immune cells	Controlled and appropriate way activation of immune cells

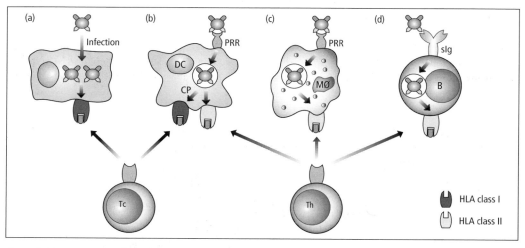

Figure 2.10 Presentation of antigenic peptides associated with HLA class I or II determined by antigen processing pathway and antigen-presenting cell type. (a) Infection of cells leads to processing of cytosolic antigens to generate peptides that associate with HLA class I for recognition by CD8+ Tc cells. (b) Dendritic cells (DC) take up antigens into vesicles by binding to pattern recognition receptors (PRR) as illustrated here, by macropinocytosis, or via Fc receptors and complement receptors if the antigens are opsonized by antibodies and complement (see Fig 7.3), leading to the generation of peptides that are presented by HLA class II to CD4+ Th cells. Dendritic cells also divert antigens into the class I processing pathway (CP, cross-presentation) for priming of Tc cells. (c) Macrophages bind antigens via PRRs as illustrated here, or via Fc receptors and complement receptors if the antigens are opsonized by antibodies and complement (see Fig 7.3): this leads to class II-associated presentation. (d) B cells bind antigens specifically to surface immunoglobulins (sIg), leading to endocytosis and presentation by HLA class II.

The route or processing pathway whereby antigenic peptides are generated for binding to HLA class I molecules is shown in Fig. 2.11. These peptides are produced endogenously, being generated from proteins synthesized in the cell and transported to the cytosol. They signal to the Tc cells that the target cell is a source of antigens (e.g. infectious viral particles) and should therefore be killed. Protein antigens present in the cytosol are degraded in an enzyme complex called a proteasome, which is present in all cells. The physiological role of proteasomes is to degrade cellular proteins that are marked for disposal by conjugation with ubiquitin, e.g. because they have misfolded during synthesis or have been chemically damaged. In virally infected cells, a large proportion of the proteins synthesized are of viral, rather than cellular origin, but some of these viral antigens will again be earmarked for proteasomal degradation. Some of the antigenic peptides generated by the proteasomes are transferred to the endoplasmic reticulum via peptide transporter proteins. Peptides of appropriate length (eight or nine amino acids) and amino acid sequence associate with newly synthesized HLA class I molecules that are held in the endoplasmic reticulum adjacent to the peptide transporters by stabilizing proteins (calreticulin, Erp57 and tapasin). The HLA class I molecules then serve as couriers to deliver the peptide fragments of the endogenous antigens to the cell surface and present them to specific Tc cells, thus focusing cytotoxic activity where it is most needed.

Th cells are usually activated by dendritic cells and their role is then to help other cells of the immune system, such as macrophages and B lymphocytes, to become activated in order to fulfil their effector functions. These **professional antigen-presenting cells** (dendritic cells, macrophages and B cells) express HLA class II molecules, whereas most tissue cell types do not. Th cells express CD4, thereby restricting them to the recognition of antigen associated with HLA class II and directing them to interact with these other cells of the immune system (Table 2.2; Fig 2.10).

The processing pathway for antigens that associate with HLA class II molecules is shown in Fig. 2.12. This requires protein antigen to enter a cytoplasmic vesicle called an **endosome**, which occurs when exogenous antigen is engulfed by a process termed **endocytosis**. This is initiated when antigenic material is bound to specialized cell surface receptors; for dendritic cells and macrophages these include pattern recognition receptors (e.g. DEC-205 and macrophage mannose receptor) that are widely expressed by these innate cell types

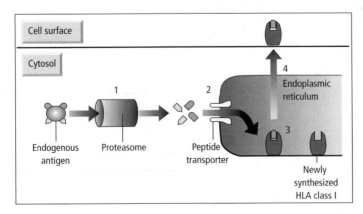

Figure 2.11 Processing of antigen for presentation by HLA class I. (1) Protein antigens present in the cytosol are degraded in an enzyme complex called a proteasome; (2) some of the peptides generated are transferred to the endoplasmic reticulum via peptide transporter proteins; (3) peptides of appropriate length (eight or nine amino acids) and amino acid sequence associate with newly synthesized HLA class I molecules; (4) the peptide–HLA complexes are transported to the cell surface where they are available for recognition by T cells.

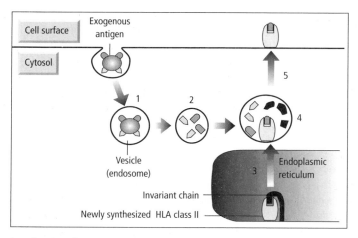

Figure 2.12 Processing of antigen for presentation by HLA class II. (1) Endocytosis of exogenous protein antigen leads to its internalization into a vesicle; (2) enzymes entering the vesicle degrade the antigen; (3) newly synthesized HLA class II molecules in the endoplasmic reticulum associate with the invariant chain and are transported to the vesicle; (4) the invariant chain is degraded and antigen peptides of the appropriate length and amino acid sequence associate with the class II molecules; (5) the peptide–HLA complexes are transported to the cell surface where they are available for recognition by T cells.

(Fig 2.10); in addition, both dendritic cells and macrophages express Fc receptors and complement receptors that enable them to bind and phagocytose antigens that have been opsonized (i.e. coated) with antibodies and/or complement proteins (this is described in Chapter 7 and illustrated in Fig 7.3). Dendritic cells also continually engulf large quantities of surrounding fluid (which may contain antigens) by a process called **macropinocytosis**. By contrast, B cells endocytose antigens that bind with high affinity to their specific surface immunoglobulins, i.e. antigens are processed and presented only by those B cell clones that recognize them specifically (Fig 2.10). Peptides are generated by degradation of the antigens in the endosomes by enzymes called **cathepsins**. Newly synthesized HLA class II migrates to the vesicle from the endoplasmic reticulum in association with a protein called the **invariant chain**, part of which occupies the peptide-binding groove; this is why HLA class II molecules, unlike HLA class I, do not bind peptides within the endoplasmic reticulum. In the vesicle, the invariant chain is itself degraded, apart from a fragment occupying the peptide-binding groove called the CLIP peptide.

The release of CLIP and loading of antigenic peptide into the peptide-binding groove is facilitated by an HLA class II-like molecule called HLA-DM (see p. 25). The class II molecule then transports the peptide to the cell surface for presentation to Th cells.

Because naïve T cells are initially activated (primed) by dendritic cells, the question arises as to how CD8⁺ Tc cells are primed because most microbes do not infect dendritic cells to generate endogenously produced antigens for presentation by HLA class I. The answer is that dendritic cells have the specialized property of **cross-presentation** or **cross-priming** whereby exogenous antigens or their peptides are diverted into the class I processing pathway for presentation to CD8⁺ T cells (Fig 2.10). Once activated in this way, Tc cells can interact with and kill infected tissue cells presenting copies of the same peptides. The reason why dendritic cells are particularly good at activating naïve Th and Tc cells is because, as well as presenting antigenic peptides, they are a potent source of additional co-stimulatory signals when activated, as discussed in Chapters 3 and 4.

The HLA complex of genes

The genes encoding HLA molecules form a cluster or complex of loci on chromosome 6 (Fig. 2.13). The first genetic loci encoding HLA molecules to be described were HLA-A and HLA-B followed by HLA-C. These genes encode the α chains of three class I molecules that are expressed on most cells (β_2-microglobulin is encoded elsewhere in the genome). Other class I genes have been identified in the class I region and are termed **MHC class IB genes**. The functions of the proteins they encode are not fully understood but include presenting relatively invariant and, in some cases, non-peptide antigens to particular subsets of T cells (see Chapter 3). In addition, some MHC class IB proteins (e.g. HLA-G, which is expressed on placental extravillous trophoblast during fetal gestation, and HLA-E) may be involved in protecting certain tissues from attack by **natural killer cells** (see Chapter 9), whereas others (MICA and MICB) promote natural killer activity.

Three HLA class II molecules (HLA-DP, HLA-DQ and HLA-DR) are encoded by genes for their α and β chains within the HLA complex (Fig. 2.13). The HLA-DR locus contains three functional genes: one α and two β genes, whereas the HLA-DQ and -DP loci each have genes encoding one α and one β chain.

The HLA complex also contains genes coding for other immunological components (Fig. 2.13). Within the HLA class II region are genes encoding proteasome components (LMP-1 and LMP-2), peptide transporter proteins (TAP-1 and TAP-2) and tapasin (TAPBP) involved in the MHC class I antigen-processing pathway; also HLA-DM, an HLA class II-like molecule involved in the MHC class II antigen-processing pathway (see p. 24), and HLA-DO (DNαDOβ) which is a negative regulator of HLA-DM. Within what is termed the HLA class III region, there are also genes coding for complement proteins C2, factor B (Bf) and C4 (see Chapter 6), and the cytokines tumour necrosis factor (TNF) α and β (see Chapter 4).

HLA polymorphism

The genes for both HLA class I and II molecules exist in a much larger number of allelic forms than is the case for most tissue proteins, and are therefore said to be **polymorphic**. The regions of the HLA molecules in which this variability mainly occurs form the antigen-binding groove, which interacts with both antigenic determinants and the antigen receptors of T cells. It is for these reasons that the MHC molecules, expressed in tissue transplanted from one individual to another, are recognized as foreign by T cells of the recipient, leading to an antigraft immune response (see Chapter 17). By contrast, T cells that would react with self HLA in the absence of a foreign antigen are eliminated as part of the censoring process which occurs in the thymus (see pp. 31–3).

Because allelic HLA molecules have differences in their binding grooves, they show preferences for interaction with particular antigenic peptides and T cell receptors. In extreme cases, an individual may be unable to make an immune response to a particular antigenic determinant because this peptide may not bind to the MHC molecules of the individual (Fig. 2.14b); alternatively, T cells capable of recognizing the MHC–antigen combination

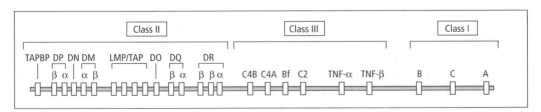

Figure 2.13 Genetic map of the human major histocompatibility complex located on chromosome 6. See text for further details.

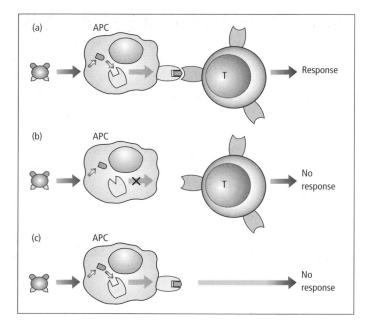

Figure 2.14 Possible ways in which HLA molecules may influence immune responsiveness. Antigen is processed in an antigen-presenting cell (APC) and antigen peptide interacts with the binding groove of an HLA molecule. This complex is transported to the cell surface where it can stimulate a T cell with receptors specific for the antigen (a). (b) No response will occur if the HLA-binding groove has a structure incompatible for association with the antigen peptide, or (c) no T cells are available with receptors specific for this antigen–HLA combination.

may have been deleted during T cell development in the thymus (see Chapter 3) because this particular combination looks very similar to tissue components of the individual, i.e. the T cells would be autoreactive (Fig. 2.14c). By contrast, other individuals expressing different MHC alleles may mount good responses to the determinant because it binds well to their MHC molecules and specific T cells are available to recognize it (Fig. 2.14a). This may help to explain why the MHC system has evolved extensive polymorphism: it ensures that at least some members of a population will be able to make a good immune response to any possible antigen, so it is unlikely that a pathogen could arise to which no individuals can mount an effective immune response. A corollary of this is that individuals who do mount a good response to major, potentially lethal, pathogens will have a selective advantage favouring the transmission and expanded representation of their protective HLA alleles in the gene pool. An example is the high prevalence of the HLA-B53 allele in West Africa where malaria is endemic. Possession of this allele is associated with protection against a lethal form of malaria; HLA-B53 is much less common in other parts of the world where malaria is not present. It is also not surprising that many immunopathological diseases are associated with particular HLA types (see Chapter 15).

Key points

1 Antigens that induce immune responses are termed immunogens, whereas those that induce non-responsiveness are known as tolerogens.

2 The specificity and affinity of interaction between an antigen receptor and an antigenic determinant (epitope) are dependent on complementarity of shape and charge.

3 The antigen receptors of B and T cells are related to other members of the immunoglobulin superfamily and the B-cell receptor is a cell-bound form of secreted immunoglobulin.

4 The specificity of an immune response is ensured by the clonal selection of lymphocytes whose receptors bind the antigen with high affinity.

5 B-cell antigen receptors and antibodies can bind antigen in its native, unmodified form, recognizing accessible surface epitopes. T cell receptors recognize antigenic peptides bound to HLA molecules expressed on the surface of antigen-presenting cells or target cells; this requires processing (fragmentation) of the antigen, and epitopes may be derived from any part of the antigen.

6 HLA class I and II molecules are also members of the immunoglobulin superfamily and possess a groove that accommodates antigenic peptides for presentation to T cells.

7 Most mature T cells express either CD8 or CD4, which restricts them to recognize antigen associated with HLA class I or II, respectively.

8 Cytotoxic function is associated with $CD8^+$ T cells and HLA class I-associated antigen recognition. This facilitates T cell recognition and killing of tissue cells bearing antigens derived from cytosolic processing (e.g. following viral infection).

9 Helper function is associated with $CD4^+$ T cells and HLA class II-associated antigen recognition. This facilitates T cell help by interaction with cells such as interdigitating dendritic cells, macrophages and B cells. The antigens are processed by endocytosis and degradation in cytoplasmic vesicles in these antigen-presenting cells.

10 There are three major class I molecules (HLA-A, -B and -C) and three major class II molecules (HLA-DP, -DQ and -DR) encoded by genes within the HLA complex on chromosome 6.

11 HLA class I and II genes exist in a large number of allelic forms (i.e. they are polymorphic). Each of them preferentially binds different antigenic peptides and this causes variation in immune responsiveness to particular antigens between different individuals.

Chapter 3

Lymphocyte development and activation

Little was known about the function of lymphocytes until the early 1960s when experiments performed by Gowans demonstrated that the lymphocyte was the immunocompetent cell without which the immune system lost its ability to recognize and respond to antigen. He showed that rats depleted of their lymphocytes by continuous thoracic duct drainage failed to reject foreign grafts and lost the ability to develop delayed hypersensitivity reactions and antibody responses. Each of these activities could be restored by returning the lymphocytes intravenously. Thus, lymphocytes are the cells responsible for conferring on the immune response the cardinal features of specificity, memory and self-discrimination.

The main features of lymphocyte development and differentiation are depicted in Fig. 3.1. Lymphocytes are derived from haemopoietic stem cells present, sequentially during ontogeny, in the yolk sac, liver and bone marrow. Lymphoid stem cells, like the precursors of the myeloid and erythroid lineages, are replenished from the **pluripotent stem cells** throughout life.

The primitive lymphoid cells, which originate from bone marrow, develop into two major lymphocyte populations. Some lymphocytes require a period of differentiation in the thymus and are called **T cells**. In birds, the other lymphocytes were found to differentiate in a lymphoid component of the hind gut—the bursa of Fabricius—and were named **B cells**. Mammalian B cells, however,

continue to differentiate in the bone marrow and emerge as mature lymphocytes. Bone marrow and thymus, being tissues in which lymphocytes constantly arise and develop throughout life, are known as **primary lymphoid organs**.

Mature lymphocytes leave the primary lymphoid organs and circulate round the body and migrate through lymphocyte-rich tissues where lymphocyte activation is most likely to occur. These **secondary lymphoid organs** include lymph nodes, the white pulp of the spleen and mucosa-associated lymphoid tissue (MALT). B and T cells preferentially home to different parts of these tissues known as B- and T-dependent areas, respectively.

B cell development

The earliest cells of the B lymphocyte lineage can be detected in fetal liver and are present in bone marrow throughout life (Fig. 3.1). The progenitor cells committed to this lineage randomly select variable region genes encoding the combining site of their antigen receptors and their secreted antibodies. The variety and arrangement of these genes is such that a vast number of different specificities (of the order of 10^8) can be generated within an individual (see p. 56), and the immune system can thus recognize many different antigens. However, all the antigen receptors of a single B cell have identical combining sites.

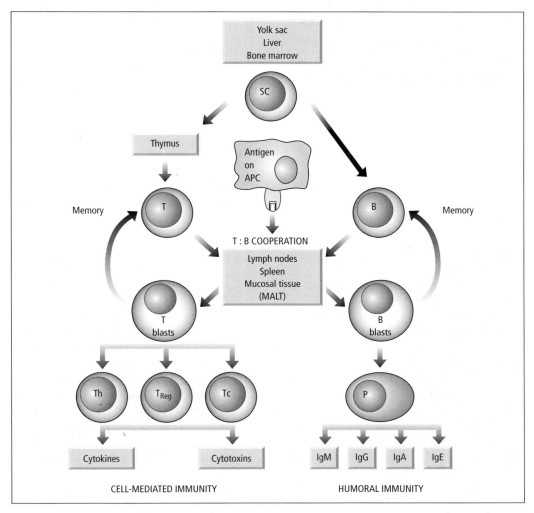

Figure 3.1 Lymphocyte development and differentiation pathways. APC, antigen-presenting cell; Ig, immunoglobulin: P, plasma cell; SC, stem cell; Th, T$_{Reg}$ and Tc, T lymphocytes with helper, regulatory and cytotoxic activities, respectively.

B cell antigen receptors and secreted antibodies occur as five **immunoglobulin classes**, designated IgM, IgD, IgG, IgA and IgE, which differ in the amino acid sequences of their heavy chains (see Chapter 5). The B cell precursors, or **pre-B cells**, produce IgM heavy chains (μ chains) which are transiently expressed in association with two smaller polypeptide chains (V$_{pre-B}$ and λ5) as the **pre-B cell receptor** that is involved in promoting further development. The pre-B cells then produce light chains that associate with cytoplasmic μ

chains, which are expressed as antigen-specific surface IgM on the **immature B cells**.

B cell precursors require a variety of signals to guide them along the developmental pathway; these are provided by bone marrow stromal cells through surface and secreted molecules (e.g. stem cell factor and interleukin-7). However, some B cell precursors do not emerge from this pathway, but undergo a process of programmed cell death called **apoptosis** in which they degrade their own DNA. This may be because they do not rearrange the genes to encode functional antigen receptors (as described in Chapter 5). Alternatively, they may generate receptors that are specific for tissue components in their surroundings. Binding these self antigens triggers their deletion by apoptosis or inactivation (**anergy**) and thus helps to limit autoreactivity. Some autoreactive B cells undergo further light chain rearrangements which may result in a new receptor that no longer recognizes self antigens, thus rescuing these B cells: this is called **receptor editing**.

B cell activation and maturation

Most of the mature, unactivated (i.e. virgin) B cells that leave the bone marrow express both IgM and IgD on their surface; they are small cells, with only a thin rim of cytoplasm. The activation of B cells by most protein antigens requires help from T cells, which is facilitated by the expression of HLA class II molecules by B cells. Such responses are said to be **thymus-dependent** in view of their requirement for thymus-derived T cells. By contrast, some antigens (particularly certain carbohydrates, glycolipids and polymeric proteins) are able to stimulate B cells directly without the involvement of conventional T cells, and are therefore called **thymus-independent (TI)**. These are of two types: **TI-1 antigens** are **mitogens** which directly stimulate B cell proliferation (e.g. bacterial lipopolysaccharide), whereas **TI-2 antigens** possess repeating antigenic determinants which enable them to cross-link the receptors of B cells to which they are specifically bound (e.g. bacterial flagellin).

B cell activation by antigens that cross-link their surface receptors is mediated by two polypeptides associated with the surface immunoglobulins, called **Igα** and **Igβ**. These interact with cytoplasmic tyrosine kinase enzymes, triggering an intracellular signalling cascade resulting in gene activation.

When activated by antigen, B cells enlarge and become **lymphoblasts** (Fig. 3.1). Some of their progeny mature into **plasma cells**, which lack surface immunoglobulin, but synthesize large quantities of immunoglobulin molecules which are secreted as free antibody; the plasma cells have highly developed arrays of rough endoplasmic reticulum. Other B lymphoblasts revert to a resting state and form a **memory population** specific for the antigen that induced the primary response. It is these cells that, upon re-exposure to the same or a very similar cross-reactive antigen, generate a rapid and more vigorous secondary response, as exemplified in Fig. 1.3.

Virgin B cells express IgM and IgD but lose surface IgD expression following stimulation by antigen. Memory B cells also lack this class of immunoglobulin. Some of the B cells activated in a primary response mature into IgM-secreting plasma cells, but others, including many that become memory cells, switch the class of immunoglobulin they synthesize (to IgG, IgA or IgE) with little or no change in their antigenic specificity (Fig. 3.2). Thus, the majority of antibodies produced in a secondary response are of classes other than IgM. The immunoglobulin gene rearrangements that enable variable domains to be combined with different heavy chain constant regions in the various immunoglobulin classes are described in Chapter 5.

A subpopulation of B cells are distinguished from the majority by expressing a protein called **CD5**. These **B-1 cells** arise earlier in fetal develop-

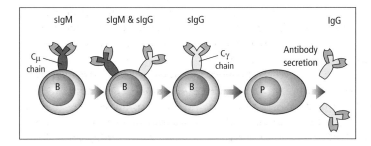

Figure 3.2 Immunoglobulin class switching in an activated B cell exemplified by a change from IgM to IgG production. This involves switching the C_H domains expressed, while the V_H domain and light chain (V_L and C_L domains) are unchanged. P, plasma cell.

ment than conventional **B-2 cells** and produce mainly **polyspecific** IgM antibodies which bind to numerous ligands with relatively low affinity, particularly TI-2 antigens such as bacterial polysaccharides. They may contribute to the early phases of immune responses, bridging innate and adaptive immunity.

T cell development and education

The precursors of T lymphocytes leave the bone marrow at a very early stage of their development and migrate to the thymus (Fig. 3.1), which they enter at the outer margin of the cortex, and are then known as **thymocytes**. The thymic cortex is densely packed with actively proliferating, immature thymocytes, whereas the inner medulla is more sparsely populated by mature cells (derived from cortical thymocytes), which are destined to migrate to secondary lymphoid tissues. The medulla also contains complex aggregates of epithelial cells—Hassall's corpuscles—the function of which is unknown.

Soon after entering the thymus, each thymocyte starts to express the β chain of its T cell receptor for antigen (TCR) in association with a polypeptide chain called pTα (although some are selected for expression of alternative TCR polypeptides called γ and δ chains, which are discussed below). Similar to the pre-B cell receptor described on p. 29, this pre-TCR is involved in promoting further development leading to expression of both α as well as β TCR chains specific for antigen plus HLA (see p. 17). The variable region genes of the TCR α and β chains are randomly selected from the large number available in a manner analogous to that employed by B cells in generating their surface immunoglobulins (see p. 59). Thus, although all the antigen combining sites of a single thymocyte are identical, these cells collectively express a large repertoire of specificities.

Associated with the TCR on the cell surface are several polypeptides (γ, δ, ε and ζ), which are collectively called **CD3** (see Table 2.1); these are analogous to Igα and Igβ of B cells in that, when the TCRs bind to antigen plus HLA on antigen-presenting cells, CD3 interacts with cytoplasmic

tyrosine kinase enzymes to trigger intracellular signalling leading to gene activation. At this stage, each thymocyte also bears both of the T cell surface glycoproteins **CD4** and **CD8**, which are members of the immunoglobulin superfamily (see Figs 2.3 and 2.8). However, cells that survive to become mature T cells continue to express only one of these two molecules. T cells are central to the activation and regulation of immune responses. It is therefore important that they interact efficiently with foreign antigens presented on self HLA molecules, but do not react against other components of 'self'. These restrictions on the T cell repertoire of antigenic specificities are determined by the selective development of precursors in the thymus—a process known as **T cell education**—during which more than 95% of developing thymocytes are eliminated, generating **central tolerance** of T cells to many potential autoantigens.

The stromal framework of the thymus includes an epithelial component, which develops from the third and fourth pharyngeal pouches, and bone marrow-derived interdigitating dendritic cells and macrophages. The stromal cells express both HLA class I and II molecules whose antigen-binding grooves bear 'self' peptides derived by natural degradation of the body's own proteins (as is the case for all cell-surface HLA molecules in the absence of foreign antigens). The interaction of a thymocyte's TCR with these cells plays a large part in determining whether or not it will be selected to become a fully developed T cell (Fig. 3.3).

Any thymocytes that do not interact with the stromal cells, either because they have failed to develop functional TCR or because their TCR cannot bind to self HLA, undergo programmed cell death by apoptosis. Thymocytes whose TCR interact with HLA molecules on mainly bone marrow-derived stromal cells with high avidity (and/or undergo TCR clustering), thereby showing specificity for the self antigens, are also eliminated by apoptosis (Fig. 3.4).

The thymocytes that are selected for continued development are those whose TCR interact with HLA molecules bearing self-peptides (mainly on cortical epithelial cells) with low avidity (and/or do not undergo TCR clustering), inferring that they

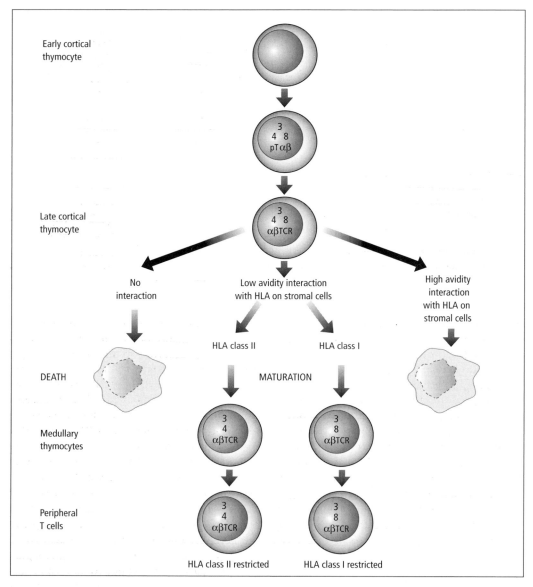

Figure 3.3 Stages of T cell differentiation and selection in the thymus.

would bind more strongly to specific foreign peptides bound to self HLA (Fig. 3.4). Furthermore, those thymocytes whose TCRs interact with HLA class I maintain expression of CD8 but lose CD4, and vice versa for those interacting with HLA class II. Thus, the medullary thymocytes, which have survived passage through the cortex and which become mature recirculating T cells, express either CD4 or CD8 and are mainly specific for foreign antigens bound to self HLA molecules.

A special property of medullary epithelial cells of the thymic stroma is that they synthesize not only ubiquitous proteins (which are present in all tissues of the body), but also **tissue-specific**

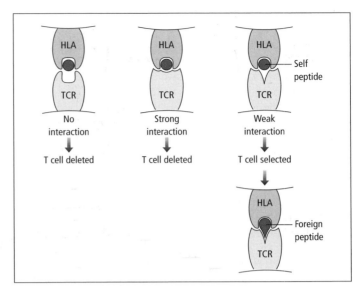

Figure 3.4 T cell selection in the thymus is governed by interactions of T-cell antigen receptors (TCR) with self peptides bound to HLA. Only those showing weak interactions are selected for survival and maturation because these will have strong interactions with foreign peptides bound to HLA.

antigens (TSAs) whose production is otherwise restricted to particular tissues and organs, such as insulin and thyroglobulin which are specifically produced in the pancreatic islets and the thyroid, respectively. Presentation of TSA-derived peptides by the thymic medullary epithelium can eliminate T cells that recognize them, thus inducing organ-specific tolerance. The production of these TSAs in the thymus is regulated by a transcription factor called AIRE (autoimmune regulator), mutations of which are associated with autoimmune polyendocrine syndrome type 1. A variety of organ-specific autoimmune diseases (discussed in Chapter 14) occur in this syndrome, presumably because of defective induction of central T cell tolerance to TSAs.

T cell subpopulations

Mature T cells show heterogeneity in their functional properties as well as in their expression of CD4 and CD8 (Fig. 3.1). T cells that are able to kill virus-infected or allogeneic cells, i.e. cells expressing foreign antigenic determinants on their surface, are called **cytotoxic T cells** (Tc). **Helper T cells** (Th) help other cells to mount immune responses; for example, they stimulate antibody production by B cells, promote the development and/or maintenance of memory Tc cells and enhance the phagocytic activity by macrophages. Most Th cells express CD4, whereas Tc cells are mainly CD8⁺. However, this correlation of function with phenotype is not absolute because a minority of CD4⁺ T cells have cytotoxic activity.

The majority of T cells possess TCR composed of α and β chains (called αβ T cells), express CD8 or CD4, and recognize antigenic peptides bound to HLA class I or II molecules, respectively. By contrast, a minority of T cells bind to antigens either directly (i.e. not associated with HLA molecules) or associated with MHC class IB molecules (see p. 25). Furthermore, some of the antigens recognized are not peptides or proteins but can be glycolipids, phospholipids or unusual nucleotides. Three subpopulations of T cells with these properties have been identified:

1 CD4⁺ αβ T cells that express a molecule called NK1.1, which is also present on natural killer cells (see Chapter 9) and are therefore called NKT cells;
2 αβ T cells that express neither CD4 nor CD8; and
3 γδ T cells whose TCRs are composed of peptides termed γ and δ (analogous to the TCR α and β chains, respectively), and some of which also lack CD4 and CD8.

Some of these T cells arise earlier in fetal development than conventional αβ T cells; have limited variability in the antigen-combining sites of their TCR; and accumulate in mucosal epithelial tissues (e.g. gastrointestinal and reproductive tracts). They may have regulatory functions in the early stages of immune responses and bridge innate and adaptive immunity in a manner analogous to the B-1 cells discussed on p. 30. HLA class 1B molecules called **CD1**, which are encoded outside the HLA gene complex, are particularly important in presenting bacterial lipids to NKT cells.

Some T cells inhibit, rather than activate, immune responses. T cell-mediated suppression was originally described in the 1970s, but technical limitations at the time impaired its elucidation. More recently, a variety of **regulatory T cells (T$_{Reg}$)** have been described within the populations of CD4$^+$ or CD8$^+$ αβ T cells, the γδ T cells and the NKT cells (Fig 3.1). Many T$_{Reg}$ cells produce suppressive cytokines as discussed in Chapter 4. An important function of CD4$^+$CD25$^+$ T$_{Reg}$ cells that arise in the thymus is to suppress autoimmune and allergic reactions, because mutations in a gene required for the development of these T$_{Reg}$ cells are associated with a syndrome in which patients develop type 1 diabetes, thyroiditis and allergies.

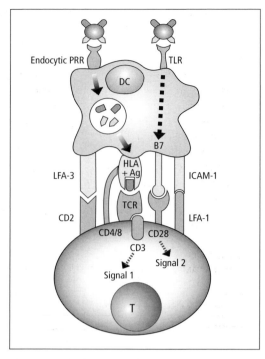

Figure 3.5 The formation of an immunological synapse between cell-surface molecules of an antigen-presenting dendritic cell and a T cell generates signals 1 and 2 for T cell activation. See text for details.

Co-stimulation of lymphocyte activation

Although the activation of T lymphocytes is governed primarily by interactions with antigen and HLA (often termed 'signal 1'), other co-stimulatory signals are also required for efficient activation. Some are the soluble mediators called **cytokines** (discussed in Chapter 4), while others involve adhesive interactions between surface molecules of the communicating cells (Fig 3.5). In particular, the activation of T cells requires 'signal 2', which involves binding of CD28 expressed on the T cell surface with B7 molecules (CD80 and CD86) which are expressed particularly by activated dendritic cells. Antigen recognition by T cells in the absence of the CD28–B7 interaction causes the T cells to become **anergic** (i.e. unresponsive) to further stimulation, or even to die by apoptosis. In the absence of the strong activating signals generated by infec-

tion and inflammation, dendritic cells are in an immature state in which they take up and process antigens, but do not express B7. Thus, presentation of tissue autoantigens by immature dendritic cells induces T cell inactivation and is an important mechanism of maintaining self-tolerance amongst autoreactive T cells that escape clonal deletion in the thymus.

Inflammatory mediators (e.g. cytokines) and microbial pathogen-associated molecular patterns (PAMPs) induce dendritic cell maturation, which involves down-regulation of antigen uptake, up-regulation of HLA and B7 expression, and migration to secondary lymphoid tissues where they are potent stimulators of naïve T cells because they can deliver both signals 1 and 2. An important stimulus for maturation of dendritic cells is the interaction of their **Toll-like receptors (TLRs)** with PAMPs that trigger B7 expression and cytokine production. A variety of TLRs bind different PAMPs, including those listed in Table 3.1.

Various other adhesion molecules are involved in the interactions of T cells with APCs (Fig 3.5). These include the binding of CD2 (expressed by T cells) to lymphocyte function-associated antigen 3 (LFA-3), and LFA-1 to intercellular adhesion molecule type 1 (ICAM-1). All these adhesive interactions between T cells and APCs form an **immunological synapse** with the TCR, CD28 and CD4 or CD8 at the centre of the synapse, surrounded by CD2 and LFA-1 (Fig 3.5). (Adhesion molecules are also involved in leucocyte interactions with endothelial cells, as described in Chapter 10.)

Table 3.1 Examples of pathogen-associated molecular patterns (PAMPs) that interact with Toll-like receptors (TLRs).

Type of microbe	PAMP
Bacterial	Lipopolysaccharide
	Lipoarabinomannan
	Lipoprotein
	Peptidoglycan
	Lipoteichoic acid
	Flagellin
	Unmethylated CpG DNA
Viral	Double-stranded RNA
	F-protein (respiratory syncytial virus)
Fungal	Zymosan (yeast)
Protozoal	Glycophosphoinositol (*Trypanosoma cruzi*)

Regulation of lymphocyte responses

The ability of the adaptive immune system to switch off responses when they are no longer needed is essential for purposes of economy, to allow for responses to other antigens which may be encountered, and to prevent the benefits of eliminating an invading antigen being overshadowed by unacceptable damage to self tissues (see Chapters 13–15). All immune responses can be regarded as a balance between help and suppression. Clearance of antigen can result in apoptosis of the antigen-specific T cells caused by the removal of stimulating survival signals, and some forms of antigen–antibody complexes inhibit lymphocyte activation. Antibody-secreting plasma cells are end-stage cells and some undergo apoptosis within a few days or weeks of their formation, although others survive and secrete antibodies over very long periods, thus accounting for the persistence of circulating antibodies specific for previously encountered antigens.

Activated T cells can be down-regulated because they (unlike resting T cells) express a molecule called **CTLA-4**, which binds to B7 molecules on APCs more strongly than does CD28. Whereas the CD28–B7 interaction activates resting T cells, the binding of CTLA-4 to B7 inhibits T cell activity. In addition, T cells can undergo **activation-induced cell death** whereby apoptosis is triggered, e.g. by surface interactions of Fas and Fas-ligand (described in Chapter 9). The nature and role of T_{Reg} cells has been described above.

Key points

1 Stem cells in the bone marrow give rise to precursors which, in the case of B cells, mature in the bone marrow. T cell precursors migrate to the thymus for their development. The sites in which lymphocytes develop are known as primary lymphoid organs.

2 Antigen receptor diversity is generated during lymphocyte development by random selection of variable region genes in different lymphocytes.

3 Lymphocyte precursors that recognize self antigens are deleted through interactions with stromal cells, whereas those that can recognize foreign antigens develop fully. T cells are also selected for expression of CD8 or CD4, which restricts them to recognize antigen associated with HLA class I or II, respectively.

4 Mature lymphocytes migrate to secondary lymphoid tissues (lymph node, spleen, mucosa-associated lymphoid tissues), which are the main sites of stimulation by antigens.

5 When activated by antigen, a lymphocyte becomes a proliferating lymphoblast, some of whose progeny become memory cells and others effector cells. B lymphoblasts can switch the class of immunoglobulin that they express.

6 Antibody-secreting plasma cells arise from B cells, while effector T cells have regulatory or cytotoxic functions.

7 Primary T cell activation requires a variety of signals delivered by mature dendritic cells, with whom the T cells form an immunological synapse.

8 A variety of regulatory mechanisms cause a decline in specific lymphocyte activity once the stimulating antigens have been eliminated.

Chapter 4

Lymphocyte interactions, cytokines and the lymphoid system

The regulation of immune responses by T helper (Th) cells is dependent both on direct interactions with other cells and on the T cells secreting regulatory molecules called **cytokines**. Although T cells are a major source of cytokines, many cell types can produce them and they have a wide range of functions extending beyond the immune system (e.g. in wound healing). Cytokines are all proteins (which are often glycosylated) and have various roles in regulating the amplitude and duration of immune and inflammatory responses. They are usually produced transiently, exert their effects at very low concentrations, and act on cells within close range of the cells from which they are secreted. They mediate their actions by binding to specific cell-surface receptors, leading to changes in gene expression that modify cell behaviour.

Table 4.1 gives examples of the main cytokines with immune functions. Many are termed **interleukins** (IL-1, IL-2, IL-3, etc.), although this does not necessarily indicate similarities between these cytokines in structure or functions. Others have functional names; however, because most cytokines have a variety of functions, these names do not always indicate their main biological roles. For example, **tumour necrosis factor** (TNF) has certain antitumour properties, but is also a major proinflammatory cytokine, and **γ-interferon** (IFN-γ) 'interfers' with viral replication but is also a major macrophage activating cytokine.

IL-8 is one member of a large family of 'chemoattractant cytokines' called **chemokines**. They induce chemotaxis of various leucocytes (and other cells), induce leucocyte adhesion by activating integrins, promote mediator release by leucocytes, and influence blood vessel growth. Over 40 chemokines and approximately 20 chemokine receptors exist in humans. The chemokines are divided into four sub-families according to the pattern of distinctive cysteine residues in their structures; namely, CCL, CXCL, CL and CX$_3$CL, where 'X' indicates other amino acids, and 'L' indicates that they are ligands for the corresponding chemokine receptors, CCR, CXCR, etc. For example, IL-8 is also known as CXCL8 and it binds to CXCR1 and CXCR2.

Cytokine production by T cell subpopulations

Th cells vary in their ability to produce the combinations of cytokines that preferentially stimulate either cell-mediated or antibody-mediated immunity. As indicated in Table 4.2, **Th1 cells** secrete cytokines that predominantly induce cell-mediated immunity by activating macrophages, T cells and NK cells. They also stimulate B cells to produce opsonizing IgG antibodies that activate complement and phagocytes. Thus, Th1 cells promote immunity to cell-associated microbes, e.g. intracellular viruses, and bacteria that can be killed intracellularly by phagocytes. By contrast, **Th2**

Table 4.1 Cytokines: their sources and immunological functions.

Cytokine	Immune cells	Other cells	Immunological effects
IL-1α,β	Monocytes/macrophages	Endothelial, epithelial and neuronal cells, fibroblasts	Activation of T and B cells, macrophages and endothelium. Stimulation of acute phase response
IL-2	T cells	—	Proliferation and/or activation of T and B cells and NK cells
IL-3	T cells, mast cells, thymic epithelium	Keratinocytes, neuronal cells	Proliferation of pluripotent stem cells. Production of various blood cell types
IL-4	T and B cells, macrophages, mast cells and basophils, bone marrow stroma	—	Activation of B cells. Differentiation of Th2 cells and suppression of Th1 cells
IL-5	T cells, mast cells	—	Development, activation and chemoattraction of eosinophils
IL-6	T cells, monocytes or macrophages	Fibroblasts, hepatocytes, endothelial and neuronal cells	Activation of haemopoietic stem cells. Differentiation of B and T cells. Production of acute phase proteins
IL-7	Bone marrow stroma	—	Growth of B cell precursors. Proliferation and cytotoxic activity of T cells
IL-8	T cells, monocytes, neutrophils	Endothelial and epithelial cells, fibroblasts	Chemoattraction of neutrophils, T cells and basophils. Activation of neutrophils
IL-10	T and B cells, macrophages	Keratinocytes	Suppression of macrophage functions and Th1 cells. Activation of B cells
IL-12	B cells, macrophages, dendritic cells	—	Differentiation of Th1 cells. Activation of NK and T cells
IL-13	T cells	—	Activation of B cells. Suppression of Th1 cells. Increased epithelial mucus production
IL-15	Macrophages	—	Induces lymphocyte proliferation
IL-18	Macrophages	—	Induces IFN-γ production by T and NK cells
TNF-α	Macrophages, lymphocytes, neutrophils, mast cells	Astrocytes, endothelium, smooth muscle	Activation of macrophages, granulocytes, cytotoxic cells and endothelium. Enhanced HLA class I expression. Stimulation of acute phase response. Antitumour effects
TNF-β	T cells	—	Similar to TNF-α
IFN-α,β	T and B cells, monocyte or macrophages	Fibroblasts	Antiviral activity. Stimulation of macrophages and NK cells. Enhanced HLA class I expression
IFN-γ	T cells, NK cells	—	Antiviral activity. Stimulation of macrophages and endothelium. Enhanced HLA class I and II expression. Suppression of Th2 cells
G-CSF	T cells, macrophages, neutrophils	Fibroblasts, endothelium	Development and activation of neutrophils
M-CSF	T cells, macrophages, neutrophils	Fibroblasts, endothelium	Development and activation of monocytes/macrophages
GM-CSF	T cells, macrophages, mast cells, neutrophils, eosinophils	Fibroblasts, endothelium	Differentiation of pluripotent stem cells. Development of neutrophils, eosinophils and macrophages
TGF-β	T cells, monocytes	Chondrocytes, osteoblasts, osteoclasts, platelets, fibroblasts	Inhibition of T and B cell proliferation and NK cell activity

CSF, colony-stimulating factor; G, granulocyte; IFN, interferon; IL, interleukin; NK, natural killer; M, macrophage; TGF, transforming growth factor; TNF, tumour necrosis factor.

Table 4.2 Th1 and Th2 cytokines and their effects.

T cell subset	Cytokine produced	Stimulation of macrophages	Stimulation of B cells	Stimulation of other immune cells	Cells inhibited
Th1	IFN-γ	+	+ (IgG1–3)	NK cells	Th2
	GM-CSF	+			
	TNFα/β	+	+	Endothelium	
	IL-2		+	T and NK cells	
Th2	IL-4/IL-13		+ (IgG1–4, IgE)	Mast cell growth	MØ/Th1
	IL-5		+ (IgA)	Eosinophils	
	IL-6		+		
	IL-10		+		MØ/Th1

cells produce cytokines that principally induce B cell activation and maturation, and promote the production of IgE and IgA antibodies as well as IgG (Table 4.2). They also promote the growth of mast cells and eosinophils. It seems likely that this combination of immune components which is orchestrated by Th2 cells has evolved to defend the body against larger extracellular parasites (i.e. parasitic worms) in particular. Although such parasites have been largely eradicated from developed countries, they still infect hundreds of millions of people worldwide, and have doubtless been a major influence in the evolution of the immune system. In the absence of metazoan parasite infestations, these same immune components generate atopic disorders in response to environmental allergens in an increasingly high proportion of the population (see Chapters 13–15). Activated cytotoxic T cells show a similar dichotomy of cytokine production to Th cells, and have been subdivided into Tc1 and Tc2 cells.

The Th1 and Th2 subpopulations are mutually inhibitory through the cytokines they produce (Table 4.2): IFN-γ inhibits the proliferation of Th2 cells whereas IL-10, IL-4 and IL-13 inhibit macrophages and Th1 cells. Also, the different types of T_{Reg} cells described in Chapter 3 variously produce IL-4 and IL-10, thus inhibiting cell-mediated immunity, and some produce transforming growth factor-β (TGF-β) which inhibits the proliferation of both T and B lymphocytes. However, some inhibitory activities of T_{Reg} cells may require cell–cell contact rather than being cytokine-mediated.

Th1 and Th2 cells arise from common precursors designated Th0 cells, which can be committed in either direction depending on the 'polarizing' signals that they receive at the time of their activation by dendritic cells. A naïve Th0 cell is initially stimulated by TCR–antigen peptide (signal 1) and CD28–B7 (signal 2) interactions with a dendritic cell (see Fig 3.5), which then also delivers a polarizing signal that may be prompted by CD40L on the T cell interacting with CD40 on the dendritic cell (Fig 4.1). The nature of the polarizing signal depends on the types of microbial and tissue factors that act on the dendritic cell itself. Thus, 'type 1' inducing factors include viral, bacterial and fungal pathogen-associated molecular patterns (PAMPs) that bind to Toll-like receptors, and inflammatory cytokines such as interferons, IL-18 and CCR5-binding chemokines. These stimulate dendritic cells to produce IL-12, which promotes Th1 polarization (Fig 4.1). Factors that promote 'type 2' orientation of dendritic cells include components of parasitic worms and inflammatory mediators such as histamine, prostaglandin E_2 and CCR2-binding chemokines. These induce little IL-12 production by dendritic cells, leading to Th2 polarization (Fig 4.1). In addition, the so-called Notch pathway, which regulates lineage choices in various cells, may influence T cell polarization. Dendritic cells can be induced to express different Notch ligands which bind to Notch on T cells and promote either Th1 or Th2 development. IL-4, possibly derived from NKT cells or mast cells, also stimulates the development of Th2 cells. Furthermore, antigens that are presented at high concentrations or that bind

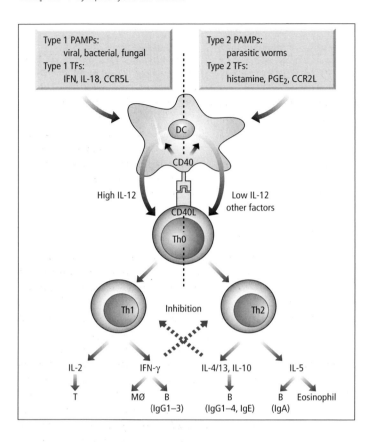

Figure 4.1 Th0 differentiation into Th1 and Th2 cells dependent on type 1 and type 2 polarizing signals produced by dendritic cells as a consequence of their interaction with type 1/type 2 pathogen-associated molecular patterns (PAMPs) and tissue factors (TFs) and CD40 stimulation. See text for details. The factors produced by dendritic cells that directly promote Th2 polarisation are unclear.

Table 4.3 The influence of cytokine production on disease pathogenesis following infection of macrophages by *Mycobacterium leprae*.

Event	Development of tuberculoid leprosy	Development of lepromatous leprosy
Th activation: cytokine production	Activation of Th1: production of IFN-γ	Activation of Th2: production of IL-4
Effector cell stimulation: effects on mycobacteria	Activation of macrophages: intracellular digestion of mycobacteria in cytoplasmic vesicles	Activation of B cells: antibodies have no access to intracellular mycobacteria
Resulting pathology	Some inflammatory tissue damage, but destruction of mycobacteria	Growth of mycobacteria and severe tissue damage

to T cells with high avidity promote Th1 development, whereas low concentration and low avidity antigens favour Th2 responses.

A bias towards activation of Th1 or Th2 cells can influence the effectiveness of the immune response against different infectious pathogens. This is illustrated in Table 4.3 for *Mycobacterium leprae*, which can infect macrophages where it survives and grows in cytoplasmic vesicles. The predominance of Th1 or Th2 activity in the immune response then influences whether tuberculoid or lepromatous leprosy results.

The lymphoid system

In order for lymphocytes to maintain constant surveillance for foreign antigens throughout the body, and to mount an efficient response when an antigen is detected, a dynamic and highly organized lymphoid system is required. The estimated frequencies of T and B cells specific for a particular antigen are between 1 : 10^4 and 1 : 10^6. Thus, the probability of specific lymphocytes coming into contact with antigen and with each other purely by chance are negligible. The nature of the lymphoid system facilitates these interactions and provides an optimal environment for antigen-specific lymphocyte activation.

Secondary lymphoid tissues

Lymphoid tissues, e.g. lymph nodes, the white pulp of the spleen and mucosa-associated lymphoid tissue (MALT), are the main sites of lymphocyte activation by antigens. Both T and B lymphocytes actively recirculate and preferentially home to different parts of these tissues, known as T- and B-dependent areas, respectively.

Lymph nodes

Tissue fluid drains into the lymphatic system and carries antigens from infected tissues to lymph nodes via the **afferent lymphatics** and **subcapsular sinus** (Fig. 4.2). B lymphocytes are found predominantly in the outer cortex of lymph nodes which contains a number of dense aggregations of lymphocytes termed **follicles** (Fig. 4.2). These enlarge during an active immune response to form **germinal centres** which contain large numbers of proliferating B lymphoblasts surrounded by a mantle of resting small B lymphocytes. T lymphocytes are diffusely present throughout the **paracortex** of the lymph node. Lymphocytes leave lymph nodes via the **medulla** which drains into the **efferent lymphatics**. The cooperative events that take place within lymph nodes to generate the antigen-specific activation of lymphocytes are outlined in Figs 4.2 and 4.7 and described on pp. 45–6.

Spleen

The spleen is not a site of drainage from other solid tissues, but captures blood-borne antigens. The T- and B-dependent areas of the spleen are confined to the islands of **white pulp** surrounding arterioles (Fig. 4.3), whereas the red pulp is the site of effete red cell disposal. The **follicles** (incorporating germinal centres) and outer **marginal zones** are mostly occupied by B cells whereas the **periarteriolar lymphoid sheath** (**PALS**) consists almost entirely of T cells.

MALT

Unencapsulated MALT (which includes **tonsils**, **Peyer's patches**, **appendix**, **bronchial** and **mammary tissues**) contains many follicles. Within the wall of the small intestine, the Peyer's patches are particularly prominent with a domed B cell follicle (which may contain a germinal centre) and smaller adjacent T cell areas (Fig. 4.4). The Peyer's patches underlie **M cells** in the gut epithelium which capture antigens from the intestinal lumen and deliver them to the lymphoid tissue. Lymphocytes are also diffusely distributed in the subepithelial **lamina propria** of the intestine where many of the lymphocytes have the characteristics of large granular lymphocytes, as well as there being large numbers of activated CD4$^+$ T and B cells. The gut is also well endowed with its own variant of the mast cell, the mucosal mast cell. Many intestinal **intraepithelial lymphocytes** are CD8$^+$ T cells, and there is also a relatively high representation of T cells that possess the $\gamma\delta$ type of antigen receptor (see p. 33). MALT have several functions peculiar to their location: mucosal surfaces are a major route of entry for many pathogenic microbes, and MALT are the site of secretory IgA production (see p. 54) and have specialized T cell populations. On the other hand, mucosal surfaces are colonized by relatively harmless commensal microbes. Many other innocuous 'foreign materials' impinge on mucosal surfaces, including food in the gut, inhaled particles (e.g. pollen) in the respiratory tract, and sperm in the female reproductive tract. It is important that tolerance

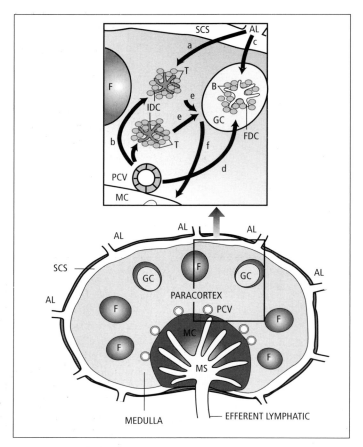

Figure 4.2 Lymph node structure and lymphocyte activation. The lower diagram shows the overall structure of a lymph node with cortical aggregations of B lymphocytes into **follicles** (F) and **germinal centres** (GC) and subdivision of the medulla into **medullary cords** (MC) and **medullary sinuses** (MS). T lymphocytes are the predominant cell in the paracortex. The upper diagram is an amplified inset of part of the cortex indicating the pathways by which antigen and lymphocytes gain access to the lymph node. This is either via **afferent lymphatics** (AL) and the **subcapsular sinus** (SCS) (a and c) or via the **postcapillary venules** (PCV) (b and d). Antigen in the form of immune complexes preferentially localizes to **follicular dendritic cells** (FDC) in the B cell-containing follicles or germinal centres, whereas antigen transported by dendritic cells in lymph (and possibly blood) is presented to Th cells in the paracortex which comes into close contact with these **interdigitating dendritic cells** (IDC). The process of T–B cooperation involves the approximation of these two kinds of cell in the paracortex, culminating in the production of B lymphoblasts which migrate to the follicles (together with some of the T cells) (e) where they undergo further maturation and selection through interaction with antigen on follicular dendritic cells in the germinal centres and further interactions with T cells before migrating (f) into the medullary cords where they can be detected as antibody-secreting cells.

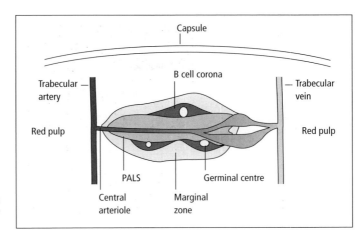

Figure 4.3 Structure of white pulp in the spleen. PALS, periarteriolar lymphoid sheath.

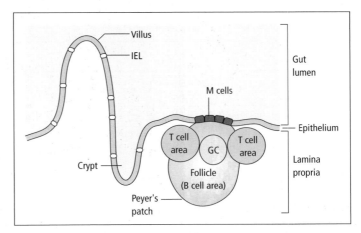

Figure 4.4 Organization of gut-associated lymphoid tissue (GALT), including Peyer's patch, lamina propria and intraepithelial lymphocytes (IEL). GC, germinal centre.

rather than immunity is induced to these substances otherwise allergic reactions result (discussed in Chapters 13–15) and, for example, a variety of T_{Reg} cells are active within MALT.

Lymphocyte recirculation and homing

Once they have left the primary lymphoid organs, mature lymphocytes continually recirculate between the blood, body tissues and secondary lymphoid organs (Fig. 4.5). There is a modest, but steady, transit of lymphocytes across the venules of most tissues in the resting state. These cells migrate into **afferent lymphatics** and gain access to lymph nodes via the **subcapsular sinus** (Fig.

4.2). However, the majority of lymphocytes that enter lymph nodes do so directly from the blood supply of the nodes, within a specialized region of the postcapillary venules lined by activated **high endothelial cells**, these being enlarged, cuboidal cells, unlike the more common, flat endothelium. Lymphocytes adhere to the high endothelial cells and migrate between them to enter the node. These processes are dependent on interactions between lymphocyte surface adhesion molecules, called **selectins** and **integrins**, and their endothelial co-ligands, some known as **vascular addressins** because they are indicative of the tissue type, e.g. lymph node, MALT or sites of inflammation (Table 4.4). Naïve lymphocytes express high levels of **L-selectin** which binds to

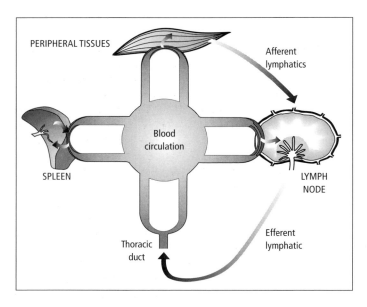

PERIPHERAL TISSUES

Afferent
lymphatics

Blood
circulation

SPLEEN

LYMPH
NODE

Thoracic
duct

Efferent
lymphatic

Figure 4.5 Lymphocyte recirculation. Lymphocytes enter lymph nodes from the blood by crossing specialized 'high endothelium' in the postcapillary venules.

Site of homing	T cell adhesion molecules	Vascular ligands
Lymph node	L-selectin	GlyCAM-1, CD34
MALT	L-selectin	MAdCAM-1
	LPAM-1 ($\alpha_4\beta_7$ integrin)	MAdCAM-1
Infected/inflamed tissues	LFA-1 ($\alpha_L\beta_2$ integrin)	ICAM-1/-2
	VLA-4 ($\alpha_4\beta_1$ integrin)	VCAM-1

Table 4.4 Adhesion molecules involved in the selective homing of T cells to different tissues.

sulphated carbohydrate residues of the glycoprotein addressins GlyCAM-1 and CD34 expressed by lymph node high endothelium. Naïve T cells also express the chemokine receptor CCR7 which directs their migration into the lymph node paracortex by interacting with chemokines produced there, whereas B cells express CXCR5 which similarly promotes their movement into follicles. T lymphocytes that home to MALT express L-selectin, but also the **integrin** LPAM-1, both of which interact with the addressin MAdCAM-1 expressed by mucosal endothelium (Table 4.4). Integrins are a family of adhesion molecules composed of two polypeptide chains (α and β), the different varieties of which combine to form integrins with specificity for different ligands: for example, LPAM-1 is $\alpha_4\beta_7$ integrin.

Lymphocytes exit from lymph nodes via the **medulla** and **efferent lymphatics** to enter the blood circulation via the **thoracic duct** (Figs 4.2 and 4.5). The spleen has no lymphatic supply and splenic lymphocytes gain direct access to the circulation via the splenic vein. Activated T cells show reduced expression of L-selectin, but up-regulate expression of the integrins LFA-1 ($\alpha_L\beta_2$) and VLA-4 ($\alpha_4\beta_1$). This facilitates their migration into sites of infection and inflammation where macrophage-derived inflammatory cytokines such as TNF-α and IL-1 induce endothelial expression of the immunoglobulin superfamily molecules ICAM-1 and ICAM-2 (ligands for LFA-1) and VCAM-1 (ligand for VLA-4).

Lymphocytes that have been stimulated by antigen in one kind of lymphoid tissue (e.g. mucosal or non-mucosal) preferentially home back to the same kind of tissue. This is of value in defence against infections acquired by a particular route. For example, it is relevant to the newborn in that mothers challenged intestinally with antigen develop antibody-secreting cells which migrate to mammary tissue and produce secretory IgA of relevant specificity in their milk.

The recirculation of lymphocytes (approximately 1–2% per hour) enables the immune system continually to monitor the whole body for many different antigens, despite the relatively small number of lymphocytes specific for each. The homing to organized lymphoid tissues brings together the various lymphocytes and APCs that must cooperate in order to mount an efficient immune response, as described in the next section.

Lymphocyte selection and maturation

The secondary lymphoid organs are the main sites of lymphocyte activation by antigen. The route of antigen access to the body determines the primary sites of interaction: antigenic material coming into contact with mucosal surfaces will localize to MALT, while blood-borne material is taken up by the spleen. Antigen in tissue fluids enters draining lymph nodes either as free antigen in the lymph, or bound to dendritic cells. In the skin, for example, immature dendritic cells called **Langerhans' cells** bind antigen, transport it to lymph nodes and become activated dendritic cells that present antigen to T cells of the paracortex. When a lymph node is stimulated by antigen there is a general increase in lymphocyte uptake across the high endothelium. This influx is not selective for lymphocytes that recognize the antigen but those that interact with antigen are retained in the node where they become activated and proliferate. Several days later some of these cells enter the medulla and efferent lymph as blast cells and, later still, there is an efflux of memory cells into the circulation.

The processes of lymphocyte cooperation and maturation induced by antigen recognition in lymph nodes are illustrated in Figs 4.2 and 4.6–4.10. In the paracortex, mature dendritic cells that arrive in the afferent lymph, having endocytosed and processed protein antigens in surrounding tissues, present HLA class II-associated antigenic peptides to Th cells (and also cross-present HLA class I-associated peptides to CD8[+] Tc cells), as described in Chapter 2. The dendritic cells also provide co-stimulatory signals as part of the immunological synapse formation (see Chapter 3), as well as the Th1/Th2 polarizing cytokines described earlier in this chapter. In addition, the dendritic cells secrete other T cell activating cytokines, e.g. IL-1 which induces T cell expression of IL-2 receptors (CD25) (Fig. 4.6). The T cells secrete IL-2 which induces their own proliferation as well as, for example, that of nearby Tc cells (Fig. 4.6). It is now thought that IL-2 is not essential for the initial replication of activated T cells, but that it contributes to the maintenance of T cell proliferation and effector functions, particularly in non-lymphoid tissues such as sites of infection. IL-2 is also necessary for the development and maintenance of CD4[+]CD25[+] T_{Reg} cells (see p. 34), and thus contributes to the regulatory control of adaptive immunity.

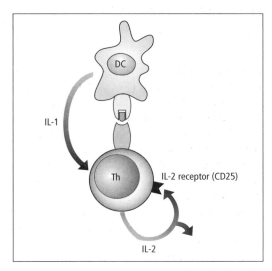

Figure 4.6 The role of cytokines in T helper cell (Th) activation. Activated T cells divide in response to IL-2; see text for further details. APC, antigen-presenting cell; DC, dendritic cell.

B lymphocytes are also present in the lymph node paracortex, either because they recently entered the tissue from the postcapillary venules, or they have migrated into the paracortex from adjacent follicles. Free antigens carried to the lymph node can then be bound and processed by the few B cells with surface immunoglobulins specific for these antigens. The B cells then present HLA class II-associated peptides to the activated Th cells that are identical copies of those presented to the T cells by the dendritic cells (Fig. 4.7). However, in order for a B cell to be stimulated by a T cell, the epitope that is recognized by the T cell must be physically linked to that bound by the surface receptors of the B cell. Only in this way will the T cell epitope be taken up efficiently by the B cell for processing and presentation to the T cell (Fig. 4.7). The B cells that present antigen also express B7 and CD40, and their interaction with the Th cells induces their activation, proliferation and maturation via CD40 signalling and cytokines. The immunological synapse that the T cell forms with the B cell induces cytoskeletal realignments within the T cell so that cytokines are released directionally at the point of contact between the two cells. Several cytokines contribute to B cell activation, replication and differentiation into plasma cells; these include IL-4 and IL-6, as illustrated in Fig. 4.8 (and others indicated in the figure legend). Some B cells mature into plasma cells within the primary focus of activation in the paracortex; these migrate to the medulla where they secrete antibodies for a few days before undergoing apoptosis. These antibodies are specific for the antigens that initiated the B cell activation (Fig. 4.7).

The other activated B cells, together with some of the activated Th cells, migrate to adjacent follicles where the B cells undergo rapid proliferation (as **centroblasts**) to form **germinal centres** (Fig. 4.9). B cells with varying affinities for the antigen are generated by **somatic mutation** of their immunoglobulin variable domains during proliferation (see Fig. 4.10 and Chapter 5). The **centrocytes** (as they are known when they have stopped dividing) with highest affinity are selected for further maturation by interacting with antigen held for long periods on the surface of **follicular dendritic cells** (FDC) in the form of **immune complexes** with antibodies and complement proteins: the FDC express Fc receptors and complement

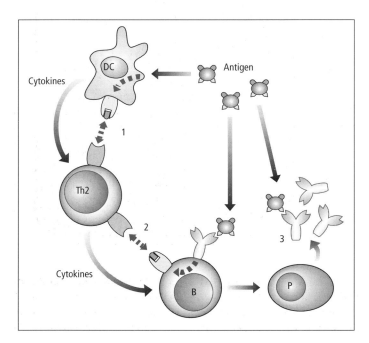

Figure 4.7 Helper T cell function for B cell activation. The stages represented are: (1) antigen processing by a dendritic cell (DC) and presentation in association with HLA class II for recognition by a specific CD4+ Th2 cell; (2) binding and processing of antigen by a specific B cell with HLA class II association for interaction with the Th2 cell; (3) activation of the B cell results in the production of antibodies specific for the antigen. Cytokines also contribute to the activation processes.

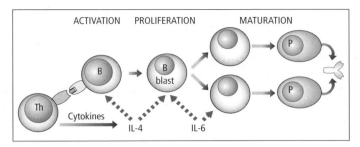

Figure 4.8 The role of cytokines in B cell activation. The differentiation of a B cell (following interaction with a Th cell via presentation of antigen associated with HLA class II) involves an increase in metabolic activity and size, giving rise to a lymphoblast that undergoes mitosis and finally matures into an antibody-secreting plasma cell (P). Cytokines secreted by Th cells (and other cells) act on the B cell at different stages of differentiation. This is illustrated with IL-4 and IL-6, but other cytokines may also be involved: e.g. IL-1 and TNF promote early activation; IL-2 and IL-13 stimulate replication; IL-13 and IFN-γ promote maturation to plasma cells.

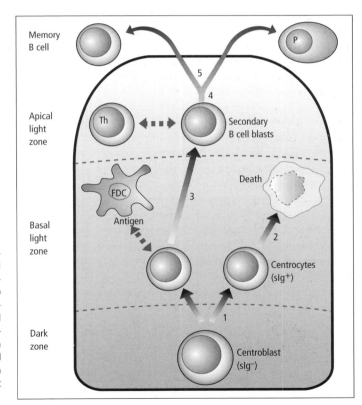

Figure 4.9 The maturation of antigen-specific B cells in the germinal centre of a lymph node. (1) Clonal expansion and somatic mutation; (2) failure to interact with antigen on follicular dendritic cells (FDC) leads to cell death; (3) selection for further maturation is driven by interaction with antigen on FDC; (4) proliferation and isotype switching is stimulated by Th cells; (5) B memory cell development or maturation to plasma cells (P).

receptors which bind the immune complexes. The centrocytes with lower affinity for antigen, which do not interact with FDC, undergo apoptosis and die. This process of selecting B cells with highest affinity for antigen is termed **affinity maturation**. FDC, like the dendritic cells that stimulate T lymphoctes, have dendritic processes but, in other respects, are very different. For example, in

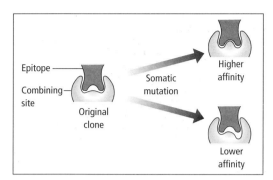

Figure 4.10 Somatic mutation of immunoglobulin variable domains involves point mutations resulting in amino acid changes that effectively increase or decrease the affinity of interaction with the antigen epitope.

accordance with their antigen-presenting function for B cells, but not T cells, FDC lack expression of HLA class II molecules.

The selected B cells undergo further interactions with antigen-specific Th cells, which stimulate proliferation, and immunoglobulin class switching (from IgM to IgG, IgA or IgE) according to their profile of Th1 or Th2 cytokine production as discussed on page 37 (Table 4.2). The interactions with Th cells also lead to the formation of plasma cells and memory cells. The plasma cells formed in lymph node germinal centres recirculate to the bone marrow where they secrete antibodies into the circulation for periods of months or even years. (Similarly, long-lived plasma cells formed in the MALT migrate to the lamina propria.) The memory cells remain quiescent until the body is re-exposed to the same antigens when the adaptive memory response is then induced, as described in Chapter 1.

Laboratory methods

Identification and isolation of lymphocytes

A variety of molecules expressed on the surface of lymphocytes are not found on other cell types. These **differentiation markers** are often utilized in the identification and isolation of lymphocytes. The CD nomenclature for these markers is outlined in Table 2.1. A number of techniques use antibodies (monoclonal or polyclonal; see p. 61) that specifically bind to a particular marker. For example, anti-CD3 antibodies specifically bind to T cells, but not to other leucocytes. If a fluorescent molecule (e.g. fluorescein or phycoerythrin) has been conjugated to the antibodies, the T cells can then be identified by the fluorescence observed in a UV microscope or detected in a **flow cytometer** (also known as a **fluorescence-activated cell sorter**), which will separate the fluorescent from the unlabelled cells (Fig. 4.11). The isolation of a particular type of lymphocyte can also be achieved by interaction with antibodies (against a surface marker) bound to a plastic dish (a technique called **panning**) or to particles (e.g. magnetic beads or red blood cells—known as **rosetting**; Fig. 4.11). The CD2 molecules on T cells will bind to LFA-3 molecules on sheep red blood cells and this property is also used in the formation of rosettes (Fig. 4.11).

The above techniques can be used to select cells positively, i.e. those that bind to a particular antibody, or to select negatively all the cells that are not bound. Another method for negative selection is to add complement (see Chapter 6), so that all the cells that have bound the antibody are lysed.

Stimulation of lymphocytes

Within a population of lymphocytes only a very small proportion specifically react to one particular antigen. These can be detected by the changes they undergo and the effects they mediate when stimulated by antigen. The activation of T lymphocytes results in metabolic activity and rapid proliferation, which can be quantified *in vitro* by the incorporation of a radioactively labelled precursor into the newly synthesized DNA, RNA or protein. This is known as the **lymphocyte transformation test**. Activated T cells can also be identified by the *de novo* expression of activation markers (e.g. CD25, described on p. 45) or by the production of cytokines.

The cytotoxic activity of Tc cells and NK cells can be determined in the **chromium release assay**. Target cells are incubated with a radioactive

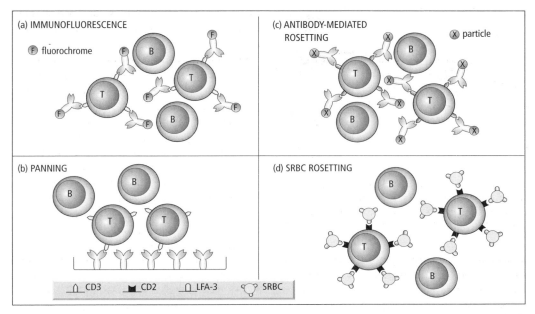

Figure 4.11 Techniques for the identification and separation of lymphocytes, as applied to T cells. (a–c) show methods employing anti-T cell antibody (e.g. anti-CD3) with the antibody conjugated to (a) a fluorescent probe; (b) a plastic dish; or (c) microscopic particles. The direct rosetting of T cells with sheep red blood cells (SRBC) is illustrated in (d).

chromium compound which they take up into their cytoplasm. Lysis of the targets by killer cells can be measured by the release of radioactivity into the extracellular fluid.

The activation of B cells by antigen results in their maturation into plasma cells, which can be detected by the specific antibodies they secrete.

Key points

1 The cytokine and chemokine proteins secreted by various cell types regulate the amplitude and duration of immune and inflammatory responses.

2 Th1 and Th2 cells secrete cytokines that promote principally cell-mediated immunity and antibody-mediated immunity, respectively, and are mutually inhibitory.

3 The generation of Th1 and Th2 cells is determined by polarizing signals, mainly derived from dendritic cells, which are dependent on the microbial and tissue factors that activate the dendritic cells.

4 The polarization of T cells towards Th1 or Th2 influences the effectiveness of the response against particular microbes, e.g. in leprosy.

5 Mature lymphocytes are found mainly in secondary lymphoid tissues, consisting of the spleen, lymph nodes and MALT. These have specific areas enriched in T or B cells.

6 Lymphocytes recirculate between blood, body tissues and secondary lymphoid tissues. The homing of different lymphocytes to different lymphoid tissues is determined by adhesive interactions with high endothelial cells.

7 T cells interact with antigen on presenting cells in the T-dependent areas of secondary lymphoid tissues. B cells activated by these T cells then form germinal centres in the lymphoid follicles where they undergo proliferation, selection and maturation to become plasma cells and memory cells.

8 Lymphocytes and their subpopulations can be identified and isolated by virtue of their cell-surface differentiation molecules. The stimulation of specific lymphocytes by antigen results in measurable activities, e.g. proliferation and cytokine production, cytotoxicity and antibody production.

Chapter 5

Immunoglobulins

All vertebrates possess immunoglobulin-like molecules. They are synthesized and secreted by end cells of the B cell lineage, i.e. plasma cells. These serum proteins were first discovered a century ago by Paul Ehrlich and his colleagues by virtue of their ability to confer protection, i.e. immunity, against a number of important bacterial infections. Their function as antigen-recognition molecules gave rise to the alternative term, antibodies. They are largely confined to the broad and heterogeneous band of γ-globulins observed on electrophoresis (Fig. 5.1) and show considerable diversity of structure and function.

Structure

The typical immunoglobulin molecule is asymmetrically composed of four polypeptide chains linked by disulphide bridges (Fig. 5.2). The larger chains are designated **heavy** and the smaller **light**: it is the combined amino-terminal ends of these two chains that create the two antigen combining sites of the molecule. Within a given immunoglobulin molecule the heavy chains are identical with each other, as are the light chains, so that the two antigen combining sites have the same specificity for antigen. The carboxy-terminal portions of the heavy chains trigger various effector functions following combination of the immunoglobulin molecule with its specific antigen. Several immunoglobulin fragments can be prepared using proteolytic enzymes and these have been of value in unravelling the functional activities of different parts of these molecules. Digestion with papain cleaves on the amino-terminal side of the inter-heavy chain disulphide bonds, yielding two **Fab** fragments, thus designated because they retain the ability to recognize antigen (i.e. **f**ragment **a**ntigen-**b**inding). The other fragment can be readily crystallized and was thus termed **Fc** (i.e. **f**ragment **c**rystallizable). Pepsin digestion cleaves the molecule to the carboxy-terminal side of the inter-heavy chain disulphide bonds and this generates a Fab dimer designated F(abc′)$_2$, leaving a rather smaller Fc fragment designated pFc′.

Variable and constant domains

Figure 5.3 illustrates the immunoglobulin molecule in a Y configuration and emphasizes the flexible hinge region which permits considerable movement of the Fab arms. Both light and heavy polypeptide chains consist of a series of similar globular subunits or **domains**. Each domain consists of a stretch of approximately 110 amino acids of polypeptide chain folded into two layers of β-pleated sheet held together by a single intrachain disulphide bridge giving a roughly cylindrical conformation. Although there is considerable overall similarity between the various light and heavy chain domains, the amino-terminal domain shows a marked degree of variation in many of its amino acid residues and is termed **variable** in contrast to the other domains, which vary comparatively little from each other and are termed **constant**. Light chains contain one variable and one constant domain (V_L and C_L), whereas heavy chains contain one variable domain (V_H) and three or four constant domains (C_H1, C_H2, C_H3 and C_H4) depending on the class of immunoglobulin. The domain structure of immunoglobulins is very similar to the

pattern of polypeptide looping found in T cell receptors as well as that seen in both kinds of HLA glycoprotein and other cell-surface adhesion molecules (see Fig. 2.3). This suggests that they have all developed as specializations of an ancestral recognition molecule present upon the surface of most kinds of cell. They are together regarded as members of the **immunoglobulin superfamily**.

The antigen combining site

Much of the variation found between immunoglobulins of different antigenic specificities is located within three 'hot spots' or **hypervariable regions** (HVR1, -2 and -3; Fig. 5.3), which lie in close proximity to each other within the folded structure of the variable domain. Thus, the most variable parts of this domain are brought together to form the **antigen combining site** or cleft consisting of the three hypervariable regions from the light chain and a further three from the adjacent heavy chain (Fig. 5.4a).

The specific chemistry and shape of this combining site is complementary to the specific chemistry and shape of the **antigenic determinant** or **epitope** (Fig. 5.4b; see Chapter 2); thus, the HVR lining the combining site are also referred to as **complementarity-determining regions**. The term 'combining site' is confined to that part of the molecule that specifically interacts with the epitope, whereas the entire area of surface

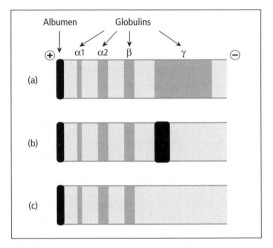

Figure 5.1 Protein electrophoresis of (a) normal serum, (b) serum showing a compact band of monoclonal immunoglobulin (from a case of myeloma) and (c) serum from a patient with hypogammaglobulinaemia.

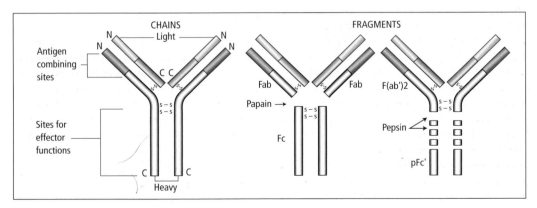

Figure 5.2 Immunoglobulin chains and the fragments formed by proteolytic digestion. C, carboxy-terminus; N, amino-terminus.

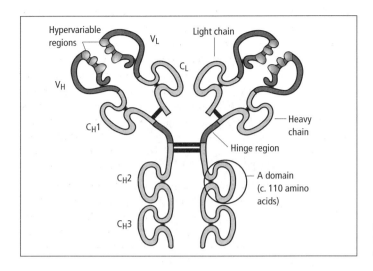

Figure 5.3 The domain structure of immunoglobulin molecules, with the domains shown as peptide loops.

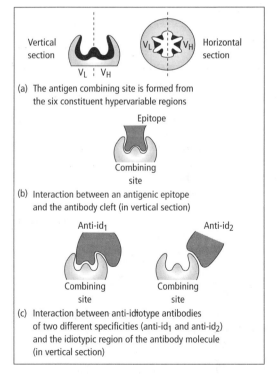

(a) The antigen combining site is formed from the six constituent hypervariable regions

(b) Interaction between an antigenic epitope and the antibody cleft (in vertical section)

(c) Interaction between anti-idiotype antibodies of two different specificities (anti-id$_1$ and anti-id$_2$) and the idiotypic region of the antibody molecule (in vertical section)

Figure 5.4 Spatial configuration of the antigen combining site or cleft and its interaction with epitopes and anti-idiotypes.

conformation that is unique to an immunoglobulin molecule of particular antigenic specificity is known as the **idiotype** (from the Greek *idios*, meaning 'private'). These unique shapes and surfaces can themselves be recognized by other antibodies which are then referred to as having **anti-idiotype** specificity (Fig. 5.4c). If they interact sufficiently with the antigen combining site, they may block the combination of antigen epitope with it (e.g. anti-id$_1$) or, if they react with a more peripheral part, they may not inhibit epitope combination (e.g. anti-id$_2$).

Affinity and avidity

The strength of binding or association of a single epitope for a single combining site in a homogeneous system is termed **affinity**. The more usual situation whereby an antigen bearing several epitopes combines with a variety of specific antibody molecules, each with their own combining sites, is a very heterogeneous system and the term **avidity** is used to indicate the average strength of this association. The former is as easy to measure as the strength of binding of a hormone for its receptor; the latter is a much more complicated affair. Avidity also refers to the combined affinities of the two (or more) antigen combining sites of a single antibody molecule, as illustrated in Fig. 5.5. The number of combining sites defines the **valency** of the antibody (e.g. two for IgG, 10 for IgM), and the equivalent valency of the antigen is the number of repeats of the particular epitope it carries.

Classes and subclasses

There are five classes of immunoglobulin in humans: IgG, IgA, IgM, IgD and IgE (Table 5.1; Fig. 5.6). These show important structural and

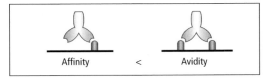

| Affinity | < | Avidity |

Figure 5.5 A comparison of the affinity and avidity of binding of a monomeric antibody molecule.

functional differences within the constant regions of their heavy chains and, in the case of IgG and IgA, subdivide further into subclasses. Each of these structural variants is present in all normal individuals. They can be identified and quantified by specific antisera raised in another species and are referred to as **isotypes**. Other, single amino acid, variations occur as heritable polymorphisms and are known as **allotypes**. These have been identified within IgG (the Gm system), IgA (the Am system) and on κ chains (the Km system).

Each class (or subclass) of immunoglobulin consists of four-chain units as depicted in Figs 5.3 and 5.6. In IgG, IgD and IgE these are monomeric, whereas IgA often occurs as a dimer and IgM almost always as a pentamer. The heavy chains of each class are given the equivalent Greek letter, e.g. γ for IgG (Table 5.1). The light chains can be of two

Table 5.1 Physical and biological characteristics of immunoglobulins.

	IgG	IgA	IgM	IgD	IgE
Physical properties					
Molecular weight	150 000	160 000 (monomer)	900 000	180 000	190 000
Number of four-chain units	1	1 or 2	5	1	1
Heavy chains	γ	α	μ	δ	ε
Light chains	κ or λ	κ or λ	κ or λ	κ or λ	κ or λ
Other peptide chains	–	J ± S	J	–	–
Subclasses	γ1, γ2, γ3, γ4	α1, α2	–	–	–
Serum concentration (g L^{-1})	c. 10 (65%, 25%, 6%, 4%)	c. 2 (85%, 15%)	c. 1	c. 0.03	c. 0.0002 (i.e. 200 ng mL^{-1})
Biological activities					
Complement fixation:					
Classical pathway	γ1, γ2, γ3	–	++	–	–
Alternative pathway	+*	+	–	–	–
Phagocyte binding	γ1, γ3	+†	–	–	+†
Mast cell binding	–	–	–	–	++
NK cell binding	γ1, γ3	–	–	–	–
Eosinophil binding	γ1, γ3, γ4	–	–	–	+
Extravascular diffusion	γ1, γ2, γ3, γ4	+	–	–	+
Mucosal transfer	–	++	+	–	–
Placental transfer	γ1, γ2, γ3, γ4	–	–	–	–

J, J chain; NK, natural killer; S, secretory piece.

* See text.

† See Table 7.2.

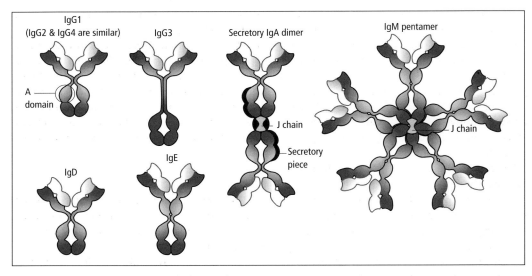

Figure 5.6 Structure of immunoglobulin isotypes, with the domains shown as globular units.

types, kappa (κ) or lambda (λ) and the two light chains of a single immunoglobulin molecule are of the same type, i.e. *either* κ or λ. Both polymeric forms (IgA and IgM) contain an additional peptide known as **J chain** (15 000 Da molecular weight), which plays a part in holding the monomeric subunits together. Dimeric IgA, present in secretions, contains a further component known as **secretory piece** (70 000 Da molecular weight), which is derived from cells of the secretory epithelium through which IgA is transported.

IgG

This is the most plentiful immunoglobulin in internal body fluids and is produced particularly during secondary immune responses. The γ chains contain three constant regions ($C_\gamma 1$, $C_\gamma 2$ and $C_\gamma 3$) which are involved in the different effector functions of the molecule (Table 5.1). The three most plentiful subclasses (IgG1, IgG2 and IgG3) activate the classical complement pathway via the $C_\gamma 2$ domain (see Chapter 6). IgG in aggregated form can enhance existing activation of the alternative complement pathway but the particular involvement of individual subclasses and domains is unclear.

The subclasses IgG1 and IgG3 (and, to some ex-

tent, IgG4) also interact with three Fc receptors expressed on various cell types. The high-affinity $Fc_\gamma RI$ and $Fc_\gamma RII$ bind in the lower hinge region close to the $C_\gamma 2$ domain, whereas both $C_\gamma 2$ and $C_\gamma 3$ may be involved in binding to $Fc_\gamma RIII$. The interaction of microbe-associated IgG with macrophages and neutrophils facilitates the phagocytosis and killing of the bound microbe (see Chapter 7), while IgG interacting with the surfaces of eosinophils (see Chapter 8) and natural killer cells (see Chapter 9) facilitates the lysis of extracellular targets. The bacterium *Staphylococcus aureus* produces Fc-binding proteins (protein A and protein G) which, by inhibiting the Fc-dependent functions of IgG, may aid bacterial survival (see Chapter 10).

All four subclasses of IgG interact with Fc receptors in the placenta (FcRn) and are transported into the fetal circulation. FcRn is structurally similar to HLA class I proteins, and binds IgG in the $C_\gamma 2$–$C_\gamma 3$ junction.

IgA

This is the major immunoglobulin of external secretions. It is particularly evident during the secondary immune response to antigen gaining access via mucosal surfaces. It does not activate complement by the classical pathway but is able to stabilize the alternative pathway C3 convertase (see Chapter 6). It also has an affinity for phagocyte surfaces through interaction with Fc$_\alpha$RI, although this is less than that of IgG1 and IgG3. Much of its protective value may be a result of its direct combination with and neutralization of pathogenic microorganisms in the gut and respiratory tract without necessarily involving any other effector systems.

IgA dimers and their associated **J chains** are produced by submucosal plasma cells. They gain access to the lumen of the gut and other mucosal sites by complexing with a receptor for polymeric immunoglobulin present on the surface of enterocytes and hepatocytes. This receptor has a high affinity for J chains and, after combination with it, dimeric IgA is transported across the cell by endocytosis and then released with the outer portion of the poly-Ig receptor still attached. This component is designated the **secretory piece** and may protect secretory IgA from proteolytic cleavage.

Dimeric, J chain-containing IgA also gains access to the portal circulation and is transported into bile via the poly-Ig receptor present on hepatocytes. The secretion of IgA antibodies in breastmilk provides protection to the gastrointestinal tract of newborns. As most circulating IgA in humans (in contrast to mice and rats) is present in monomeric form it is unlikely that this is an important route for the transport of secretory IgA into the gut under normal conditions.

IgM

This is the key immunoglobulin of the primary response and is a large pentameric molecule containing 10 antigen combining sites, giving the potential for high avidity binding to antigen. The five monomeric units are linked together with a single J chain molecule. Its heavy (μ) chains have four constant domains (Fig. 5.6). IgM is an efficient activator of the classical complement pathway (see Table 5.1). The level of specific antibody belonging to this class fades with progressive exposure to specific antigen in favour of other isotypes, e.g. IgG and IgA. T cells have a role in governing the mechanism of isotype switching, and the nature of the immunoglobulin gene arrangements that mediate this event are described below. Owing to its relatively large size, IgM does not normally escape from the circulation into tissue fluids. However, J chain-containing IgM has an affinity for the poly-Ig receptor and when there is a relative dearth of IgA, as in IgA deficiency, then IgM can appear in secretions linked to the secretory piece.

IgD

This is normally present in minute concentrations in blood and other body fluids but is readily detected on the surface of many early B cells in conjunction with IgM. It is thought not to mediate any of the usual effector functions attributed to other immunoglobulins but may have a role as antigen receptor on early B cells.

IgE

This monomeric immunoglobulin has four constant domains (like IgM) and, although it is the least plentiful of all immunoglobulins, its presence can be dramatically felt by its ability to bind to high-affinity Fc receptors (Fc$_\varepsilon$RI) on the surface of mast cells and basophils that interact with the C$_\varepsilon$2–C$_\varepsilon$3 domains (see Table 5.1) and, when complexed with specific antigen, to trigger the release of inflammatory mediators (see Chapter 8). Its physiological role may be to function with mast cells as a 'gatekeeper' regulating the exit of cells and plasma into extravascular sites. Certain other cell types express a lower affinity receptor for IgE (Fc$_\varepsilon$RII) that binds to the C$_\varepsilon$3 domains; IgE binding to these receptors on eosinophils may be important in immunity to parasitic worms.

Triggering of effector systems

In some situations antibodies can act alone, e.g. neutralization of bacterial toxins and viruses, and inhibition of flagellar motility. However, their effect is most striking when they are able to trigger and recruit the assistance of other effector molecules and cells, e.g. complement and phagocytes (see Table 5.1). Clearly, it would be inappropriate for this event to be mediated by uncomplexed immunoglobulin and strict requirements have to be fulfilled before the appropriate signal is generated. For activation of the classical complement pathway by IgG, two adjacent IgG molecules have to be stabilized within an immune complex or IgG aggregate and at an appropriate distance from each other such that a minimum of two of the six heads of the first complement protein (C1q) can interact with the $C_\gamma 2$ domain which then causes a steric rearrangement of the C1 complex with activation of C1r and C1s (see Chapter 6). Each of the other domains in the IgG molecule is stabilized by a hydrophobic interaction with its homologous partner, whereas the $C_\gamma 2$ domains are partly masked by carbohydrate and protrude outward, facilitating their interaction with C1q. A single IgM molecule, with five Fc regions, can interact with C1q by itself. However, this again only occurs when the antibody is complexed with antigen, which is thought to distort the molecule so as to expose the Fc-binding sites for C1q within the $C_\mu 3$ domains.

Each of the other effector functions, e.g. phagocyte activation and mast cell degranulation, is also triggered by the approximation and stabilization of Fc domains within complexed antibody. The requirement for cross-linking of surface IgE on the mast cell has been shown by the demonstration that mast cell degranulation can be produced by intact divalent anti-IgE but not with monovalent Fab fragments.

Immunoglobulin genes

It was a source of puzzlement for many years how, if each protein (or polypeptide chain) is encoded by a single gene, immunoglobulin molecules with identical constant regions but a vast repertoire of different variable domains could be synthesized. The discovery of non-expressed intervening sequences or **introns**, as well as peptide coding sequences or **exons** within chromosomal DNA, and the realization that rearrangements of these sequences were possible have helped to clarify this problem.

It was difficult to comprehend how up to 10^8 different antibody specificities could be encoded by genes inherited in the germline but it is now clear that many of the rearrangements of DNA and RNA that take place during B cell differentiation make significant contributions to the total diversity of the antibody molecules that are produced. Figure 5.7 illustrates the way in which rearrangements are made in the germline DNA coding for κ light chain proteins. Each variable domain is encoded by two gene segments (i.e. exons): a variable (V) gene segment makes the larger contribution (including HVR1 and HVR2), and a small joining (J) segment.

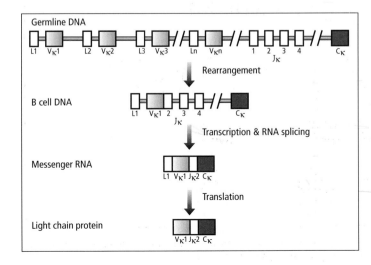

Figure 5.7 Organization and rearrangement of genes coding for κ light chains. The notation for individual exons is as follows: C_κ, constant regions; L, leader; J, joining; $V_\kappa 1 \ldots V_\kappa n$, variable regions.

The germline DNA contains approximately 40 functional V_κ exons and five expressable J_κ exons on chromosome 2. During B cell development in the bone marrow, random selection for expression of a V_κ and a J_κ exon takes place in each pre-B cell by rearrangement of the DNA to link any one of the V_κ exons with any one of the J_κ exons (e.g. $V_\kappa 1$ and $J_\kappa 2$ in Fig. 5.7). The recombined V–J junction encodes the HVR3 of the variable domain. The single exon for the κ light chain constant domain (C_κ) is located near the J segments (Fig. 5.7). Following transcription of the whole genetic locus into RNA, the RNA between the V–J and C exons is spliced out to yield the uninterrupted V–J–C message which is then translated into the light chain protein (Fig. 5.7).

The λ light chain locus is on chromosome 22 and the processes of rearrangement and expression of the λ genes are similar to those described above for κ light chains. There are approximately 30 functional V_λ exons and four functional J_λ exons, each associated with a different C_λ exon.

Further diversity is possible with the rearrangements that take place in the DNA coding for heavy chains on chromosome 14 (Fig. 5.8). As well as 65 functional V_H exons and six J_H exons there is an additional group of approximately 27 exons in between, termed the diversity (D) segments. The first step in DNA rearrangement involves the random selection and joining of a D and a J exon, followed by rearrangement to one of the V_H exons. In this case it is the V–D–J junction that forms the heavy chain HVR3. The recombination of exons which generates the variable region genes is catalysed by the **V(D)J recombinase** enzyme complex. The first stage of recombination involves an endonuclease encoded by two **recombination-activating genes** (**RAG1** and **RAG2**). These are expressed together only in developing lymphocytes and their deficiency inhibits lymphocyte development (see Chapter 12). A number of other DNA modifying proteins are also involved in the recombination events.

In a naïve B cell (i.e. that has not been activated by antigen), RNA splicing joins the transcribed variable domain gene to the C_μ or C_δ constant

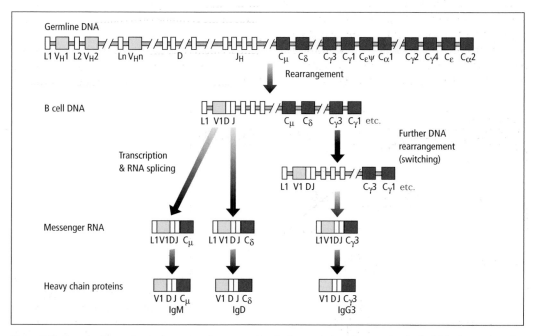

Figure 5.8 Organization and rearrangement of genes coding for heavy chains. The notation for individual genes is as for Fig. 5.7 with the following addition: D, diversity. $C_{\varepsilon\psi}$ is a non-expressed pseudogene.

region RNA to be translated into the heavy chains for IgM and IgD, respectively.

Thus, three genetic elements code for a light chain (V, J and C) and four encode a heavy chain (V, D, J and C), i.e. a total of seven genetic elements encode a complete immunoglobulin protein. Furthermore, within the DNA that encodes each heavy chain constant region, there are separate exons for each C_H domain, i.e. three each for C_δ, C_γ and C_α, and four each for C_μ and C_ϵ. The genetic mechanism whereby a B cell switches the class of immunoglobulin it produces is described below. The production of both surface and secreted immunoglobulins by a B cell (i.e. antigen receptors and antibodies) is brought about by the differential expression of an additional exon which encodes the membrane-spanning portion of the surface-bound immunoglobulin.

The origins of diversity

Several factors contribute to the enormous range of antibody diversity present in higher vertebrates, as listed in Table 5.2. The diversity already encoded within the diploid genome and generated by the random selection of V, D and J exons in each B cell precursor have been considered above. Further diversity within HVR3 is generated during the joining of V and J, or V, D and J segments by the random formation of variations in nucleotide sequence at the junctions. These are produced by slight imprecisions of alignment in the DNA sequences being joined and/or the insertion of additional nucleotides. In either case, this can result in the coding of different amino acids at the exon junctions.

The selection and rearrangement of heavy chain V, D and J exons and light chain V and J exons occur independently of one another. This leads to greater binding site diversity because, for example, two B cells expressing identical V_H domains could employ entirely different V_L domains and so have different antigenic specificities.

A final level of diversification occurs in activated proliferating B cells during the course of an immune response. This involves point mutations (i.e. single nucleotide substitutions during DNA replication), particularly within HVR-encoding sequences, which can result in changes in the antigen contact amino acid residues. In some cases, this **somatic mutation** produces B cells with receptors of higher affinity for the antigen which are therefore selected in germinal centres for maturation into plasma cells or memory cells (see Chapter 4).

Allelic exclusion and clonal selection

The rearrangement of immunoglobulin genes during B cell development is not always successful, i.e. non-productive arrangements can occur that do not encode functional heavy or light chains. However, each B cell precursor has several opportunities to generate productive rearrangements by virtue of having two alleles of each gene within the diploid genome, together with the possibility of utilizing either type of light chain (i.e. κ or λ). The developmental order of rearrangements starts with each heavy chain allele followed by the κ alleles and finally, if necessary, the λ alleles. A productive rearrangement blocks further rearrangements of a similar type. For example, if one heavy chain allele is successfully rearranged, the other heavy chain allele is never used in that B cell, and a λ chain allele will only be used if both attempts to rearrange the κ chain alleles are non-productive.

Table 5.2 Mechanisms that contribute to the diversity of immunoglobulin variable domains.

Multiple germline genes	Multiple V, D and J exons
Exon rearrangements	Random selection of the V, D and J exons rearranged for expression
Junctional diversity	Imprecise nucleotide alignment and/or insertion of nucleotides at the V–D–J junctions
H–L chain combinations	Independent selection of heavy and light chain variable region genes in each B cell
Somatic mutation	Point mutations in the variable region genes of activated B cells

This **allelic exclusion** ensures that all the surface and secreted immunoglobulins made by a single B cell have the same V_H and V_L domains and hence the same antigenic specificity. This explains the genetic basis of how an antigen-specific response is mounted by **clonal selection**, as described in Chapter 2. In essence, this means that those lymphocytes bearing receptors that fit the epitope best are preferentially stimulated to divide and produce more cells of the same specificity. It is extremely unusual for only one kind of receptor, i.e. specificity, to be stimulated with the result that a hierarchy of cells is triggered, giving rise to a **polyclonal** response consisting of antibody molecules with a range of affinities for the epitopes concerned. The antibodies produced in a secondary response are likely to be of higher affinity in view of preferential expansion of those clones that best fit the antigen.

Monoclonal or **oligoclonal** responses are usually seen in abnormal situations, e.g. myelomatosis, during recovery following a bone marrow graft or when antibody-producing cells are fused experimentally with plasmacytoma cells to form a monoclonal hybridoma (see p. 61).

The sequential rearrangement of light chain genes is utilized to rescue some autoreactive B cells by a process called **receptor editing**. If a B cell develops autoreactive sIgM, it has the opportunity to perform further light chain gene rearrangements to change its receptor's antigenic specificity to one that is no longer autoreactive, thus avoiding clonal deletion.

Isotype switching

The heavy chain constant region genes occur in three groups adjacent to the J_H exons on chromosome 14 (Fig. 5.8). C_μ and C_δ are closest to the J segments, and the others occur in two groups of four (although one of the C_ϵ genes is a non-productive pseudogene). They are likely to have arisen by tandem gene duplication during evolution and the primordial gene cluster probably took the form C_μ/C_δ followed by C_γ, C_ϵ and C_α. Production of IgM and IgD with the same variable domains involves differential RNA splicing, whereas switching to ex-

pression of the same V–D–J combination with any of the other constant region genes (i.e. $C_\gamma 3$ through to $C_\alpha 2$) requires further DNA rearrangements. This is controlled by 'switch' sequences of DNA in the introns adjacent to each constant region gene, which enable loops of DNA to be removed and constant region genes for IgG, IgE and IgA to be located in close proximity to the variable region genes (Fig. 5.8). It is not yet clear what causes one switch sequence to have preference over another, although T lymphocytes and/or their cytokines are involved in the process: for example, IL-4 promotes switching to IgE synthesis, and IL-5 to IgA.

T cell receptor genes

The genes that encode the T cell receptor α and β polypeptide chains are similar to the immunoglobulin genes. The variable domains are encoded by V and J exons for the α chain, and V, D and J exons for the β chain. Most of the variability is focused at the V–J and V–D–J junctions, which form the regions of the combining site that interact most fully with the antigenic peptide held in the binding groove of an HLA molecule. Thus, T cell receptor diversity is generated by the same mechanisms that give rise to the diversity of B cell receptors and antibodies, with the exception that somatic mutation does not occur in T cell receptor genes. Further differences from immunoglobulins concern the constant domains of T cell receptors in that there is no isotypic variation and there is no secreted form of T cell receptors lacking the transmembrane domain.

Exploiting the properties of immunoglobulins: laboratory methods

Antigens and antibodies do not combine in fixed proportions, i.e. their union is not stoichiometric. This is illustrated in a standard **quantitative precipitation test** (Fig. 5.9) in which increasing concentrations of antigen are added to a series of tubes containing a constant concentration of antibody. A maximum amount of precipitate is formed at an optimum point but antigen–antibody complexes form at other numerical proportions of antigen

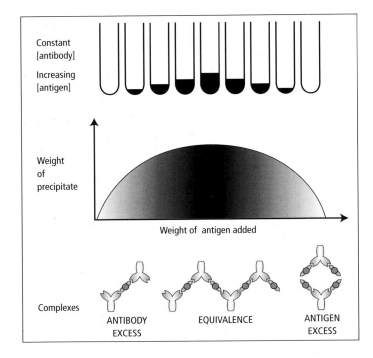

Constant
[antibody]

Increasing
[antigen]

Weight
of
precipitate

Weight of antigen added

Complexes

ANTIBODY
EXCESS

EQUIVALENCE

ANTIGEN
EXCESS

Figure 5.9 The quantitative precipitation test showing the variation in amount of precipitate formed and the size of complexes at different antigen : antibody ratios.

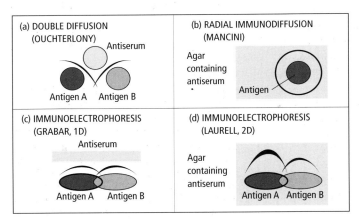

(a) DOUBLE DIFFUSION
(OUCHTERLONY)

Antiserum

Antigen A   Antigen B

(b) RADIAL IMMUNODIFFUSION
(MANCINI)

Agar
containing
antiserum

Antigen

(c) IMMUNOELECTROPHORESIS
(GRABAR, 1D)

Antiserum

Antigen A   Antigen B

(d) IMMUNOELECTROPHORESIS
(LAURELL, 2D)

Agar
containing
antiserum

Antigen A   Antigen B

Figure 5.10 Immunodiffusion techniques for characterizing specific antigens or antibodies.

and antibody. These **immune complexes** vary in their composition: complexes formed near the point of optimal proportions or **equivalence** are largest and tend to form a lattice, whereas those formed in antibody or antigen excess are smaller and precipitate less readily. This method can be used to determine the amount of antibody present in an antiserum as well as the valency of the antigen.

These principles underlie many different kinds of **immunodiffusion** techniques in which antigens and antibodies diffuse toward each other through a transparent support medium, e.g. agar, to form lines of precipitation in the equivalence zone (Fig. 5.10). These methods are used to detect and characterize solutions or extracts of antigens or antibodies (e.g. **double diffusion**), to measure the concentration of a particular protein antigen

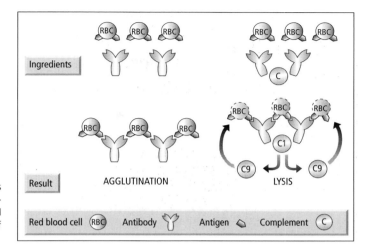

Figure 5.11 Agglutination and lysis techniques for detecting specific antibodies. Results are often reported as a titre, i.e. the weakest dilution of serum that gives a positive result.

(e.g. **radial immunodiffusion**), to detect qualitative differences in proteins present in serum or other fluids (e.g. **immunoelectrophoresis**; see also Fig. 16.2) and to quantify proteins differentially (**two-dimensional immunoelectrophoresis**).

The coupling of antigens to the surface of red cells or other particles provides greater sensitivity for the detection of specific antibodies by **agglutination**, **lysis** or **complement fixation** (Fig. 5.11). These techniques still form the mainstay of blood grouping, cross-matching and the detection of many microbial and autoantibodies.

Immunofluorescence, and techniques using enzyme-labelled (**ELISA**) and radiolabelled (**RIA**) reagents are also widely used to determine the specificity of antigen–antibody reactions (Fig. 5.12) and to examine tissues for the presence of immunological components. Their applications are legion but, as with all laboratory methods, the accuracy and precision of the results obtained depend on the regular use of internal and external standards and the rigorous application of quality control protocols.

Monoclonal antibodies from hybridomas

The production of antibodies by continuously growing **B cell hybridomas** was first described by Köhler and Milstein in 1975. **Monoclonal**

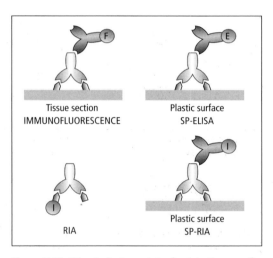

Figure 5.12 Other indicator systems for detecting specific antibody. Immunofluorescent techniques involve the reaction of antibody with sections of antigen-containing tissue. After suitable washing, the antibody can be detected using a fluorescein-labelled second antibody (i.e. antiglobulin) and UV microscopy. The solid phase enzyme-linked immunosorbent assay (SP-ELISA) utilizes antigen-coated plastic tubes or wells. Antibody binding is detected using an enzyme-conjugated antiglobulin and the colour generated on addition of substrate is read visually or with a spectrophotometer. Radioimmunoassay (RIA) is used more often to determine amounts of antigen (e.g. hormone) and is a measure of how much a standard amount of radiolabelled antigen is displaced from antibody binding in the presence of the unknown material. Solid phase RIA is exactly comparable to SP-ELISA except that a radiolabelled antiglobulin is used and the amount of antibody bound is determined by γ counting.

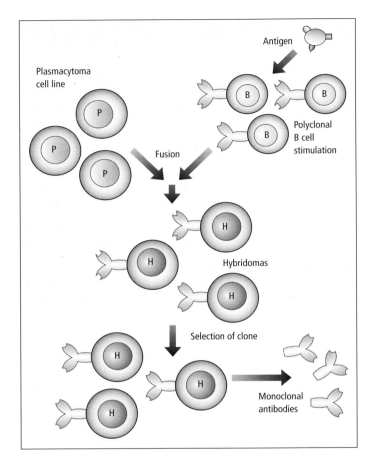

Figure 5.13 Formation of B cell hybridomas for the production of monoclonal antibodies.

antibodies derived from hybridoma cell lines are now of great importance in basic and clinical medicine as well as many other areas of biology. Figure 5.13 illustrates the method of hybridoma production. B cells, induced to divide and produce antibody by stimulation with a particular antigen, are fused with the cells of a plasmacytoma line (usually antibody non-secreting) adapted to continuous growth in culture. The resulting hybridoma cells possess properties of both partners in the fusion and thus can divide repeatedly but also secrete antibodies specific for the immunizing antigen. These hybridomas, like the original antigen-specific B cells, will be polyclonal, but individual clones can be isolated by culturing the cells singly and identifying the resulting monoclonal cell lines producing antibody of the desired specificity.

The usefulness of monoclonal antibodies derives from their clearly defined specificity, potentially limitless supply, and ease of production from established hybridomas. Examples of their uses include assays for the detection of microbes and the enumeration of cells expressing particular surface markers (e.g. the CD molecules of leucocytes; see Table 2.1). Monoclonal antibodies are also used clinically, e.g. administration of anti-CD3 antibody to kidney transplant patients to inhibit T cells causing acute rejection (see pp. 176 and 187).

Key points

1 A typical immunoglobulin is composed of two identical heavy chains and two identical light chains. The amino-terminal variable domains of a heavy and a light chain form an antigen combining site within one of the two Fab portions of the molecule. The Fc portion is composed of the heavy chain constant regions on the carboxy-terminal side of the hinge region.

2 The variable domains constitute the idiotype of an immunoglobulin, and form the antigen combining site lined by hypervariable regions which are complementary to the specific epitope.

3 Affinity defines the strength of interaction between a single antigen combining site and an epitope, whereas avidity refers to the cumulative interactions of several combining sites with an antigen.

4 Immunoglobulin isotypes (i.e. classes and subclasses) are defined by differences in their heavy chain constant regions. These determine their biological characteristics, e.g. complement activation, cellular association via Fc receptors and tissue distribution.

5 Immunoglobulin variable domains are encoded by numerous V, D and J exons whose diversity of selection, junctional variation, V_H/V_L combination and somatic mutation among different B cells generates the enormous repertoire of antigen combining sites. Similar mechanisms (with the exception of somatic mutation) generate the diversity of T cell receptors for antigens.

6 DNA rearrangements to bring the expressed heavy chain V–D–J exon combination into proximity with a different heavy chain constant region gene result in switching to the immunoglobulin class encoded by that gene.

7 The ability of antibodies to cross-link with antigens to form immune complexes is utilized in precipitation and agglutination assays. Other assays to detect antibody binding involve complement fixation or other measurable detection systems (e.g. involving fluorescent dyes, enzyme activities or radioisotopes).

8 The technology to produce monoclonal antibodies from B cell hybridomas has facilitated many studies in biology and medicine.

Chapter 6

Complement

The presence of serum factors that could augment the effects of antigen–antibody combination was first detected by Jules Bordet about 100 years ago. He showed that serum containing a red cell antibody would cause lysis of red cells when it was fresh but only agglutination when aged (Table 6.1). The material that complemented the effect of antibody could be restored by the addition of fresh non-antibody-containing serum and is now known to consist of a number of different plasma proteins which operate as an enzyme cascade similar to the coagulation system.

Most attention used to be focused upon the lytic ability of the complement system but this is now known to be one of several important biological effects of complement activation. Most of these involve the activation or fixation of the third complement component (C3) and this can be achieved in two different ways: by **activation** of the **classical pathway** and the **lectin pathway**, or by **stabilization** of the **alternative pathway** (Fig. 6.1). If these initial steps take place on a cell or basement membrane then complement activation will proceed via the **membrane attack pathway** with the production of lytic lesions. Figure 6.2 gives an overview of the complement cascade.

The classical pathway (Fig. 6.3) and the lectin pathway

The first step involves the generation of an enzyme, C1 esterase, following a complex interaction between the three subunits of the first complement component C1 (C1q, C1r and C1s). The C1q molecule resembles a bunch of tulips and the critical requirement for C1 activation is that at least two of the six 'flower heads' of the C1q molecule interact with the $C_\lambda 2$ domain of two adjacent IgG molecules (Fig. 6.4a) or two comparable complement-activating sites in the $C_\mu 3$ domain of two adjacent subunits of a single pentameric IgM molecule (Fig. 6.4b). In either case, these critical requirements are only fulfilled when the immunoglobulin is in complexed (i.e. antigen-bound) or aggregated form and this prevents the inappropriate activation of C1 by uncomplexed antibody.

The conformational change induced results in activation of C1r, which then activates C1s to form the esterase ($\overline{C1s}$). This enzyme acts on the next component in the sequence, C4, to yield a small fragment C4a and a larger fragment C4b. The latter binds covalently to membranes in the immediate vicinity but with a short half-life. C4b binds C2 in the presence of magnesium ions, causing the C2 molecule to become susceptible to the action of $\overline{C1s}$, which cleaves it to form C2a and C2b. C2a remains attached to C4b on the surface membrane and this complex, designated $C\overline{4b2a}$, functions as a

Table 6.1 Incubation of red cells with combinations of antibody and complement.

RBC	RBC antibody	Complement	Result
Present	Present	—	Agglutination
Present	Present	Present	Lysis
Present	—	Present	No effect

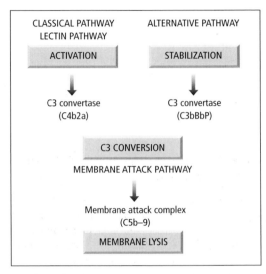

Figure 6.1 Pathways of complement activation. See Fig. 6.2 and text for greater detail.

C3 convertase with a half-life of approximately 5 min at 37°C (Fig. 6.3).

Strict control of complement activation is necessary to limit complement-mediated tissue damage. Classical pathway activation is regulated by several inhibitors (Table 6.2), e.g. **C1 esterase inhibitor** (C1INH), which inactivates C$\overline{1r}$ and C$\overline{1s}$ as well as other serine esterases present in plasma. The combined activities of a **C4-binding protein** (C4BP) and **factor I** limit the effect of C$\overline{4b2a}$. C4BP accelerates the dissociation of C$\overline{4b2a}$ and facilitates the cleavage of C4b by factor I (Fig. 6.3 and Table 6.2).

The classical pathway can be activated by factors other than immunoglobulins, e.g. C-reactive protein, lipid A of bacterial endotoxins, polyanions, polycations and some virus membranes. In particular, the lectin pathway is initiated by **mannan-binding lectin** (MBL), which has a structure

similar to that of C1q and both are members of the **collectin** family: indeed, other collectins may also activate complement. However, the six globular 'flower heads' of MBL do not bind to immunoglobulins but interact directly with mannose residues (and certain other sugars) expressed on microbial surfaces (Fig. 6.4c). The interaction of MBL with microbes activates two MBL-associated serine proteases (MASP-1 and MASP-2) , which are homologous to C1r and C1s, and these cleave C4 and C2 to generate C3 convertase (Fig. 6.2).

C3 conversion

This is the bulk reaction of the complement pathway during which several biological activities are generated. **C3 convertases** (C$\overline{4b2a}$ or C$\overline{3bBbP}$ described below) cleave C3 to give a small C3a fragment and a larger C3b fragment. C3a stimulates inflammation by causing degranulation of basophils and mast cells and is chemotactic for neutrophil polymorphs (Table 6.3); for these reasons C3a (together with C5a and C4a, which have similar properties) is referred to as an **anaphylatoxin** (anaphylaxis being a term used to describe the acute effects of mast cell degranulation; see Chapter 8).

C3b has a transient ability to form covalent bonds with membrane surfaces where it can act in concert with either of the two C3 convertases (C$\overline{4b2a}$ or C$\overline{3bBbP}$) to trigger the membrane attack pathway by interacting with C5 (Fig. 6.2). C3b is inactivated by a combination of **factor I** and **factor H**, which yields iC3b. This converts, after cleavage by trypsin-like enzymes, to C3d and C3c (Table 6.2).

C3b and iC3b also mediate the phenomenon of **immune adherence** by their ability to bind to **C3 receptors** on phagocytes (neutrophils and macrophages). In this way, the coating or

65

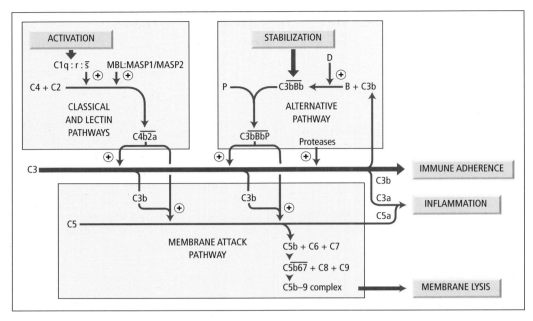

Figure 6.2 Overall plan of the classical, lectin, alternative and membrane attack pathways of complement activation. Individual components have numbers or capital letters, e.g. C4 or P. Lower-case letters indicate complement fragments, e.g. C3b. A horizontal bar above a component indicates that it has become activated, e.g. C̄3b. ⊕ indicates enzymatic activity.

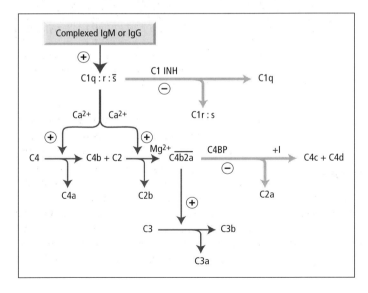

Figure 6.3 Detailed plan of the classical pathway of complement activation. Ca^{2+} and Mg^{2+} indicate a requirement for divalent calcium and magnesium ions. See Table 6.2 for the full names of inhibitors. ⊕ indicates enzymatic activity; ⊖ indicates the action of inhibitory proteins.

Table 6.2 Inhibitors of complement activation.

Mechanism of inhibition	Mediator of inhibition
Dissociation of the C1q : r : s complex	C1 inhibitor (C1 INH)
Dissociation of C4b2a	C4-binding protein (C4BP) *also* Complement receptor 1 (CR1) *also* Decay-accelerating factor (DAF)
Dissociation of C3bBb	Factor H (H) *also* Complement receptor 1 (CR1) *also* Decay-accelerating factor (DAF)
Breakdown of C4b and C3b	Factor I (I), with membrane cofactor protein (MCP), C4BP, factor H (H) and CR1
Inhibition of C9 assembly with C5b–8	CD59

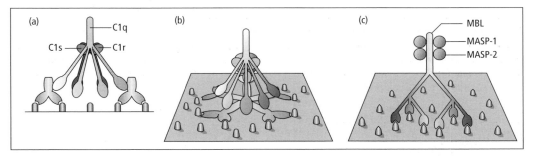

Figure 6.4 Interaction between C1 and antigen-bound antibodies, or mannan binding lectin and microbial polysaccharides. (a) Binding of C1q to the $C_\lambda 2$ domains of two adjacent IgG molecules. (b) Binding of C1q to the $C_\mu 3$ domains of a pentameric IgM molecule. (c) Binding of MBL to mannose residues as constituents of a microbial surface.

opsonization of antigens by C3b facilitates their phagocytosis (see Chapter 7).

Solubilization of immune complexes

Immune complexes have a greater tendency to aggregate if formed under conditions of complement depletion. The presence of an intact classical pathway retards precipitation, and activation of the alternative pathway and the interposition of C3b into the antigen–antibody lattice is required for solubilization to persist. Complexes containing C3b bind to complement receptors on red blood cells which transport them to the liver and spleen where macrophages remove the complexes from the red cell surface. The complement system thus has an important role in the processing of immune complexes to enable them to be cleared by the mononuclear phagocyte system. It also promotes the generation of B cell memory following the binding of complexes to follicular dendritic cells in germinal centres. This role of complement may also explain the link between genetically determined complement deficiencies and a predisposition to immune complex disease.

The alternative pathway (Fig. 6.5)

Another kind of C3 convertase can be formed by the stabilization of a different set of proteins (but

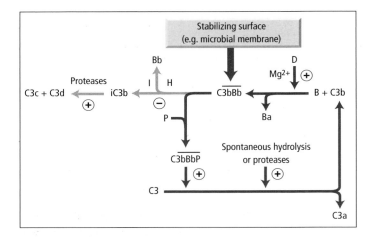

Figure 6.5 Detailed plan of the alternative pathway of complement activation. Mg^{2+} indicates a requirement for divalent magnesium ions. See Table 6.2 for the full names of inhibitors. ⊕ indicates enzymatic activity; ⊖ indicates the action of inhibitory proteins.

which includes C3b itself—a product of the classical pathway). Even in the absence of classical pathway activation, a degree of C3 conversion occurs resulting from spontaneous hydrolysis and this is enhanced by other proteases, e.g. plasmin, or other inflammatory products. This low level or **tickover** C3 conversion makes it possible for the alternative pathway to operate without activation of earlier components of the classical pathway. However, the complex that C3b forms with factor B in the presence of the protease factor D, i.e. C3bBb, rapidly dissociates unless factors are present that can stabilize it. These factors include microbial polysaccharides such as endotoxin, zymosan, sialic acid-deficient erythrocytes, nephritic factor, aggregrated forms of IgA and some subclasses of IgG (see Table 5.1).

The inhibitory factor H constantly acts to dissociate C3bBb (Table 6.2) but its affinity for C3b is considerably reduced when these stabilizing factors are present. They offer a protected surface which shields C3bBb from the inhibitor and permits its interaction with another alternative pathway protein—**properdin** (P)—to form the stable **alternative pathway convertase** C3bBbP, which then acts on C3 (and C5) in equivalent fashion to C4b2a. Indeed, C4 and C3 are structurally and functionally homologous, as are C2 and factor B. Thus, the alternative pathway takes the form of a feedback loop that operates whenever C3b is

formed and is sustained when factors are present to stabilize the assembly of its C3 convertase.

The membrane attack pathway (Fig. 6.2)

When C3b binds to either of the two C3 convertases described above, the membrane attack pathway is set in train following cleavage of C5. However, only the first step, in which C5 is cleaved to form C5a and C5b, is enzymatic.

C5a is the most potent of the anaphylatoxins and activates neutrophil polymorphs as well as mediating mast cell degranulation and neutrophil chemotaxis (Table 6.3). Both C3a and C5a are inactivated by a carboxypeptidase.

C5b has a labile binding site for cell membranes and binds C6 to form the stable complex C5b6, which then combines spontaneously with C7 to form C5b67. C5b67 has a short half-life but will bind to lipid membranes in the immediate vicinity. C8 binds to this complex, which inserts itself into cell membranes. Incorporation of C9 into the complex causes further penetration of the lipid bilayer may result in osmotic lysis of the cell. The fully developed lytic lesion—known as the **membrane attack complex** (MAC)—is a polymerized form of 10–16 C9 molecules and has the appearance of a plug or rivet in the electron microscope (Fig. 6.6). This mechanism of cell

Table 6.3 Biological sequels to complement activation.

Function	Mediators	Mechanisms
Inflammation	C5a > C3a > C4a	Stimulation of mediator release by mast cells
		Attraction of neutrophils
		Activation of neutrophils
Immune adherence	C3b, iC3b > C4b	Binding to complement receptors
		Stimulation of phagocytosis
		Clearance of immune complexes
Membrane damage	C5b–9	Insertion of the membrane attack complex into lipid membranes

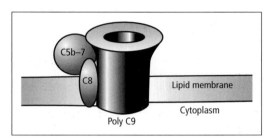

Figure 6.6 The membrane attack complex of complement.

disruption shows interesting similarities with cell-mediated cytotoxicity (see Chapter 9). The promiscuous binding of C5b67 to cell membranes can result in tissue damage, known as **reactive lysis**. However, this is limited by a protein called **CD59** expressed on tissue cells which inhibits the association of C9 with C5b–8.

Inadequate regulation of complement activation

Hereditary angio-oedema

C1 esterase inhibitor acts on various serine esterases including C$\overline{1r}$, C$\overline{1s}$, plasmin and kallikrein. A deficiency of this enzyme is associated with acute attacks of angio-oedema which may follow minor trauma. C1 esterase inhibitor is important in controlling the action of plasmin and kallikrein in extravascular sites and in its absence the uncontrolled activation of C4 and C2 or of kininogen to bradykinin will occur with major effects on capillary permeability. This process does not cause effective C3 conversion as it mostly occurs in a fluid phase without the generation of a stable membrane-bound C3 convertase.

Paroxysmal nocturnal haemoglobinuria

This disease occurs in patients with deficiencies in expression of decay-accelerating factor and CD59. The inadequate control of C3 convertase activity and MAC assembly results in intravascular red cell lysis.

Nephritic factor

This is an IgG molecule with specificity for C$\overline{3bBb}$ and is present in the sera of most patients with mesangiocapillary glomerulonephritis or partial lipodystrophy. Its presence is usually associated with marked depletion of C3, evidence of alternative pathway activation and normal levels of C1, C4 and C2. As the reactivity of this antibody resides in its Fab portion it is regarded as an autoantibody although purified nephritic factors have been shown to be larger than normal IgG and have an increased carbohydrate content. IgG antibodies reactive with the classical pathway C3 convertase C$\overline{4b2a}$ have been described in postinfective nephritis and systemic lupus although the link between infection and the development of these autoantibodies is unclear.

Complement polymorphisms and deficiencies

Heritable allotypic variation has been identified for many of the complement components (e.g. C4, C2, C3, C5, C6, C7, C8, factor B and factor D) and the loci for genes coding for C4, C2 and factor B are found in close association within the HLA complex (see Chapter 2). It is possible that some of the associations between certain HLA haplotypes and particular diseases may operate through functional differences in these variant complement proteins, particularly when there is little or no functional activity, e.g. as with the C4 null gene (see Chapter 15). Deficiencies of most of the individual complement components have been described and are briefly reviewed in Chapter 12.

Key points

1 Complement consists of a number of plasma proteins that operate as an enzyme cascade giving rise to various biological activities.

2 The complement system can be triggered via the classical pathway of C1 activation by antigen–antibody complexes, and the lectin pathway that involves mannan-binding lectin interacting with microbial surfaces, leading to formation of the C3 convertase $C\overline{4b2a}$, or via the alternative pathway involving stabilization of the C3 convertase $C\overline{3bBbP}$ on microbial surfaces.

3 The central event in complement activation is the conversion of C3 into C3a and C3b, which then activates the membrane attack pathway.

4 The biological activities resulting from complement activation are immune adherence (C3b binding to complement receptors), inflammation (C5a and C3a stimulating mast cells and neutrophils) and membrane lysis (by the membrane attack complex C5b–9).

5 Regulatory proteins limit inappropriate complement activation by causing dissociation or degradation of activated components. Inadequate regulation or inappropriate activation of complement can damage host tissues.

Chapter 7

Phagocytes

Metchnikoff coined the terms 'macrophage' and 'microphage' for the two main varieties of phagocyte and believed that they had a more important role in protective immunity than Ehrlich's serum factors (i.e. immunoglobulins). However, in 1903 Almroth Wright demonstrated that the effector function of phagocytes is triggered by immunoglobulins—a similar state of affairs to that already described for the interaction between complement and immunoglobulin molecules. The clearance function of phagocytic cells—studied largely by the use of vital dyes—was emphasized in the definition of the 'reticuloendothelial' system, but in recent years this misleading term has been replaced by a return to a Metchnikovian division into **mononuclear phagocytes** and **neutrophil polymorphs**. Mononuclear phagocytes are given different names in different tissues (Table 7.1) and are often referred to, collectively, as the **mononuclear phagocyte system**. They differ in size and morphology from neutrophils and, in addition to their role as phagocytes, are also able to present antigen to T cells (see Chapter 2). When activated, they secrete many proteins.

Macrophages

Macrophages are released from bone marrow as immature monocytes and mature in various tissue locations where they reside for weeks or years. They accumulate slowly at sites of infection, respond to a variety of stimuli (including cytokines) and have considerable potential for synthesis, secretion and regeneration. **Azurophilic lysosomal granules**, which are more evident in monocytes than in mature macrophages, contain lysozyme, myeloperoxidase and acid hydrolases (Fig. 7.1). Macrophages also possess a non-specific esterase and produce various neutral proteases, e.g. collagenase, elastase and plasminogen activator. Other **secreted products** include many complement components (and inhibitors), coagulation factors, fibronectin, cytokines and prostaglandins, e.g. PGE_2 and $PGF_{2\alpha}$.

Neutrophils

Polymorphonuclear neutrophil leucocytes mature and are stored in bone marrow and are released rapidly into the circulation in response to various stimuli, notably bacterial infection. Neutrophils are 'end cells' and only remain in the circulation for a few hours before they migrate into tissues where they die within 1–2 days. The functions of the neutrophil are mostly directed toward the killing and degradation of bacteria and are the major constituent of what, in the pre-antibiotic era, was known as 'laudable pus'. Their primary **azurophil lysosomal granules** contain several cationic proteins with antibacterial properties (the **defensins** and **serprocidins**) in addition to lysozyme, myeloperoxidase and acid hydrolases

Table 7.1 Cells of the mononuclear phagocyte system.

Cell	Tissue
Monocyte	Blood
Macrophage	Bone marrow, spleen, lymph node medulla, lung (alveolar and pleural), peritoneum
Langerhans' cell	Skin
Veiled cell	Lymph
Interdigitating dendritic cell	Lymph node paracortex
Kupffer cell	Liver
Osteoclast	Bone
Type A cell	Synovium
Mesangial cell	Kidney
Microglial cell	Brain

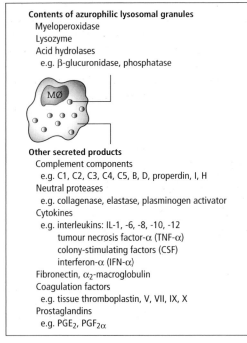

Contents of azurophilic lysosomal granules
  Myeloperoxidase
  Lysozyme
  Acid hydrolases
    e.g. β-glucuronidase, phosphatase

Other secreted products
  Complement components
    e.g. C1, C2, C3, C4, C5, B, D, properdin, I, H
  Neutral proteases
    e.g. collagenase, elastase, plasminogen activator
  Cytokines
    e.g. interleukins: IL-1, -6, -8, -10, -12
      tumour necrosis factor-α (TNF-α)
      colony-stimulating factors (CSF)
      interferon-α (IFN-α)
  Fibronectin, α_2-macroglobulin
  Coagulation factors
    e.g. tissue thromboplastin, V, VII, IX, X
  Prostaglandins
    e.g. PGE_2, $PGF_{2\alpha}$

Figure 7.1 Stored and secreted products of the macrophage.

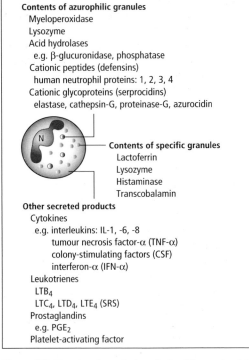

Contents of azurophilic granules
  Myeloperoxidase
  Lysozyme
  Acid hydrolases
    e.g. β-glucuronidase, phosphatase
  Cationic peptides (defensins)
    human neutrophil proteins: 1, 2, 3, 4
  Cationic glycoproteins (serprocidins)
    elastase, cathepsin-G, proteinase-G, azurocidin

Contents of specific granules
  Lactoferrin
  Lysozyme
  Histaminase
  Transcobalamin

Other secreted products
  Cytokines
    e.g. interleukins: IL-1, -6, -8
      tumour necrosis factor-α (TNF-α)
      colony-stimulating factors (CSF)
      interferon-α (IFN-α)
  Leukotrienes
    LTB_4
    LTC_4, LTD_4, LTE_4 (SRS)
  Prostaglandins
    e.g. PGE_2
  Platelet-activating factor

Figure 7.2 Stored and secreted products of the neutrophil.

(a vitamin B_{12}-binding protein). Neutrophil polymorphs can also produce cytokines and are a potent source of leukotrienes, e.g. LTB_4 (a chemotactic agent for polymorphs and monocytes) and LTC_4, LTD_4 and LTE_4, which together constitute **slow reacting substance** (SRS). They also produce prostaglandins, e.g. PGE_2, and platelet-activating factor (PAF).

Common features of phagocyte responses

Both kinds of cell respond to infective stimuli with the following sequence of activities: chemotaxis, target recognition, ingestion, killing and degradation.

Chemotaxis

Phagocytes exhibit directed movement along concentration gradients of chemotactic agents, e.g.

(Fig. 7.2). Unlike macrophages, they also possess **secondary specific granules** which contain lactoferrin (an iron-binding protein) as well as lysozyme, histaminase and transcobalamin II

anaphylatoxins (C3a, C5a), **leukotriene B4**, **chemokines** (e.g. interleukin-8) and phospholipids and peptides derived from bacteria. Neutrophils respond rapidly to these inflammatory stimuli by marginating to the walls of small blood vessels, adhering to endothelial cells and exiting into sites of inflammation (see Chapter 10).

Target recognition

Phagocytes can interact with targets hydrophobically or via specific sugar residues, e.g. mannose and glycan, or lipopolysaccharide for which they have receptors. These pattern recognition receptors (discussed on p. 6) are expressed by macrophages in particular and include scavenger receptors, mannose receptor, glucan receptor, CD14 and Toll-like receptors. In addition, secreted recognition molecules such as **collectins** (e.g. mannan-binding lectin, which also activates complement; see Chapter 6) and **pentraxins** (e.g. C-reactive protein) can also coat microbes (a process termed **opsonization**) to facilitate their uptake by macrophages.

Target recognition is greatly enhanced when specific antibody of class IgG and/or C3b opsonizes the target surface (Fig. 7.3). Both neutrophils and macrophages possess **Fc receptors** specific for IgG1 and IgG3. Human polymorphs have 20 times as many receptors as macrophages and these receptors are more scarce on the immature monocyte. Neutrophil polymorphs also possess receptors of lower affinity for the Fc of IgA (Table 7.2). Both cells have receptors for C3b (**CR1**) and C3bi (**CR3** and **CR4**), which mediate the **immune adherence** phenomenon. CR3 and CR4 are members of the family of leucocyte integrins (see Chapter 10). The effective binding of complexed IgG to Fc receptors on phagocytic cells is caused by a co-operative effect between adjacent IgG molecules brought together in an immune complex or other aggregated form as well as a conformational change in the immunoglobulin Fc region with the expression of a new binding site. The C3 receptors, on the other hand, react with the converted C3b or C3bi fragments (and C4b in the case of CR1). C3 receptors are particularly effective in promoting the attachment of phagocytes to targets, whereas Fc receptor binding induces both phagocytosis and the

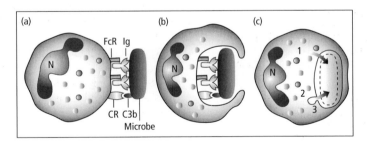

Figure 7.3 Microbial phagocytosis and killing by a neutrophil. (a) Recognition of a target opsonized by IgG antibodies and complement; (b) ingestion of the target resulting in phagosome formation; (c) degradation of the target in the phagolysosome: 1, neutral pH—toxic oxygen compound; 2, alkaline pH—cationic proteins; 3, acidic pH—lysosomal enzymes. FcR, Fc receptor.

Table 7.2 Fc receptors on macrophages, neutrophils and eosinophils.

	IgG1	IgG2	IgG3	IgG4	IgA1	IgA2	IgE
Macrophages	++	−	++	−	−	−	+
Neutrophils	++	+	++	+	+	+	−
Eosinophils	+	+	+	+	−	−	+

respiratory burst that generates toxic oxygen compounds.

Ingestion

Phagocytosis is a form of localized endocytosis and contrasts with the exocytotic process by which mast cells degranulate. It is an energy-dependent process in which the plasma membrane gradually envelops the ingested particle and buds off the surface membrane internally to form a phagosome (Fig. 7.3). This then fuses with lysosomal granules to form the **phagolysosome** in which many of the processes take place that kill and degrade the ingested material (Fig. 7.3).

Killing and degradation

Oxygen-dependent mechanisms

Phagocytes contain both oxygen-dependent and oxygen-independent mechanisms for microbial attack (Table 7.3). Phagocytosis is accompanied by a burst of respiratory activity initiated by a membrane oxidase that reduces molecular oxygen to the **superoxide** anion (O_2^-) (Fig. 7.4). Most of the respiratory activity takes place within the hexose monophosphate shunt which provides NADPH as a fuel for the reduction of molecular oxygen. This process, which is initiated at the cell surface, continues on the inner surface of the phagolysosome.

Table 7.3 Lytic mechanisms of the phagocyte.

Oxygen-dependent
Hydrogen peroxide
Singlet oxygen
Hydroxyl radical
Hypohalite
Nitric oxide
Oxygen-independent
Lysozyme
Lysosomal products
cationic proteins (defensins, serprocidins)
acid hydrolases
Lactoferrin (bacteriostatic)
Neutral proteases

Superoxide is converted to **hydrogen peroxide** (H_2O_2) by spontaneous dismutation (predominantly at the cell surface) with the production of **singlet oxygen** ($^1O_2$) or by the action of superoxide dismutase (SOD) (present intracellularly) giving rise to molecular oxygen. Singlet oxygen is a highly reactive and unstable molecular species that emits light as it returns to ground state. This process can be measured by the technique of chemiluminescence. Hydrogen peroxide and superoxide also interact to form another extremely reactive species—the **hydroxyl radical** ($\cdot$OH). A major source of microbicidal activity develops in the phagolysosome when hydrogen peroxide interacts with halide (Cl^- in the neutrophil and I^- in the macrophage) in the presence of **myeloperoxidase** (MPO) to form **hypohalite** and water. Hypohalite can then further react with hydrogen peroxide to form more singlet oxygen.

A variety of toxic materials are produced during the oxidative burst. Several processes limit the spread of these toxic effects. **Catalase**, largely present in peroxisomes, converts hydrogen peroxide to water and oxygen; **superoxide dismutase** converts singlet oxygen to hydrogen peroxide; and hydrogen peroxide is also broken down by the

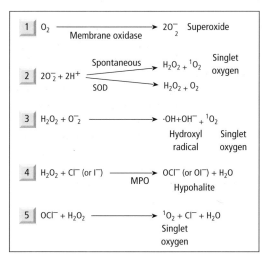

Figure 7.4 Sequential production of cytotoxic oxygen compounds in phagocytic cells. MPO, myeloperoxidase; SOD, superoxide dismutase.

glutathione redox system involving glutathione peroxidase. The chief extracellular antioxidant is caeruloplasmin, which has an equivalent role to that of superoxide dismutase within the cell. Caeruloplasmin is one of several acute phase proteins whose synthesis is considerably increased by the liver following the release of interleukin-1 (see pp. 102–3).

Nitric oxide is another cytotoxic compound for which oxygen is a substrate. It is generated by neutrophils and some tissue cells via the action of nitric oxide synthetase (NOS) and the cofactor tetrahydrobiopterin (THBT) on L-arginine and O_2.

Oxygen-independent mechanisms

Ingested microbes become exposed to the contents of lysosomal granules when these fuse with the phagocytic vesicle. In the neutral to alkaline conditions of the newly formed phagolysosome, the most active components are the families of **basic cationic proteins** which act against both Gram-positive and Gram-negative organisms. The **defensins** (human neutrophil proteins-1, -2, -3 and -4) are cyclic peptides of 29–43 amino acids which insert into the membranes of their targets. The **serprocidins** are elastase, cathepsin G, proteinase G and azurocidin. Some, but not all of them, are serine esterases and their antibacterial properties are not dependent upon their enzymatic activity.

The pH drops within 10–15 min of phagosome–lysosome fusion. This acidic environment is itself detrimental to many microorganisms, and lysosomal enzymes become active: **lysozyme** hydrolyses the peptidoglycan of Gram-positive cell walls and **acid hydrolases** digest many constituents. **Lactoferrin** has a bacteriostatic effect because of its ability to bind iron strongly, thus making it unavailable to bacteria.

The killing activity of phagocytes is enhanced in the presence of certain cytokines. γ-Interferon (IFN-γ), a product of activated T cells and large granular lymphocytes, is particularly active and tumour necrosis factor α (TNF-α) can act in conjunction with IFN-γ: TNF-α is produced by activated T cells, but also by macrophages when stimulated by certain bacterial products, e.g. lipopolysaccharide.

When macrophages and neutrophils encounter targets that are too large to phagocytose, they may release their digestive products, referred to as **frustrated phagocytosis**, causing inflammatory damage to surrounding tissues (see Chapter 14).

Deficiency disorders

The identity of the membrane oxidase that initiates the respiratory burst in phagocytic cells has been characterized as an NADPH oxidase and an associated flavin–cytochrome b complex. Patients with **chronic granulomatous disease** (CGD) lack this important enzyme and although their cells can phagocytose normally they are unable to kill most catalase-positive microorganisms, e.g. *Staphylococcus aureus* and *Serratia marcescens*. Catalase-negative organisms, e.g. streptococci, pneumococci and *Haemophilus influenzae*, are killed inside CGD phagocytes as they produce their own hydrogen peroxide which, as it is not broken down by microorganism-derived catalase, is able to join forces with the phagocyte's myeloperoxidase to generate hypohalite and a cidal effect.

C3 receptor deficiency has been described in individuals whose phagocytes can mount a normal respiratory burst and show normal IgG-dependent phagocytosis (e.g. of *Staph. aureus*) but impaired complement-dependent phagocytosis (e.g. of opsonized yeast). The C3bi (CR3) receptor is deficient whereas the C3b receptor (CR1) is normal, indicating the importance of the former in promoting this form of phagocytosis. Both these deficiencies are discussed further in Chapter 12.

Key points

1 Macrophages and neutrophils are called phagocytes because of their ability to ingest and destroy microbes.

2 Phagocytes produce a range of antimicrobial and inflammatory mediators. Some are stored in vesicles, e.g. azurophilic granules in both macrophages and neutrophils, and specific granules in neutrophils. Others are secreted.

3 Phagocytes migrate to sites of infection and inflammation in response to chemotactic signals.

4 Efficient target recognition by phagocytes involves binding to opsonized particles via Fc receptors and complement receptors, as well as direct interactions of pattern recognition receptors with microbes.

5 Ingestion of microbes and formation of phagolysosomes activates oxygen-dependent and oxygen-independent mechanisms of killing. Secretion of these mediators can cause inflammatory tissue damage.

6 Defects of the respiratory burst or complement receptor expression by phagocytes cause increased susceptibility to infection.

Chapter 8

Mast cells, basophils and eosinophils

Three kinds of granulocyte—mast cells, basophils and eosinophils—are distinguished from neutrophils by the differential staining characteristics of their granules. In mast cells and basophils this is caused by the presence of an acidic proteoglycan; in eosinophils the characteristic granules contain several basic proteins. The basophil is a circulating cell whereas the mast cell is sessile and present throughout the body but chiefly in perivascular connective tissue, epithelia and lymph nodes. There is heterogeneity within the mast cell population and dye binding is considerably affected by the method of fixation as well as the individual stains used. In appropriately fixed sections, the granules of mucosal and connective tissue mast cells differ in their staining properties. Mucosal mast cells have some features in common with basophils (which contrast with connective tissue mast cells), i.e. they are smaller, short lived, have chondroitin sulphate as acidic proteoglycan, are resistant to the inhibitory effect of sodium cromoglycate and require T cells for their growth and differentiation. Basophils have been identified in some forms of T cell mediated immune responses, e.g. Jones–Mote or cutaneous basophil hypersensitivity (see Chapter 14), and the vagaries of fixation and staining techniques have probably caused them to be overlooked in other situations.

Mast cell **degranulation** has a general role in immunity by regulating the egress of inflammatory cells and molecules through endothelial tight junctions whenever a local inflammatory response is required to deal with a focus of infection (see Fig. 1.6 and Table 8.1). This increase in capillary permeability may be partly a result of the contraction of endothelial cells similar to the effect on smooth muscle fibres elsewhere. It is likely that the remarkable variation in permeability that occurs in the postcapillary venule of the lymph node is regulated by a similar process of IgE or complement-mediated mast cell degranulation as mast cells are found plentifully at the corticomedullary junction of lymph nodes, when appropriate fixation and staining methods are used. There is evidence that, in particular, mast cell derived tumour necrosis factor is important in promoting the lymph node enlargement that accompanies an immune response. By contrast, the inappropriate activation of mast cells is one of the principal causes of allergic inflammation (see Chapters 13 and 14).

Triggering of mast cells and basophils

Mast cells and basophils possess surface **Fc receptors** with a high affinity for IgE (FcεRI). Mast cells become activated either when surface-bound IgE molecules become cross-linked by antigen (or experimentally by anti-IgE) or following the local release of the **anaphylatoxins** C3a or C5a for which mast cells also bear receptors. In either case, a complex series of events follows in which various membrane enzymes are activated, calcium ions enter the cell, and granules and their preformed mediator contents are released by exocytosis (Fig. 8.1). New mediators generated from arachidonic acid metabolism are released over a longer time-scale, and were traditionally referred to as **slow reacting substance** of anaphylaxis (SRS).

The initial step involves the activation of a serine esterase followed by the activation of methyl transferases acting on membrane phospholipids, on the one hand, and adenyl cyclase which generates an increase in intracellular cyclic adenosine monophosphate (cAMP) and protein kinase activity, on the other. Phospholipid methylation and the action of phospholipases also lead to protein kinase activation (through the generation of diacyl glycerol) and are associated with three other important events:

1 the opening of membrane **calcium channels** and the release of **intracellular calcium** (the latter occurring via the generation of inositol triphosphate);

2 the generation of **fusagenic lipids** which encourage the fusion of perigranular and cell surface membranes; and

3 the production of a supply of **arachidonic acid** from which various newly synthesized mediators are derived.

The activation of adenyl cyclase is critical for mediator release although its inhibition does not prevent phospholipid methylation. Once calcium enters the cell it is bound by calmodulin, which increases the activity of various enzymes (including protein kinases) and promotes the processes by which cytoskeletal proteins cause the contraction of microfilaments, leading to the extrusion of the granules and their contents. The antiallergic drug **sodium cromoglycate** blocks mast cell degranulation and is thought to act by preventing the transmembrane influx of calcium ions.

Mast cell mediators

Preformed mediators

The preformed mediators present within mast cell granules consist of **histamine**, eosinophil and neutrophil **chemotactic factors** (ECF and NCF), heparin proteoglycan, acid hydrolases (e.g. aryl sulphatase and β-glucuronidase) and neutral proteases (e.g. tryptase and chymase; Fig. 8.2). Histamine is a small molecule that contracts smooth

Table 8.1 Inflammatory effects of mediators released by mast cells.

Vasodilatation
Vascular permeability
Smooth muscle contraction
Leucocyte chemotaxis

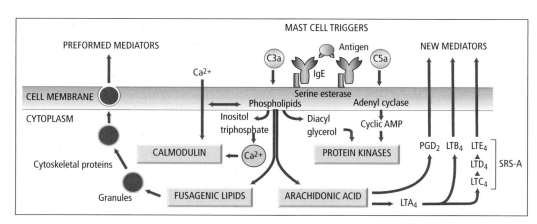

Figure 8.1 Processes involved in mast cell triggering and mediator release. See text for further details. LT, leukotriene; PG, prostaglandin.

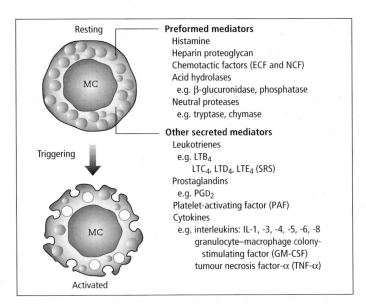

Resting

Preformed mediators
Histamine
Heparin proteoglycan
Chemotactic factors (ECF and NCF)
Acid hydrolases
e.g. β-glucuronidase, phosphatase
Neutral proteases
e.g. tryptase, chymase

Other secreted mediators
Leukotrienes
e.g. LTB_4
LTC_4, LTD_4, LTE_4 (SRS)
Prostaglandins
e.g. PGD_2
Platelet-activating factor (PAF)
Cytokines
e.g. interleukins: IL-1, -3, -4, -5, -6, -8
granulocyte–macrophage colony-
stimulating factor (GM-CSF)
tumour necrosis factor-α (TNF-α)

MC

Triggering

MC

Activated

Figure 8.2 Stored and secreted products of the mast cell (MC).

muscle and increases vascular permeability. It is present in mast cell granules as part of a protein complex containing the proteoglycan **heparin**. Heparin is replaced by **chondroitin sulphate** in the basophil. Heparin is anticoagulant and anti-complementary and may have a role in promoting the diffusion of mast cell mediators following de-granulation despite activation of the coagulation pathway, as well as contributing to the packaging and stabilization of mediators within the granules. The chemotactic factors released by mast cells not only attract other granulocytes, but also increase the expression of their C3 receptors and have a stimulatory effect on the respiratory burst and the generation of oxygen-derived products.

Secondary mediators

SRS release takes place at a slower tempo than histamine release, the latter being a preformed mediator whereas the former has to be freshly syn-thesized. These 'secondary' mediators are lipid de-rivatives of **arachidonic acid** formed via two different pathways of metabolism under the con-trol of cyclo-oxygenase and lipoxygenase enzymes (Figs 8.3 and 8.4). They include **SRS** (now known to consist of a combination of three different

leukotrienes: LTC_4, LTD_4 and LTE_4); LTB_4 (a po-tent chemotactic agent); the prostaglandins PGE_2, PGD_2 and $PGF_{2\alpha}$; and platelet-activating factor (PAF). The microsomal enzyme **cyclo-oxygenase** (also called prostaglandin synthetase) converts arachidonic acid to unstable intermediate cyclic endoperoxides (PGG_2 and PGH_2) which are then further metabolized to form stable prostaglandin mediators specific for each cell type. The predomi-nant prostaglandin formed in mast cells is PGD_2, which causes vasodilatation, contracts smooth muscle and is chemotactic for neutrophils. PGE_2 is produced in neutrophils, macrophages and lym-phocytes and is a potent vasodilator. Macrophages also synthesize $PGF_{2\alpha}$ which contracts smooth muscle. Other stable prostaglandins produced by this pathway include thromboxane (TXA_2), formed in platelets, and prostacyclin (PGI_2), which is produced by endothelial cells.

The leukotrienes are derived from the metabolic oxidation of arachidonic acid by the **lipoxyge-nase** pathway in which the unstable 5-hydroperoxyeicosatetraenoic acid (HPETE) is con-verted initially to the leukotriene LTA_4, which, de-pending on the cell concerned, either metabolizes to LTB_4 (e.g. in neutrophils) or is converted by the SRS pathway to LTC_4, LTD_4 and LTE_4 (Fig. 8.4). This

79

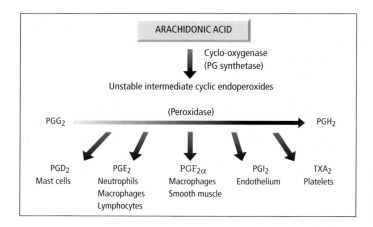

Figure 8.3 Products of the cyclo-oxygenase pathway and the cell types in which they are formed. PG, prostaglandin; TXA$_2$, thromboxane.

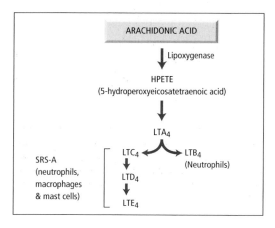

Figure 8.4 Products of the lipoxygenase pathway and the cell types in which they are formed.

latter process occurs in various granulocytes and mononuclear cells and it is possible that at least two cell types are required for the full expression of leukotriene synthesis. SRS is a particularly potent constrictor of smooth muscle and a vasodilator; it also causes mucus secretion. PGD$_2$ is the major arachidonic acid metabolite formed in connective tissue mast cells whereas LTC$_4$ production is prominent in mucosal mast cells and basophils.

Platelet-activating factors are phospholipids that cause calcium-dependent release of histamine and 5-hydroxytryptamine (5HT) from platelets and are also able to degranulate neutrophils and contract smooth muscle. Platelets

themselves may have more of an immunological role than previously thought. They have Fc receptors for both IgG and IgE. Activation via the IgG receptor causes release of 5HT whereas triggering by IgE generates oxygen metabolites which have a lytic effect on some parasites, e.g. schistosomes.

Cytokines

Activated mast cells secrete a number of proinflammatory cytokines, including tumour necrosis factor-α and chemokines (e.g. interleukin-8). They also produce IL-4, which promotes the switching of B cells to IgE production as well as Th2 cell development, and IL-5 which promotes the differentiation and activation of eosinophils.

Eosinophils

Eosinophils are distinguished by the striking affinity of their granules for acid or aniline dyes. They form a small proportion of peripheral blood leucocytes (1–5%) but are more prevalent in tissues. They probably share a common precursor with the basophil and show a later differentiation stage in the blood comparable to macrophage activation. They become more plentiful (in blood and relevant tissues) in allergic and parasitic diseases and their functions can be divided into effects on parasites and the inflammatory process.

Various factors have been identified that promote eosinophil proliferation and differentiation, e.g. granulocyte–macrophage colony-stimulating factor (GM-CSF), IL-3 and IL-5 and other eosinopoietic factors. Eosinophils also show a brisk chemotactic response to several materials liberated during the immune response, e.g. **ECF** (from mast cells), C5a and certain chemokines. ECF and C5a display synergism in their chemotactic effects on eosinophils.

Eosinophils phagocytose poorly but degranulate promptly in the presence of chemotactic factors and when membrane-bound IgG or IgE is cross-linked by antigen, i.e. exocytosis is more marked than endocytosis following triggering of their surface membrane, in contrast to the neutrophil. Eosinophils have Fc receptors for both IgG and IgE isotypes (see Table 7.2): they express low-affinity receptors for IgE (Fc$_\varepsilon$RII), as well as high-affinity receptors (Fc$_\varepsilon$RI) when activated. Like neutrophils, they also possess C3b receptors. They are able to form phagolysosomes following membrane triggering but this phenomenon is much less marked than in the neutrophil, and eosinophils display only limited proteolytic activity. A prominent role of neutrophils is the intracellular digestion of microbes (e.g. bacteria) which are readily phagocytosed. Eosinophils are more effective in the extracellular digestion of infectious agents that are too large to be engulfed (e.g. parasitic worms such as schistosomes and helminths) (Fig. 8.5). Some of the contrasting features of mast cells, eosinophils and neutrophils are summarized in Table 8.2.

Eosinophil products (Fig. 8.6)

Eosinophils display an oxidative burst with generation of H$_2$O$_2$ and, probably, superoxide, but it is uncertain whether they produce the other more

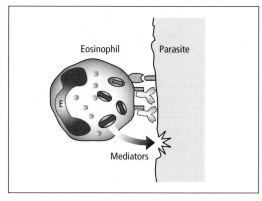

Figure 8.5 Extracellular digestion by an eosinophil. The eosinophil is targeted to the surface of a parasitic worm opsonized by IgG or IgE antibodies and C3b. Lytic mediators are exocytosed onto the parasite surface (see text and Fig. 8.6).

Table 8.2 Contrasting features of connective tissue mast cells, eosinophils and neutrophils.

	Mast cells	**Eosinophils**	**Neutrophils**
Lifespan	Long lived	Long lived	Short lived
Dynamics	Sessile	Mobile	Mobile
Chemotactic response	–	+++ (ECF, C5a, chemokines)	+++ (NCF, C5a, chemokines)
Degranulation response (exocytosis)	+++	+++	+
Phagocytosis (endocytosis)	–	+	+++
Lytic ability	–	+++ (basic proteins, O radicals)	+++ (lysosomal enzymes, O radicals)
Receptors for cell triggering	IgE C3a C5a	IgE IgG C3b	IgG IgA C3b
Biological role	Gatekeeper, proinflammatory	Antihelminth, pro- or anti-inflammatory	Antibacterial

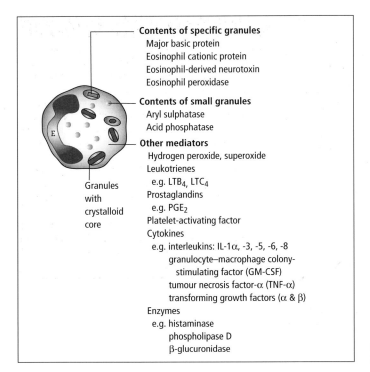

Contents of specific granules
Major basic protein
Eosinophil cationic protein
Eosinophil-derived neurotoxin
Eosinophil peroxidase

Contents of small granules
Aryl sulphatase
Acid phosphatase

Other mediators
Hydrogen peroxide, superoxide
Leukotrienes
    e.g. LTB_4, LTC_4
Prostaglandins
    e.g. PGE_2
Platelet-activating factor
Cytokines
    e.g. interleukins: IL-1α, -3, -5, -6, -8
        granulocyte–macrophage colony-
            stimulating factor (GM-CSF)
        tumour necrosis factor-α (TNF-α)
        transforming growth factors (α & β)
Enzymes
    e.g. histaminase
        phospholipase D
        β-glucuronidase

Granules with crystalloid core

E

Figure 8.6 Stored and secreted products of the eosinophil.

lytic oxygen radicals found in the neutrophil (see Fig. 7.4). Eosinophil peroxidase (EPO) is different from myeloperoxidase (MPO) but may be able to work in concert with hydrogen peroxide and iodide or chloride ions to lyse some microorganisms, e.g. *Trichinella*. However, the major source of lytic activity in the eosinophil is the basic or **cationic proteins** contained within characteristic granules which are freely exocytosed during the degranulation response and are directly toxic to parasites, e.g. schistosomes, as well as to host cells.

The characteristic granules have a crystalloid core consisting largely of a **major basic protein** and a peripheral matrix containing other basic proteins, e.g. eosinophil cationic protein, and eosinophil-derived neurotoxin, as well as eosinophil peroxidase. Separate smaller granules contain aryl sulphatase and acid phosphatase. Eosinophil granules do not contain lysozyme. The exact location of other enzymes released by the cell, e.g. histaminase, β-glucuronidase and phos-

pholipase D, is unclear. The protein, which forms Charcot–Leyden crystals in various tissues and body fluids subjected to eosinophil degranulation, is a lysophospholipase that resides in the plasma membrane of eosinophils (and basophils). Eosinophils also metabolize arachidonic acid to produce large amounts of PAF leukotrienes, e.g. LTB_4 and LTC_4, and PGE_2. The cationic proteins and arachidonic acid metabolites derived from eosinophils contribute, together with mast cell products, to the acute and chronic phases of allergic inflammation. However, several of the other eosinophil products have an inhibitory effect on mast cell mediators (Table 8.3), and so may be anti-inflammatory.

Eosinophils also produce a number of cytokines (Fig. 8.6). Some of these act as autocrine growth factors (i.e. GM-CSF, IL-3 and IL-5), whereas others may have proinflammatory activity (e.g. IL-1, IL-6, IL-8, TNF-α) or anti-inflammatory effects (e.g. TGF-β).

Table 8.3 Interactions between mast cell and eosinophil products.

Inflammatory mediators produced by mast cells	Inhibitory factors produced by eosinophils
Histamine	Histaminase
	PGE_2
Heparin	Major basic protein
SRS	Aryl sulphatase
LTB	Peroxidase
PGD_2	
PAF	Phospholipase

Hypereosinophilic syndrome

The release of inflammatory mediators can have serious complications in patients with the **hypereosinophilic syndrome**. These consist of endomyocardial fibrosis and thromboembolic disease, largely associated with the liberation of toxic basic proteins and PAF, respectively.

Key points

1 Mast cells and basophils are activated by multivalent antigens cross-linking surface-bound IgE molecules, or by anaphylatoxins (C3a and C5a); this induces the release of inflammatory mediators.

2 Some mast cell mediators are preformed and stored in granules (e.g. histamine) and are exocytosed immediately upon activation. Other mediators are synthesized *de novo* (e.g. leukotrienes and prostaglandins). Mast cells also secrete cytokines.

3 Eosinophils possess granules containing lytic mediators (e.g. major basic protein), which are exocytosed upon interaction with IgE or IgG molecules bound to the surface of, for example, parasitic worms.

4 Eosinophils also secrete some mediators, that promote inflammation (e.g. arachidonic acid metabolites and cytokines), whereas others have anti-inflammatory effects on mast cell mediators.

Chapter 9

Killer cells

Various cells of the immune system are able to inflict mortal damage on other living cells, e.g. bacteria, protozoa, the component cells of foreign grafts and even, in some circumstances, host tissues themselves. The ability of macrophages, neutrophils and eosinophils to release lytic oxygen radicals, lysosomal enzymes and toxic basic proteins has been reviewed in earlier chapters. Other cells, referred to here as **killer cells**, specialize in inflicting damage on **target cells** that represent a threat to the body, e.g. tissue cells that undergo malignant change or become infected. The latter applies particularly to viruses, but also to some intracellular bacteria (e.g. *Listeria monocytogenes*) and protozoa (e.g. *Toxoplasma gondii*). Killer lymphocytes may be of two types: **cytotoxic T cells** (Tc cells) and **natural killer cells** (NK cells) which are also known as **large granular lymphocytes** (LGL). They differ in their mechanisms of target cell recognition but employ identical lytic mechanisms.

Mechanisms of target cell recognition

Cytotoxic T cells

Tc cells bear specific antigen receptors which bind to antigen associated with HLA molecules on the surface of target cells, as described in Chapter 2. Most Tc cells express CD8 and therefore interact with antigen bound to HLA class I molecules (Fig. 9.1a), but some CD4$^+$ T cells can be cytotoxic for cells expressing HLA class II-associated antigens.

The differentiation of cytotoxic precursor T cells (Tcp) into active Tc cells is stimulated mainly by dendritic cells that can 'cross-present' HLA class I-associated peptides derived from exogenous antigens (see p. 24) together with the co-stimulatory signals that are necessary for T cell activation. This co-stimulatory ability of dendritic cells is usually triggered by infecting pathogens, but Th cells can also activate, or 'license', dendritic cells via CD40–CD40-ligand interactions (see p. 39). Activating signals, such as provided by interleukin-2 (IL-2), are necessary for the maintenance of Tc cell proliferation and effector function (see p. 45). Th cells are also required for the generation and/or maintenance of memory Tc cells. Tc cells have a key role in the lysis of host cells infected with budding viruses, i.e. those viruses that do not have a significant extracellular phase and are thus not amenable to the effects of antibodies working in conjunction with complement and phagocytes. The T cell killing of target cells involves three distinct phases.

1 *Adhesion and recognition*. A Tc cell initially binds to a potential target by adhesion molecules, i.e. CD2 and lymphocyte function-associated antigen-1 (LFA-1) on the former binding to LFA-3 and intercellular adhesion molecule-1 (ICAM-1), respectively, on the latter (see p. 35). If the target cell

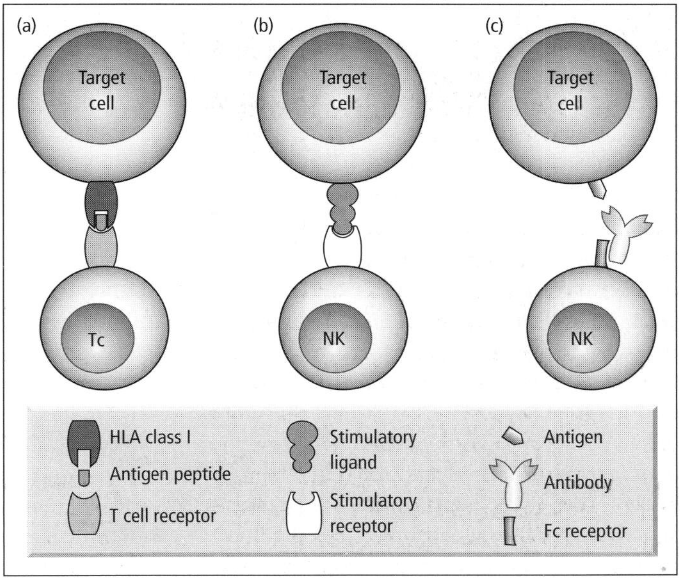

Figure 9.1 Comparison of target cell recognition by cytotoxic T (Tc) cells (a) and natural killer (NK) cells mediating natural killer activity (b) and anti-body-dependent cellular cytotoxicity (ADCC) (c). (a) The majority of Tc cells are CD8+ and recognize antigen associated with HLA class I. (b) The stimulatory receptor–ligand interaction involved in NK cell recognition is illustrated further in Fig. 9.2. (c) ADCC requires antibody to link the target to the killer cell by binding to antigen on the surface of the former and to the Fcγ receptor on the latter.

expresses antigen–HLA complexes that can engage specific antigen receptors on the Tc cell, then the cellular interaction becomes sufficiently strong and stable for killing to occur.

2 *Lethal hit*. The Tc cell contains cytotoxic mediators stored in cytoplasmic vesicles. Binding of T cell receptors to antigen–HLA causes these granules to reorientate to the area of contact with the target cell and release their contents onto the target cell surface. Thus, although the cytotoxic mediators are not antigen-specific, they are directed against cells bearing the specific target antigens (e.g. viral components) so that innocent bystander cells are not damaged. Interactions between surface molecules of the Tc cell and the target cell also contribute to the death of the latter. These processes are detailed later in this chapter.

3 *Target cell death*. The mechanisms leading to the death of the target cell involve **apoptosis**, and possibly **osmotic lysis**, which are described later in this chapter.

Once it has delivered the lethal hit, the Tc cell does not need to remain in contact with the target cell for death to ensue. Instead, the Tc cell can detach and repeat the process of killing against other cells expressing the target antigen.

Natural killer cells

Natural killer cells are identified morphologically as **large granular lymphocytes** (LGL) by virtue of having more cytoplasm than resting T and B lymphocytes, and one or two large azurophilic granules (Table 9.1). Their presence and activity is

Table 9.1 Characteristics of large granular lymphocytes (LGLs).

Large azurophilic granules
Secondary lysosomes containing acid phosphatase
Absent peroxidase and non-specific esterase
Well-developed Golgi apparatus
Fc receptors for IgG1 and IgG3 (FcγRIII or CD16)
C3b receptors (CR3)
CD56, CD94
NK and ADCC activity
Non-T suppressor activity
Respond to IL-2, IL-12 and IFN-α/β
Produce cytokines: IFN-γ, TNF-α/β, IL-3, M-CSF, GM-CSF

ADCC, antibody-dependent cellular cytotoxicity; CSF, colony-stimulating factor; G, granulocyte; IFN, interferon; IL, interleukin; M, macrophage; NK, natural killer; TNF, tumour necrosis factor.

readily detectable in peripheral blood and, to a lesser extent, in lymphoid organs. They are called *natural* killer cells because they exhibit spontaneous killing against a variety of target cell types without the need for antigen-specific activation as required by T cells (Fig. 9.1b). However, their activity is greatly enhanced by exposure to certain cytokines, particularly type I interferons (IFN-α and -β) produced by virus-infected cells, or by IL-12 secreted by activated macrophages and B cells. Activated NK cells are themselves a potent source of IFN-γ.

NK cells do not possess antigen-specific receptors, i.e. they do not rearrange genes encoding T cell receptors or immunoglobulins, even though they are members of the lymphoid developmental lineage. The ways in which NK cells recognize their targets are still being elucidated, but require that they distinguish their targets from normal cells. This is achieved by NK cells expressing various combinations of an array of receptors for cell-surface ligands. Some of these receptors inhibit killing activity when they interact with their ligands expressed by other cells, whereas others stimulate killer function. It is the balance between inhibitory and stimulatory signals that determines whether or not a potential target cell is killed. For

normal cells, the inhibitory signals dominate so the cells are not harmed (Fig. 9.2a). In abnormal cells (e.g. infected or malignantly transformed cells) the stimulatory signals dominate because of either loss of inhibitory ligand expression (Fig. 9.2b) or increased expression of stimulatory ligands (Fig. 9.2c).

Two main types of inhibitory receptors have been identified on human NK cells: killer cell immunoglobulin-like receptors (KIRs) contain immunoglobulin-like domains and interact with HLA class I proteins (particularly HLA-C), but not in an antigen-specific manner like T cell receptors; CD94/NKG2A is a lectin-like molecule that interacts with the HLA class IB protein HLA-E, which itself presents an antigen peptide derived from the leader sequence of HLA class I proteins. Some viruses (particularly herpesviruses) have mechanisms to reduce HLA class I expression by the cells they infect and tumour cells frequently lose HLA expression (which will also affect HLA-E expression). This should help to protect the infected or transformed cells from the action of Tc cells, but enhance their susceptibility to killing by NK cells because of reduced ligation of inhibitory receptors. Some KIRs and CD94/NKG2 molecules function as NK stimulatory receptors, which is surprising given that

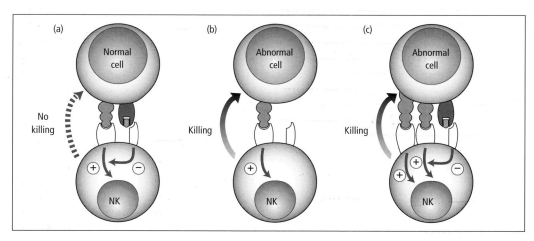

Figure 9.2 Target cell recognition by natural killer (NK) cells. Stimulatory receptors on NK cells bind to ligands on other cells. NK cells also express inhibitory receptors that bind to HLA class I. The latter interaction inhibits the triggering of cytotoxic activity against normal cells (a), but not abnormal cells with reduced or altered HLA class I expression (b) or with enhanced expression of stimulatory ligands (c). See text for further details.

they also interact with HLA class I ligands like their inhibitory counterparts; however, these stimulatory receptors may interact with different HLA ligands that are not down-regulated, or may only come into play when HLA class I expression is augmented by the action of interferons (see below). Another stimulatory receptor called NKG2D interacts with the HLA class 1B ligands MICA and MICB whose expression is induced by virus infection or malignant transformation. There are a number of other NK stimulatory receptors whose ligands have not yet been identified.

A specialized HLA class IB NK inhibitory ligand called HLA-G is expressed by fetal extravillous trophoblast cells. These placental cells invade the uterine wall during fetal development and express no HLA molecules other than HLA-G. They suppress NK cell activity by interacting with an inhibitory receptor called ILT-2, and may help to prevent an attack on the semi-allogeneic fetus by the mother's NK cells.

Antibody-dependent cellular cytotoxicity

Antibody-dependent cellular cytotoxicity (ADCC) describes an alternative mechanism used by NK cells to interact with their targets which involves the cooperation of antibodies. In addition to the adhesion molecules described above, NK cells also express receptors for the Fc portion of IgG1 and IgG3 antibodies ($Fc_\gamma RIII$). Thus, antibodies bound to surface antigens of a target cell can facilitate the adhesion of NK cells and the triggering of their cytotoxic activity (Fig. 9.1c). Although the relative importance of ADCC in immune defence is unclear, it may contribute to defence against enveloped viruses whose membrane proteins are expressed on the surface of infected cells during the process of budding.

Mechanisms of target cell killing

Secreted proteins

The cytoplasmic granules of both Tc cells and NK cells contain two types of cytotoxic proteins, called **perforins** and **granzymes**, which are rapidly se-creted onto the surface of a target cell to which a killer cell binds. The perforins are similar in structure and function to the complement protein C9 involved in the membrane attack complex (see Chapter 6). In the presence of calcium ions, the perforin molecules polymerize to form tubular structures which insert into the lipid bilayer of the target cell, thus 'perforating' its membrane. This loss of membrane integrity may lead to the death of the target cell because of the disruption of normal ion gradients, or because of the passage of water into the cell through the perforin pores leading to **osmotic lysis** (Fig. 9.3).

Granzymes are serine proteases that exert their cytotoxic effects after entry into the target cell. Their entry is assisted by the perforins, possibly because granzymes pass through the perforin pores. Alternatively, the target cell may endocytose (i.e. engulf) areas of membrane damaged by perforins in an attempt to repair its surface. By so doing, it also takes up some of the extracellular fluid containing granzymes. Once inside, granzymes induce target cell death by activating the cell's own caspase enzymes which induce an endonuclease to degrade the cell's DNA. This mechanism of cell death is termed **apoptosis** and is probably the main way in which target cells are killed (Fig. 9.3).

Tc cells and NK cells also contain tumour necrosis factor (TNF), stored in cytoplasmic vesicles, which is released onto the target cell surface where it binds to its receptor TNFR1 (also known as TNFRSF1A). This can contribute to the apoptosis of target cells by again triggering caspase activation.

Membrane ligands

In addition to the action of their granule components, killer cells are able to induce target cell death through the interaction of cell-surface ligands. Many cells express a surface receptor protein called **Fas**, and killer cells express a Fas-binding protein called **Fas-ligand** (FasL). These two proteins are structurally related to TNFR1 and the TNF cytokine, respectively. When killer cells bind to their targets, the interaction of FasL with Fas

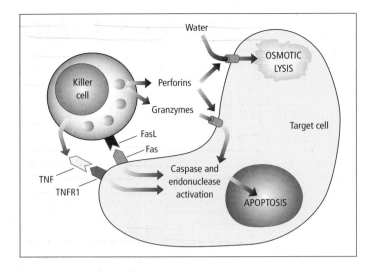

Figure 9.3 Mechanisms of target cell killing by Tc cells and NK cells. FasL, Fas-ligand; TNF, tumour necrosis factor; TNFR1, TNF receptor-1.

Table 9.2 A comparison of type I and II interferons.

Interferon type	Cell source	Antiviral activity	Cells activated	Increased HLA expression
Type I (IFN-α/β)	Virus-infected cells	+++	NK cells	Class I
Type II (IFN-γ)	Activated NK and T cells	+	Macrophages	Class I and II

induces apoptosis of the target cell (Fig. 9.3). Some CD4+ T cells, as well as all CD8+ T cells, express FasL and so can kill in this way, as well as also secreting TNF as described above.

Thus, killer cells have several weapons within their arsenal for ensuring the death of their target cells. They can 'execute' the target by damaging its surface membrane with perforins, or they can induce 'suicide' of the target through the effects of granzymes or triggering Fas or TNFR1.

Cooperation between killer cells and interferons

Effective defence against intracellular viruses requires contributions from both NK cells and Tc cells in conjunction with interferons. Tc cells are particularly efficient at killing virus-infected cells. However, the recruitment, activation and prolifer-ation of Tc cells specific for antigens of the infecting virus may take several days, whereas NK cells are spontaneously active against infected target cells. NK cells may act to limit virus spread during the early stages of infection until the Tc cells become fully activated and eliminate the virus. This is illustrated by a patient with NK cell deficiency, who suffered from repeated herpesvirus infections which were severe initially but resolved after activation of the T cell response.

Cytokines are involved in killer cell functions, and the interferons are particularly important in antiviral immunity (Table 9.2). Type I interferons (IFN-α and IFN-β) are secreted by virus-infected cells and act from the early stages of a viral infection. Type II interferon (IFN-γ) is produced by activated NK cells and T cells and contributes to the response once the killer cells become active. Both types of interferons have a direct antiviral effect by 'interfering' with the production of new virus particles. They do this by stimulating the cells to produce enzymes that degrade viral mRNA and inhibit protein synthesis.

Interferons also enhance NK cell activity and target cell recognition by Tc cells (Table 9.2). Type I interferons directly activate NK cells, whereas IFN-γ stimulates macrophages that produce another NK cell-activating cytokine, IL-12. Increased expression of HLA molecules is stimulated by interferons and enhances target cell presentation of viral antigens for recognition by Tc cells. Some viruses can suppress surface HLA expression by the cells they infect but, as described above, this makes the cells better targets for killing by NK cells.

Key points
1 There are two types of killer lymphocytes: cytotoxic T cells (Tc cells) and natural killer cells (NK cells) or large granular lymphocytes (LGL). They are cytotoxic to target cells that have become infected or malignant.
2 Most Tc cells express CD8 and interact with target cells presenting specific antigens associated with HLA class I molecules.
3 NK cells do not possess antigen-specific receptors but have surface stimulatory receptors that interact with ligands on target cells which may be up-regulated on infected or transformed cells. The killing of normal cells is prevented by simultaneous interaction of inhibitory receptors with HLA class I molecules which may be down-regulated on infected or transformed cells.
4 NK cells also have Fc receptors that can interact with antibodies bound to target cell surface antigens, leading to antibody-dependent cellular cytotoxicity.
5 Both Tc cells and NK cells possess granules containing cytotoxic proteins that are secreted onto the target cell surface. Perforins cause membrane damage and osmotic lysis, and granzymes induce apoptosis of the target cell. Tumour necrosis factor secreted by killer cells can also induce target cell apoptosis, as can Fas–Fas ligand interaction between a target cell and killer cell.
6 The spontaneous cytotoxicity of NK cells is important early on in intracellular viral infections, whereas viral clearance is dependent upon Tc cell activation. Interferons enhance killer cell functions as well as directly inhibiting viral replication.

Part 2

Immunopathology

Chapter 10

Immunity and infection

Until recently, the view had become prevalent in developed countries that scourges of infection were a thing of the past. However, a quick look at the global pattern of morbidity, and the resurgence of various forms of infectious disease among the wealthier nations of the world, indicates that infection is still a major cause of disease. The balance between the adaptive immune response and the pathogens it may face remains delicate in spite of the introduction of vaccines and many forms of antimicrobial chemotherapy. The complexity of the immune system is mirrored by the diversity of the pathogens that may interact with it. A schematic representation of host defence mechanisms, contained within their epithelial boundaries and surrounded by a universe of pathogens, is shown in Fig. 10.1. Each pathogen has its own life cycle, routes of transmission and mechanisms enhancing its survival within the hostile host environment.

Following the Second World War, and concern about infections such as poliomyelitis, influenza, malaria, smallpox and salmonellosis, various national centres were established to conduct surveillance of infectious (communicable) diseases, e.g. the Centers for Disease Control and Prevention in Atlanta, USA and the Communicable Disease Surveillance Centre in London. A reawakening of interest in, and concern about, infectious diseases has led to the appointment of specialists in communicable disease control in many countries.

The World Health Organization has coordinated measures toward the control and elimination of a number of important infectious diseases. Smallpox—already referred to in Chapter 1—was eliminated in 1980. However, there is great concern about the potential terrorist use of smallpox, and research is currently underway to improve the available vaccines. Major resources have been directed toward the elimination of poliomyelitis. However, current global estimates suggest that more than 50 million people have tuberculosis, at least 10 million are infected with malarial parasites, and approaching 50 million individuals have contracted human immunodeficiency virus (HIV) infection since it was first recognized in 1981. New vaccines, chemotherapy and effective public health measures are urgently required to combat these and other burdens of infectious disease.

A list of some important human pathogens and the diseases they cause is given in Table 10.1. However, the picture is not static and advances in microbiology, epidemiology and immunology have recently led to the identification of a number of 'new' pathogens, some of which are listed in Table 10.2.

Defence against infection

The requirements of an effective immune system are considerable and are dictated by the diversity of the pathogens that it may encounter. These

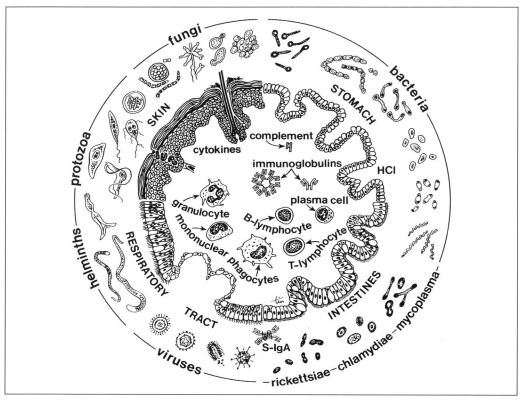

Figure 10.1 A schematic representation of host defence mechanisms and pathogenic micro- and macroorganisms. (After Van Furth R. *Review of Infectious Diseases* 1980;**2**:104–105 with permission.)

demands are met by the innate and adaptive immune system, using both cells and secreted substances such as complement and antibody, working synergistically together. The activity of these components is carefully regulated under normal circumstances to minimize damage to host tissues. However, problems arise when the regulation fails and immune-mediated disease may follow.

Thus, mammalian organisms have a powerful armoury of cells and molecules that can destroy most kinds of pathogen. These have been described in earlier chapters but are summarized diagrammatically in Fig. 10.2. They include complement-activating proteins (e.g. C-reactive protein [CRP], mannose-binding lectin [MBL] and antibodies of classes IgM, IgG and IgA); the alternative, lectin and classical complement pathways; phagocytic

cells (e.g. polymorphonuclear leucocytes and macrophages); interferons, cytokines and chemokines, T and B lymphocytes and natural killer (NK) cells.

A single defensive process may be triggered in several ways, e.g. complement can be activated by antigen–antibody complexes (via the classical pathway) or directly by microbial components such as lipopolysaccharide which activates the alternative pathway and mannose residues on the bacterial surface which activate the lectin pathway, generating inflammatory and chemotactic (C3a, C5a), opsonizing (C3b) and membrane damaging (C5b–9) activities.

Each process has its preferential targets, optima and kinetics but, in general, extracellular bacteria, viruses that have a viraemic phase (i.e. spread

Table 10.1 Some important human pathogens.

Organism	Disease
Bacteria	
Staphylococcus spp.*	Boils, septicaemia, food poisoning
Streptococcus spp.	Tonsillitis, erysipelas, scarlet fever, pneumonia
Bacillus anthracis	Anthrax
Corynebacterium diphtheriae	Diphtheria
Clostridium spp.	Tetanus, gas gangrene, botulism
Neisseria spp.	Meningitis, gonorrhoea
Escherichia coli	Urinary tract infection, gastroenteritis
Salmonella spp.	Enteric fever, food poisoning
Shigella spp.	Dysentery
Vibrio cholerae	Cholera
Proteus spp.	Urinary tract and wound infection
Haemophilus influenzae	Meningitis, pneumonia
Bordetella pertussis	Whooping cough
Yersinia pestis	Plague
Brucella spp.	Undulant fever
Mycobacterium spp.	Tuberculosis, leprosy
Legionella spp.	Legionnaires' disease
Treponema pallidum	Syphilis
Chlamydia spp.	Trachoma, pneumonia, genital tract infection
Viruses	
Polioviruses	Poliomyelitis
Hepatitis viruses (e.g. A, B, C)	Hepatitis
Rubivirus	Rubella
Measles virus	Measles
Mumps virus	Mumps
Respiratory syncytial virus	Bronchiolitis
Orthomyxoviruses	Influenza
Rhinoviruses, coronaviruses	Common cold
Rhabdovirus	Rabies
Papillomavirus	Warts
Herpes simplex virus	Herpes
Varicella-zoster virus	Chickenpox, shingles
Epstein–Barr virus	Infectious mononucleosis
Human immunodeficiency virus	AIDS
Flaviviruses	Yellow fever, dengue
Rotaviruses	Gastroenteritis
Fungi	
Candida albicans	Thrush, dermatitis
Dermatophytes (e.g. *Trychophyton* spp.)	Ringworm
Cryptococcus neoformans	Meningitis
Protozoa	
Plasmodia spp.	Malaria
Leishmania spp.	Leishmaniasis
Toxoplasma gondii	Toxoplasmosis
Trypanosoma spp.	Trypanosomiasis
Helminths	
Cestodes (e.g. *Taenia* and *Echinococcus* spp.)	Cysticercosis, hydatid disease
Trematodes (e.g. *Schistosoma* spp.)	Schistosomiasis (bilharzia)
Nematodes (e.g. *Ascaris*, *Necator*, *Wucheria*, *Onchocerca*, *Dracunculus* and *Toxocara* spp.)	Ascariasis, hookworm disease, filariasis, river blindness, guinea worm disease, toxocariasis (larva migrans)

* spp. indicates that multiple species cause disease.

Organism	Disease
Borrelia burgdorferi	Lyme disease
Campylobacter jejuni	Enteritis
Escherichia coli 0157	Haemorrhagic colitis, haemolytic–uraemic syndrome
Helicobacter pylori	Peptic ulceration, gastric cancer
Rochalimaea henselae	Cat scratch fever, bacillary angiomatosis
Cryptosporidium	Gastroenteritis
Hantaviruses	Haemorrhagic fever, renal and respiratory failure
Hepatitis D & E viruses	Hepatitis
Human herpesvirus 6–8	Rash and fever
Parvovirus B19	Rash, arthropathy and aplastic anaemia
Small round structured viruses	Gastroenteritis

Table 10.2 Recently identified human pathogens.

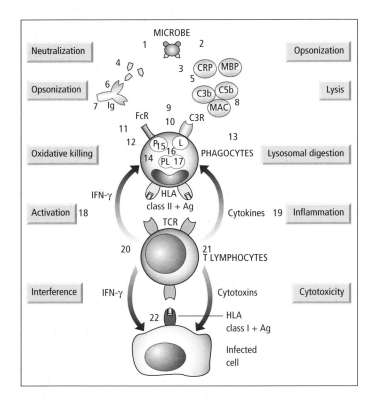

Figure 10.2 Sequential layers of defence against infection and points at which pathogens may evade these defences (see pp. 28–92 for description of mechanisms 1–22). Ag, antigen; CRP, C-reactive protein; FcR, Fc receptor; Ig, immunoglobulin; IFN, interferon; L, lysosome; MAC, membrane attack complex; MBP, mannose-binding protein; P, phagosome; PL, phagolysosome; TCR, T cell receptor.

through the bloodstream) and some fungi are susceptible to the effects of antibody, complement and phagocytes, whereas intracellular bacteria, some enveloped (or 'budding') viruses, protozoa and some other fungi can only be eliminated by the action of T cells, NK cells and macrophages. Macroparasite worms, i.e. helminths, are usually impervious to the effects of antibody and complement or lymphocyte-mediated cytotoxicity but are vulnerable to antibody-dependent reactions mediated by neutrophils, eosinophils and macrophages and to direct toxicity from granule components released by these cells such as eosinophil cationic protein (ECP). These processes lead to recovery from a primary infection. Resistance to reinfection is usually mediated by IgG or IgA antibodies, although cell-mediated immunity is required to maintain resistance to some infections, e.g. tuberculosis.

On first exposure to pathogens (e.g. bacteria), the host is dependent on the innate, pre-existing defences. These include physical barriers and non-specific bactericidal substances such as lysozyme in tears, hydrochloric acid in the stomach and surface mucus. Once the barriers have been breached, the complement system has a major role in initial damage, through direct activation of the lectin and alternative pathways by bacterial surface molecules. This process releases the **anaphylotoxins** C3a and C5a, which trigger the local inflammatory response, increasing vascular permeability and acting as chemotactic agents for the phagocytic cells, which will then engulf and digest the bacteria. Antigen processed by dendritic cells or free in the lymph can then be carried to local lymphoid tissue where it is presented to T and B cells to stimulate the production of specific antibody, initially IgM and then through class switching, IgG and, if appropriate, IgA. The release of the cytokines interleukin-1 (IL-1), IL-6 and tumour necrosis factor α (TNF-α) as a result of the inflammatory process stimulates the acute phase response, with rising levels of CRP. The activation of the complement lytic pathway leads to direct destruction of the bacteria.

Antibodies take several days to be produced and the innate mechanisms are essential to ensure survival until antibodies are available. Antibody molecules **neutralize** microbes in various ways: by inactivating microbial toxins, by preventing microorganisms attaching to receptors on host cells, by inhibiting motility or by metabolic effects. The combination of immunoglobulin molecules with an invading microbe may also lead to improved uptake by phagocytes. This process of **opsonization** may follow the interaction of antigen–immunoglobulin complexes with Fc receptors on phagocytes, but it is considerably enhanced following complement activation via the classical pathway and the interaction of C3b with C3 receptors on the phagocyte surface. Further activation of the complement sequence in this way increases the rate of destruction of the bacteria by **lysis** (see Chapter 6).

Many pathogens that survive initial contact with this array of complement-activating proteins are taken up into phagocytes and subjected to a process of **oxidative killing** within the phagosome. This is triggered by a membrane oxidase and results in the production of superoxide, singlet oxygen and hydroxyl radicals (see Chapter 7). The phagosome then fuses with lysosomal granules containing myeloperoxidase, lysozyme and acid hydrolases. Polymorph granules also contain neutral proteases and toxic cationic proteins. The presence of myeloperoxidase in the phagolysosome generates further microbicidal activity in the form of hypohalite.

The process of **lysosomal digestion** not only augments parasite killing but, in the macrophage, is a route for antigen presentation whereby antigenic epitopes are expressed on the cell surface in conjunction with HLA class II glycoproteins and provide a signal for T cell stimulation. CD4$^+$ T cells then release γ-interferon (IFN-γ) which activates macrophages and has an inhibitory effect on many viruses and some other pathogens, e.g. mycobacteria and protozoa. Interferon induces the antiviral state of **interference** by the action of two enzymes, a protein kinase and an oligoadenylate synthetase, which inhibit the translation of viral RNA and protein synthesis. IFN-γ also enhances HLA class I and II expression on the surface of virus-infected cells and **activates** the phagocytic and digestive capacity of macrophages. Activated macrophages and stimulated T, NK and B cells also produce a variety of other **cytokines** (e.g. IL-1, IL-2, IL-4, IL-6 and TNF), which add to the intensity of the **inflammatory response** (see Chapters 3 and 4). Some intracellular pathogens are eliminated by the destruction of the cells they parasitize, and this **cytotoxicity** is mediated by cytotoxins secreted by NK cells and cytotoxic T cells.

This apparent superfluity of defensive mechanisms may seem inappropriate but recent work has demonstrated the extraordinary variety of mechanisms by which successful pathogens are able to evade the actions of the immune system. This helps to explain how the tempo and severity of an infection can vary from death within 24 h (as in some cases of untreated meningococcal infection, streptococcal septicaemia or falciparum malaria), to slow but progressive infection with *Mycobacterium tuberculosis* or HIV, or an acute illness followed by complete recovery as in most cases of influenza, hepatitis A or leishmania infection, or even subclinical infection.

Mechanisms of evasion

The evolution of a successful parasite pitted against the evolution of the mammalian adaptive immune response has been described as 'a game of chess played over millennia'. Figure 10.2 pinpoints 22 mechanisms by which pathogens can evade the defensive activity of the immune system. These are described in more detail below. Some of the more successful pathogens have developed multiple mechanisms of evasion, e.g. the more virulent staphylococci and streptococci, mycobacteria, herpes simplex virus and HIV, malarial parasites, schistosomes and trypanosomes. With some infections, the battle is such that variation in the ability of the individual host to mount an effective response leads to a clinical spectrum of disease ranging from chronic and sometimes overwhelming infection to containment or destruction of the parasite and heightened immunity (e.g. lepromatous vs. tuberculoid leprosy). The immune response to larger parasites rarely eliminates the organism completely. In some protozoan infections (e.g. malaria), immunity to reinfection is only present when the initial infection persists (known as 'premunition' or non-sterile immunity) and in helminth infections (e.g. schistosomiasis) adult worms survive but reinfection with larval forms is resisted ('concomitant immunity').

Examples of evasive mechanisms
(see Fig. 10.2)

1 *Sequestration*. Wart papillomavirus in the outer epidermis, staphylococci in bone (osteomyelitis), herpes simplex virus in sensory neurones, tapeworms in hydatid cysts and retroviruses (e.g. HIV) integrated into host DNA are inaccessible to the immune response.

2 *Disguise*. Schistosomes cover their surface with various host proteins, e.g. blood group substances and HLA proteins. Cytomegalovirus adsorbs β_2-microglobulin, normally the light chain of MHC class I molecules, from serum onto its surface.

3 *Antigenic variation or drift*. The parasites that cause African trypanosomiasis possess genes that code for approximately 1000 variant forms of their surface glycoproteins; malarial parasites also display a number of surface variants, and longer term changes in influenza virus surface proteins (i.e. haemagglutinin and neuraminidase) mean that immunity is rarely sustained.

4 *Antigen shedding*. Organisms that shed surface antigens in abundance, e.g. *Streptococcus pneumoniae*, *Plasmodium falciparum* and *Schistosoma mansoni*, can neutralize the antibody response at a distance.

5 *Resistance to complement*. Bacteria with well-developed capsules (e.g. those containing sialic acid) are able to resist the effects of complement activation by enhancing the action of complement inhibitors (e.g. H and I) or by preventing interaction between C3b fixed on their surface and C3 receptors on phagocytes. Examples include *Haemophilus influenzae*, *Staphylococcus aureus* and *Streptococcus pneumoniae*.

6 *Cleavage of immunoglobulin molecules*. Several bacteria that gain access via mucosal surfaces (e.g. *Neisseria gonorrhoeae*, *Streptococcus pneumoniae* and *Haemophilus influenzae*) have a protease that cleaves IgA molecules into Fab and Fc portions. A similar activity has been demonstrated with *Trypanosoma cruzi*. This process has been called 'fabulation'.

7 *Fc binding*. Herpes simplex virus, varicella-zoster virus and some staphylococci produce a protein that binds to the Fc fragment of IgG, and some streptococci produce a substance that binds to the Fc fragment of IgA. This inhibits the ability of the Fc fragment to opsonize or activate complement.

8 *Inactivation of complement.* Herpes simplex virus has a glycoprotein that binds C3b; *Pseudomonas aeruginosa* has an elastase that inactivates C3b and C5a; and leishmania organisms are able to eject membrane attack complex from their cell membrane.

9 *Inhibition of attachment.* Some organisms, e.g. *Toxoplasma gondii*, are able to inhibit attachment to the phagocyte surface but the chemical basis for this phenomenon is not understood.

10 *Inhibition of phagocytosis.* Several organisms can resist phagocytosis as a result of the properties of their surface coat or capsule, e.g. *Streptococcus pneumoniae*, *Candida albicans* and African trypanosomes.

11 *Inhibition of chemotaxis.* The process by which phagocytes are attracted into sites of inflammation is inhibited by several organisms, e.g. *Clostridium perfringens*, *Staphylococcus aureus* and some streptococci.

12 *Blocking access of cells.* Some staphylococci liberate a coagulase that causes fibrin deposition and blocks access to inflammatory cells.

13 *Phagocyte toxicity.* Some organisms have a toxic effect on phagocytes. Staphylococcal leucocidins and streptococcal haemolysins disrupt polymorph granules and release enzymes into the cytoplasm, and some chlamydial organisms have a similar effect on macrophages. *Bordetella pertussis* releases a toxin resembling adenyl cyclase which arrests the phagocytic process, and some organisms (e.g. *Bacillus anthracis*) lyse the phagocyte on direct contact.

14 *Escape from the phagosome.* Mycobacterium leprae and *Trypanosoma cruzi* enter the phagosome but then escape from it into the cytoplasm.

15 *Resistance to killing.* Some organisms possess cell walls that resist oxidative killing, e.g. *M. tuberculosis*, *Yersinia pestis*, *Brucella abortus* and *Bacillus anthracis*. Some staphylococci produce catalase and can destroy hydrogen peroxide. Leishmania produce a superoxide dismutase and have an antioxidant effect.

16 *Inhibition of phagosome–lysosome fusion.* Several organisms, e.g. *Mycobacterium tuberculosis*, *Toxoplasma gondii* and legionella organisms are able to inhibit the process of phagosome–lysosome fusion.

17 *Resistance to digestion.* Encapsulated organisms, e.g. *Haemophilus influenzae*, and *Streptococcus pneumoniae* can resist lysosomal digestion. Some leishmania produce a lysosomal enzyme inhibitor (gp63).

18 *Impairment of the interferon response.* The interferon response is compromised by leishmania organisms and by hepatitis B virus. Epstein–Barr virus produces a molecule resembling IL-10, which inhibits IFN-γ synthesis by T and NK cells.

19 *Inhibition of cytokines.* Cytokines (e.g. IL-2 and TNF) can be inhibited by some pathogens (e.g. *Trypanosoma cruzi*).

20 *Lymphocyte activation.* Quite a few organisms, e.g. staphylococci, plasmodia, trypanosomes and Epstein–Barr virus, have been shown to activate lymphocytes polyclonally. In some instances this effect is mediated by 'superantigens' (e.g. staphylococcal enterotoxin) that bind to a broad spectrum of T cell receptors. This can prevent a specific response to the pathogen.

21 *Lymphocyte suppression.* Immunosuppression is a feature of several severe infections, e.g. measles, malaria, lepromatous leprosy and HIV infection. The mechanisms of helper T cell depletion in HIV infection are discussed on p. 109.

22 *HLA expression.* Several viruses that are able to establish latent or persistent infections, e.g. adenovirus, cytomegalovirus, herpes simplex virus and HIV, have been shown to inhibit HLA class I surface expression. In the case of herpes simplex virus this is achieved by the production of a protein that binds to the peptide transporter protein (see p. 25) and blocks the presentation of viral peptides to cytotoxic T cells. Epstein–Barr virus inhibits HLA class II-mediated antigen presentation by binding to the HLA-DRβ chain.

The inflammatory response

Pathogens are ultimately destroyed by extracellular lysis or intracellular digestion but a series of amplifying events is required to ensure that all the

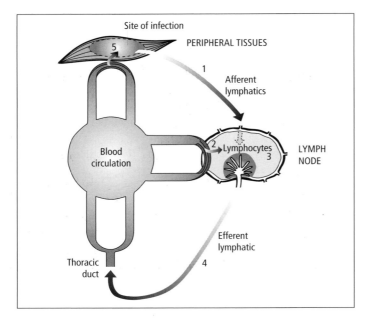

Figure 10.3 The steps involved in mounting a specific immune · response. (1) Antigen (both free and on antigen-presenting cells) is transported from the site of infection to the draining lymph node; (2) lymphocytes enter the node from the blood across high endothelial venules; (3) activation of antigen-specific lymphocytes; (4) activated lymphocytes enter the circulation; (5) cells and mediators (e.g. lymphocytes, macrophages, granulocytes, antibodies and complement) pass across the activated endothelium into the site of infection.

relevant cells and molecules arrive at the right place at the right time. This involves a modification of the normal recirculation of lymphocytes, discussed in Chapter 4 (see Fig. 4.5), to ensure that lymphocytes specific for the antigens of the invading organism are optimally activated and are targeted to the site of infection (Fig. 10.3). The secondary lymphoid tissues (e.g. lymph nodes) draining the infected tissues provide the optimal environment for interaction between antigens, antigen-presenting cells and recirculating lymphocytes, leading to the activation of specific T and B cells (discussed in Chapter 4). The recruitment of specific lymphocytes and antibodies, as well as other defensive cells and molecules, to the site of infection involves inflammatory changes in the infected tissues, particularly affecting the blood vessels, which provide the route of entry to the site (Fig. 10.3). These events include **vasodilatation**, **adhesion** of leucocytes to endothelium, increased vascular **permeability**, the chemical attraction of inflammatory cells, i.e. **chemotaxis, immobilization** of cells at the site of inflammation, and **activation** of the relevant cells and molecules to liberate their lytic products (Fig. 10.4). The clinical signs of inflammation, i.e. rubor (erythema, redness), tumor (swelling), calor (heat) and dolor (pain) were described by Celsus almost 2000 years ago.

Molecular basis of tissue inflammation

The variety of chemical mediators that promote each stage of inflammation is indicated in Fig. 10.4. These are variously derived from lymphocytes, mast cells, other leucocytes and tissue cells, complement and other serum proteins, and even microbes themselves. The apparent redundancy of several mediators exerting similar effects ensures the efficacy of the response in different types or sites of infection.

It is at sites of infection that circulating leucocytes employ cell surface **adhesion molecules** to bind to vascular endothelium and migrate into the underlying tissues (Fig. 10.5). These inflammatory processes are similar to those involved in the homing of lymphocytes to secondary lymphoid tissues during normal lymphocyte recirculation (see Fig. 4.5). Inflammatory mediators induce vascular endothelial cells to express adhesion molecules called **selectins** (P-selectin and E-selectin), which interact with heavily glycosylated proteins on

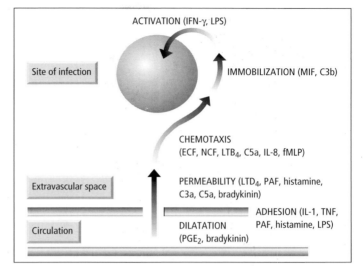

Figure 10.4 Mediators of each stage of the local inflammatory response. ECF, eosinophil chemotactic factor; fMLP, formyl-methionyl-leucyl-phenylalanine; IFN, interferon; IL, interleukin; LPS, lipopolysaccharide; LT, leukotriene; MIF, migration inhibition factor; NCF, neutrophil chemotactic factor; PAF, platelet-activating factor; PG, prostaglandin; TNF, tumour necrosis factor.

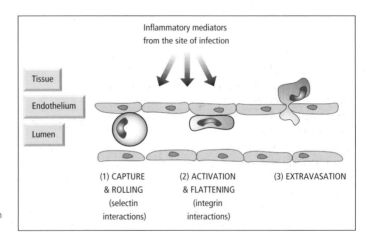

Figure 10.5 Stages in the migration of leucocytes into infected tissues.

the surface of leucocytes. Conversely, leucocytes express L-selectin which binds to endothelial **addressins**. These interactions are responsible for the initial capture of a circulating leucocyte, which then rolls along the blood vessel wall. Cytokines stimulate the endothelial cells to express other **cell adhesion molecules (CAM)**, ICAM-1 and VCAM-1, which are ligands for LFA-1 (lymphocyte function-associated) and VLA-4 (very late antigen) **integrins**, respectively. Inflammatory mediators activate these integrins on the captured leucocytes, resulting in strong adhesion to

the underlying endothelium. The leucocytes then migrate between endothelial cell junctions; secrete enzymes to digest the vascular basement membrane; and migrate towards the site of infection in response to chemotactic mediators emanating from that site.

Systemic response to infection

These defensive processes operating at local level are supported by systemic responses that enhance their effectiveness, limit tissue damage and

Effect	Mediating cytokines			Site of action
	IL-1	**IL-6**	**TNF**	
Fever	+	+	+	Hypothalamus
Leucocytosis	+	+		Bone marrow
Acute phase	+	+	+	Liver
Glucocorticoid release	+	+		Pituitary and adrenal

Table 10.3 Coordination of the inflammatory response.

promote healing. These consist of fever, leucocytosis, acute phase protein production and glucocorticoid release, and form part of the coordinated inflammatory response mediated by the cytokines IL-1, IL-6 and TNF-α (Table 10.3). These cytokines are released mostly from macrophages and lymphocytes and act locally on lymphocytes which then release other cytokines (e.g. IL-2 and IL-4), mediate cytotoxicity and synthesize antibody. Cytokines also activate neutrophils, and induce the expression of HLA glycoproteins and adhesion molecules on endothelial and other cells.

Fever

Fever is a prominent feature of many infections but can be severe, e.g. in malaria, pneumonia and septicaemia, or prolonged, e.g. in brucellosis, osteomyelitis and tuberculosis. The existence of an 'endogenous pyrogen' had been known for many years but this activity is now attributed to the cytokines, IL-1, IL-6, TNF and, possibly, interferon. These act on the thermoregulatory centre in the hypothalamus via production of the prostaglandin PGE_2. The resultant rise in body temperature enhances various cellular and biochemical processes, e.g. the bactericidal activity of polymorphs, antiviral effects of interferon, proliferative responses of lymphocytes and antibody production.

Leucocytosis

Many infections are associated with an increase in the number of polymorphonuclear leucocytes (**leucocytosis**) or lymphocytes (**lymphocytosis**) in the circulation. This is mediated by IL-1 and IL-6 and the production of colony-stimulating factors specific for these cell types. The rapid release of less mature polymorphonuclear cells from bone marrow gives rise to a preponderance of cells in peripheral blood that lack the nuclear hypersegmentation characteristic of mature neutrophils (often referred to as a 'left shift'). In severe or prolonged infection, the neutrophil azurophilic lysosomal granules stain more readily and give an appearance that has been called 'toxic granulation' although it is largely caused by increased enzyme activity. However, in very severe infections the white blood count may fall precipitately; this is a sign of overwhelming infection.

Acute phase response

A number of plasma proteins that have roles in inflammation or the healing process are produced in increased amounts by the liver during infection and after injury. This effect is mediated by the action of IL-1, IL-6 and TNF-α on hepatocytes. Human acute phase proteins can be subdivided into groups according to the magnitude of their increase (Table 10.4). Those with the shortest response time show the highest increases in concentration. Acute phase reactants operate as mediators, inhibitors or scavengers of cell-derived products. **C-reactive protein** binds to phosphorylcholine and several other molecules present on the surface of some microorganisms (e.g. *Streptococcus pneumoniae*). It also binds to DNA released from cells and enhances its removal. Bound CRP activates the classical complement pathway and may have an immunomodulatory effect. The α_1-**acid glycoprotein** also has inhibitory effects. Some acute phase proteins act as enzyme inhibitors: α_1-**antitrypsin** inhibits neutral proteases (e.g. collagenase and elastase), α_1-**antichymotrypsin** inhibits cathepsin G and

Table 10.4 Human acute phase proteins. (After Whicher JT, Evans SW, eds. *Biochemistry of Inflammation*. London: Kluwer Academic, 1992.)

Protein	Plasma concentration (g L^{-1})		Response time (h)
	Normal	In inflammation	
C-reactive protein	*c.* 0.0005	0.4	6–10
Serum amyloid A protein	*c.* 0.005	2.5	6–10
α_1-Antichymotrypsin	*c.* 0.5	3.0	10
α_1-Antitrypsin	*c.* 1.5	7.0	
α_1-Acid glycoprotein	*c.* 1.0	3.0	24
Haptoglobin	*c.* 2.0	6.0	
Fibrinogen	*c.* 3.0	10.0	
Caeruloplasmin	*c.* 0.5	2.0	
C3	*c.* 1.0	3.0	48–72
C4	*c.* 0.3	1.0	

haptoglobin inhibits other lysosomal cathepsins. Haptoglobin also conserves the iron released from haemoglobin during inflammation and **serum amyloid A** protein helps to clear cholesterol accumulated during the phagocytosis of cell debris. **Caeruloplasmin** is a scavenger of superoxide radicals and prevents the auto-oxidation of lipids. Conversely, albumin, the main serum protein, is a negative acute phase protein and falls during inflammation resulting from reduced synthesis. The acute phase response can be assessed by measuring CRP or the **erythrocyte sedimentation rate** (ESR), which is a complex measure, dependent on a number of long-lived serum acute phase proteins such as fibrinogen and fibronectin, as well as the shape, number and surface charge of the red cells.

Glucocorticoid release

IL-1 and IL-6 interact with the hypothalamic–pituitary–adrenal axis at two levels: in the hypothalamus they induce the production of corticotrophin-releasing factor which mediates adrenocorticotrophic hormone (ACTH) release, and they also act directly on the adrenal cortex. Both of these events result in the release of anti-inflammatory **glucocorticoids** (e.g. cortisol). This is a key part of the systemic response to trauma and infection and limits the destructive effects of inflammation. The release of cortisol is essential to

survival; patients unable to make this response because of pituitary disease, or damage to the adrenal gland from autoimmune destruction (e.g. Addison's disease) show a marked drop in blood pressure during infection which can be fatal.

Regulation of immune and inflammatory responses

The cells and molecules of the immune system possess considerable destructive potential which, if unleashed inappropriately, can inflict fatal effects on host tissues. It is therefore essential that immune responses to foreign pathogens are strictly regulated in magnitude and duration. This is achieved by a range of inhibitory factors, some examples of which are given in Table 10.5.

Diagnosis of microbial infection

Infection with most bacteria and some other organisms is diagnosed by laboratory culture; this allows the characterization of the organism's biochemical properties, inhibitory or toxic effects, and analysis of its antigenic structure or susceptibility to other agents (e.g. bacteriophages and antibiotics). Light or electron microscopy is preferred for some organisms in view of its speed and the characteristic appearance of some organisms. The detection of free antigen in body fluids or tissues offers advantages in some infections and usually

Inhibited components	Inhibitors
T cells	Transforming growth factor-β IL-4 and IL-10 (inhibit Th1 cells) Interferon-γ (inhibits Th2 cells) Interleukin-2 (induces T_{Reg} cells) CTLA-4
Cytokines	IL-1 receptor antagonist (competes for receptor binding) Soluble cytokine receptors (prevent binding to cell surface receptors)
Mast cell mediators	Histaminase and aryl sulphatase (from eosinophils)
Complement	C1 esterase inhibitor Decay-accelerating factor Complement receptor-1 Membrane cofactor protein Factor H Factor I

Table 10.5 Regulators of immune and inflammatory activity.

CTLA, cutaneous T lymphocyte antigen; IL, interleukin; Th T helper; T_{Reg}, T regulatory cell.

Table 10.6 The diagnosis of microbial infection.

Light or electron microscopy
Culture and identification
Antigen detection
Nucleotide analysis
Serology
Skin testing

involves the use of techniques such as agglutination, immunofluorescence, enzyme-linked immunosorbent assay (ELISA) or radioimmunoassay (RIA) methods (see Chapter 5). Nucleic acid hybridization *in situ* or involving the polymerase chain reaction (PCR) is another approach by which infection can be diagnosed without culture of the organism (Table 10.6).

Many infections are diagnosed serologically, i.e. by the identification of specific antibody in serum or other body fluids (e.g. saliva). This involves the use of techniques such as complement fixation, neutralization, agglutination inhibition, immunofluorescence, immunoperoxidase, ELISA or RIA (see Chapter 5). Skin testing is still used to measure the immune response in some circumstances, e.g. the tuberculin test for tuberculosis.

Opportunistic infection

Some individuals are especially prone to infection with recognized pathogens or may be susceptible to infection with less virulent organisms that do not cause disease in normal individuals. These so-called **opportunistic infections** are a not infrequent sequel to many of the procedures involved in modern medical care in which host defences may be bypassed or treatments given which have immunosuppressive effects (Table 10.7). The possibility of impaired immunity should always be considered when infections occur unusually frequently, in unusual locations or are caused by unusual organisms. The pattern of infection often points to the nature of the underlying defect (see Tables 12.1 and 12.10). Various diseases cause impaired immunity, e.g. chronic lymphatic leukaemia, nephrotic syndrome, uraemia, chronic infection and malnutrition (see Tables 10.7 and 12.9).

Table 10.7 Examples of conditions that favour opportunistic infection.

Bypassing host defences	Burns and other trauma
	Eczema
	Invasive procedures, e.g. intravenous lines and other indwelling devices
Primary immunodeficiency disorders	See Chapter 12
Diseases causing impaired immunity	Infections, e.g. malaria, leprosy, AIDS
	Chronic inflammatory disease, e.g. systemic lupus
	Lymphoproliferative disease, e.g. chronic lymphatic leukaemia, Hodgkin's disease, myelomatosis
	Metabolic disorders, e.g. diabetes, uraemia
	Malnutrition
	Protein-losing states
	Prematurity and old age
Treatment leading to impaired immunity	Immunosuppressive drugs or other forms of lymphoid ablation used in the management of haematological, chronic inflammatory and malignant diseases, and transplantation

Most immunosuppressive drugs inhibit T cell responses and their use may be complicated by opportunistic infection with enveloped viruses, intracellular bacteria and protozoa (see Table 17.2). Patients with severe neutropenia (i.e. having a peripheral blood leucocyte count of < 500 mm^{-3}) pose a special problem as the absence of a normal inflammatory response makes it difficult to diagnose acute infection. Here, as for many other patients with impaired defences, it is often necessary to perform microbiological screening and administer the most relevant form of antimicrobial therapy on an empirical basis. Patients who are unduly prone to opportunistic infection for long periods (e.g. after bone marrow transplantation) may require protective isolation in special units.

Chronic inflammatory diseases of unknown cause

There are a number of chronic and often severe diseases that, although they show abundant evidence of immunological stimulation, have yet to be associated with an infective agent (see Chapter 13). Examples include: rheumatoid arthritis, sarcoidosis, ulcerative colitis, type I diabetes, chronic hepatitis, various forms of glomerulonephritis and multiple sclerosis. Most of them are slow in their evolution

and show a characteristic pattern of genetic susceptibility linked to HLA class II loci (see Chapter 15). The development of diagnostic techniques that do not depend on culture of the organism (e.g. PCR), combined with advances in epidemiology, is beginning to point to microbial causes for some of these conditions. This should lead to preventive measures for these diseases, which are often resistant to treatment once they have become established.

The host–pathogen interface

The outcome of a particular infection depends on many factors that govern the ability of the pathogen to invade, evade and damage the host and the ability of the immune response to recognize and destroy the pathogen. Any weakening of the pathogen (often achieved by the administration of **antimicrobial chemotherapy**) or strengthening of the specific immune response against it (e.g. by **immunization**) will favour the immune response, whereas successful **evasion** by the parasite or the development of **immunodeficiency** (be it inherited or acquired) will tip the scales in favour of the pathogen (Fig. 10.6).

It is not surprising that the outcome for the host is often 'survival at a price' and that damage to host

105

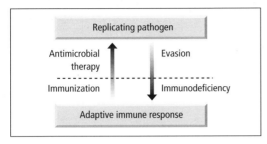

Figure 10.6 The host–pathogen interface and factors that affect it.

tissues is a common finding during the course of most infectious diseases. The pathological consequences of the endeavours of the immune response during its response to foreign material are referred to as **hypersensitivity** (in the course of an infection), **allergy** (when the trigger is inanimate) or **autoimmunity** (when the response is directed at self). These phenomena are described in more detail in Chapters 13–15.

Key points

1 Infectious diseases are still a major threat to life and health throughout the world, even though the popular impression in developed countries until recently was that scourges of infection were a thing of the past. Tuberculosis, malaria and HIV infection are just three examples of infectious diseases that each threaten the lives of tens of millions of individuals.

2 The complexity of the immune response and its multiplicity of mechanisms for destroying infectious agents reflect the many ways that pathogens have developed to evade the attentions of the immune response. Twenty-two examples of these mechanisms are cited and set against a summary of the sequential layers of host defence.

3 The inflammatory response augments the actions of the immune system. At the local level, this consists of enhanced vascular adhesiveness and permeability, associated with chemotaxis, immobilization and activation of inflammatory cells. Systemically, this is supported by the production of fever, leucocytosis, acute phase proteins and the release of glucocorticoids which are together mediated by IL-1, IL-6 and TNF released from macrophages and lymphocytes. Regulation of these processes is necessary to avoid excessive damage to host tissues.

4 Traditionally, infections have been diagnosed by culturing organisms in the laboratory from clinical samples. Increasingly, these techniques are being augmented or replaced by other methods for the detection of chemical sequences—often nucleotides—which are specific for particular groups or species of organisms, and methods that characterize the antibody response to infecting organisms. These approaches are proving of particular value in many of the chronic immunological diseases that are triggered by microbes but which do not yield culturable microbes in clinical samples.

Chapter 11

HIV infection and AIDS

The acquired immunodeficiency syndrome (AIDS) has been a major preoccupation of the lay and scientific media since it burst upon the scene in 1981. Study of the slow but relentless decay of the immune system and the pattern of infections that characterize this condition has highlighted the importance of immunology in health and disease. Public perceptions and expert assessments of the prospects for preventing, or even curing, this otherwise fatal condition have fluctuated widely but the challenge has already stimulated many innovations in basic science, laboratory diagnosis, drug and vaccine development, and approaches to patient care.

The chronology listed in Table 11.1 outlines the progress made in identifying the causative virus, in developing serological testing and the introduction of antiviral agents.

Clinical features

Those who become infected usually remain asymptomatic for many years, although 10–15% experience a febrile illness resembling infectious mononucleosis (glandular fever) around the time when the human immunodeficiency virus (HIV) antibody first becomes detectable (seroconversion). Later on, there may be persistent lymph node swelling (lymphadenopathy) without other symptoms. The addition of weight loss, fever, diarrhoea and minor opportunistic infections (e.g. oral candidiasis, herpes zoster [shingles] or tuberculosis [TB]) constitutes the **AIDS-related complex** (**ARC**) and the case definition for **AIDS** is fulfilled when more severe opportunistic infections (e.g. *Pneumocystis carinii* pneumonia, toxoplasmosis, cryptococcosis, cytomegalovirus infection and infection with both TB and non-TB mycobacteria) or tumours (e.g. lymphoma or Kaposi's sarcoma) supervene. The virus itself can cause a dementing process. Table 11.2 lists the infections to which these patients are prone. The peripheral blood CD4$^+$ T cell count declines progressively during the symptomatic phase of the illness, the more severe infections occurring when the CD4 count has fallen below 200 cells mm^{-3}. The mean incubation period from infection to the development of AIDS is 8–10 years in industrialized countries but survival times are often reduced in the developing world where death may follow less severe opportunistic infections.

Epidemiology

AIDS was first recognized among male homosexuals in California and New York but cases were soon documented throughout Europe and in sub-Saharan Africa, and have since been identified in almost every country in the world. In Africa, transmission is mostly via heterosexual contact (although blood transfusion is another important source of infection) and the number of male and

Table 11.1 Historical sequence of events.

Event	Year
First description of AIDS	1981
Discovery of HIV	1983
HIV antibody testing introduced	1985
Zidovudine (azidothymidine) approved for clinical use	1987
Combination chemotherapy introduced	1990s

Table 11.2 The spectrum of infection in AIDS.

Organism	Site of infection
Viruses	
Herpes simplex	Skin, oropharynx
Varicella-zoster	Skin
Cytomegalovirus	Gut, lung, retina
Polyomavirus	Central nervous system
Herpes virus 8	Kaposi's sarcoma
Bacteria	
Mycobacterium tuberculosis	Lung
M. avium intracellulare	Disseminated
Salmonella spp.	Gut
Rochalimea spp.	Skin, liver, central nervous system
Protozoa	
Toxoplasma gondii	Central nervous system
Cryptosporidium spp.	Gut
Giardia lamblia	Gut
Isospora belli	Gut
Fungi	
Pneumocystis carinii	Lung
Candida albicans	Oropharynx, oesophagus
Cryptococcus neoformans	Central nervous system
Coccidioides immitis	Disseminated
Histoplasma capsulatum	Disseminated
Nematodes	
Strongyloides stercoralis	Gut

female cases is almost equal. Most European cases have been attributed to infection acquired through sexual intercourse between men but the proportion infected by heterosexual contact has risen sharply in recent years. HIV is transmitted by similar routes to hepatitis B virus but has lower infectivity. The major routes of transmission are unprotected sexual intercourse, infected blood or blood products, injecting drug use or from mother to infant. The introduction of antibody screening for HIV infection in many industrialized countries has enabled fairly precise estimates to be made of the incidence and prevalence of infection. However, the long latent period before AIDS develops has led to gross underestimates of the prevalence of HIV infection in many developing countries that have not been able to introduce serological surveillance until recently, e.g. India and Thailand. It is estimated that by the end of 2003 approximately 20 million people had died of AIDS and nearly 60 million had been infected with HIV worldwide since the pandemic began. HIV infection now causes more deaths than malaria (2.9 million deaths from AIDS in 2003) and is jeopardizing the control of tuberculosis in Africa and Asia. The geographical distribution of the disease is shown in Fig. 11.1.

Virology

Only two closely related retroviruses, HIV-1 and HIV-2, have been shown to cause AIDS in humans despite much speculation to the contrary. HIV-2 infection is rare outside West Africa but both viruses are thought to have originated from a related primate virus. Several other retroviruses are known to cause immunodeficiency syndromes in other mammals, e.g. feline immunodeficiency virus in cats and simian immunodeficiency virus in macaques. Visna-maedi virus affects sheep and causes wasting and neurological features resembling those seen in AIDS but without immunodeficiency. Human T lymphotropic viruses I and II are also transmitted by blood but cause leukaemia or neurological disease without immunodeficiency.

HIV has a strong affinity for the helper T cell, but also to the macrophage. This is mediated by several of its structural components (Table 11.3). The major envelope glycoprotein (gp120) binds to the CD4 molecule as well as to the chemokine receptor, CCR5. This dual binding causes release of the glycoprotein, gp41, which fuses the viral envelope to the T cell membrane. The virus also contains an RNA polymerase (to enable it to synthesize DNA),

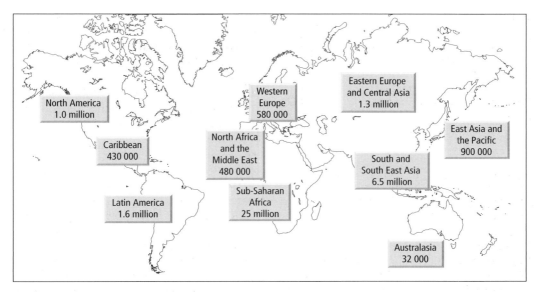

Figure 11.1 Geographical distribution of HIV-infected adults (WHO estimates for the end of 2003).

Table 11.3 Principal components of HIV.

Genes	Products
Structural	
ENV	gp160 (gp120 + gp41)
GAG	Core proteins (p24, p17, p15)
Enzymes	
POL	Reverse transcriptase, protease, integrase, ribonuclease
Regulatory	
TAT	
REV	Activating and regulatory proteins
NEF	

other enzymes and structural and regulatory proteins. Individuals who possess a non-functional variant of CCR5 are relatively resistant to HIV infection. Considerable variation occurs in the biochemical structure of the major envelope protein during the course of an infection. HIV nucleotide sequences are detectable in approximately 1 in 10 000 CD4$^+$ T cells during asymptomatic infection but the frequency rises to 1 in 100 cells when AIDS develops.

Kaposi's sarcoma is more common in patients with AIDS who have acquired their infection sex-ually, compared with those who have contracted it via infected blood or blood products. It is rarely seen in association with other immunodeficiency disorders and molecular microbiological techniques have demonstrated the presence of a new human herpesvirus (HHV8) in patients with Kaposi's sarcoma.

Immunology

In cases of HIV infection defined by seropositivity, antibodies to the envelope (gp120, gp41) or core (p24) proteins are detectable within 1–3 months of exposure. Detectable core antigen has usually disappeared by the time antibody develops. The level of core antibody falls as the disease progresses toward AIDS when the CD4 lymphocyte count falls below 500 cells mm^{-3} and opportunistic infections occur.

During the early stages of the disease there is a vigorous antiviral response involving cytotoxic CD8$^+$ T cells, and typically blood CD8$^+$ cells are markedly elevated. As the circulating free virus is reduced, the retrovirus integrates into host DNA in CD4$^+$ T cells and macrophages. This is not true latency, as there are low but detectable levels of viral particles present all the time. In the later stages of the disease, viral production increases and overwhelms the host defences. This seems to occur through mutation of the virus to generate more aggressive forms. In early and latent disease the virus tends to be macrophage-tropic, while in later stage, the virus changes to preferentially lymphocytotropic, binding specifically to the CXCR4 chemokine receptor on T cells. The biological properties also change and the late variants tend to be more destructive, although the formation of syncytia, which are formed by the combination of CD4 attachment and fusion mediated by the envelope proteins (gp120 and gp41), leads to the formation of multinuclear aggregates of T cells. This, and the internalization of CD4–gp160 complexes, have adverse effects on T cell function.

The cause of the progressive immunodeficiency that characterizes AIDS is poorly understood but there are several possibilities (Table 11.4). The virus may have a direct lytic action on the CD4$^+$ T cell although little free HIV is detectable after the initial brief viraemic phase. Infected CD4$^+$ cells will also be targets for antiviral cytotoxic T cells. In the later stages of the disease the free virus (measured as viral load) increases sharply, as T cell cytotoxiciy is unable to cope with viral mutation. The formation of syncytia is a potent mechnism for the destruction of T cells. The immune response directed to HIV-infected helper T cells may be mediated by antibody-dependent mechanisms (e.g. antibody-dependent cellular cytotoxicity or complement-mediated cytotoxicity) or by the CD8$^+$ cytotoxic T cell and in each case is likely to impair T cell function in general.

Mature T cells usually respond to receptor stimulation by cytokine secretion and proliferation but T cells taken from patients with HIV infection

Table 11.4 Possible mechanisms of helper T cell depletion in HIV infection.

Virus-induced lysis
Syncytia formation
Immune lysis (by antibody or cellular mechanisms)
Induction of apoptosis
Thymic impairment

develop apoptosis (or programmed cell death) when subjected to stimuli that would normally result in their activation. The binding of gp120 to surface CD4 molecules and their cross-linking by antibody to the envelope protein play a part in subverting the helper T cell's response to antigenic stimulation. Recent work indicates that HIV infection also causes severe damage to the thymus. This produces a marked reduction in the output of new T cells, which can be reversed by combination chemotherapy.

The HIV nef protein inhibits the expression of MHC class I antigens on the cell surface: this reduces the ability of the cells to function effectively and also impairs recognition by the antiviral cytotoxic T cells. The importance of this has been emphasized by the natural occurrence of a nef-deficient strain of HIV, which led to long-term infection but without evidence of disease progression. Under certain circumstances the activity of the CD8$^+$ T cells may be sufficient to eliminate the virus or at least maintain complete suppression.

The ability of HIV to infect antigen-presenting cells, e.g. dendritic cells and macrophages, may also impair the immune response and, by altering the pattern of cytokine secretion, may affect the balance between type 1 and type 2 helper T cell responses and cell-mediated immunity versus antibody dominance. The succession of antigenic variants of HIV that develops during the course of an infection also militates against the success of the immune response and some strains may be more effective at inducing immunosuppression.

Management

The stage of infection at which the CD4$^+$ lymphocyte count falls below 500 cells mm^{-3} and opportunistic infections develop is usually the point at which treatment with antiviral agents is commenced. The reverse transcriptase inhibitor, azidothymidine (AZT) was the drug of choice for several years but combinations (usually three or four drugs at a time) of other reverse transcriptase and protease inhibitors are currently used, particularly in patients with high plasma viral loads: this is known as **highly active antiretroviral** therapy (HAART). Such treatment is often effective in reducing plasma HIV and increasing the CD4 lymphocyte count, but requires excellent compliance with complex drug regimens. The rise in CD4$^+$ T cells and the decline in viral load, often to undetectable levels, are evidence of the effectiveness of the treatment. The new T cells have been demonstrated to be fully effective. Prophylactic treatment, usually co-trimoxazole, for *Pneumocystis carinii* infection is usually introduced when the CD4 lymphocyte count falls below 200 cells mm^{-3}; TB usually develops once the lymphocyte count falls below 50 cells mm^{-3} and other opportunistic infections are treated as they arise. With effective antiretrovrial therapy, prophylactic antibiotic therapy can be discontinued. There has also been new interest in the administration of IL-2 to stimulate the immune response to HIV.

Prevention

Public health measures and health education programmes can be effective in reducing the risk of infection by promoting safer sexual practices, by encouraging the prompt treatment of other sexually transmitted diseases, by reducing the opportunity for injecting drug users to share needles, and the provision of safe blood for transfusion and preparation of blood products.

However, control of the global epidemic of HIV infection will not be possible until an effective means of curing or preventing the disease becomes available. Considerable enterprise has been directed toward the development of an effective vaccine. The use of live attenuated HIV vaccines has lost favour after primate studies showed that such a vaccine could trigger an AIDS-like disease. Whole inactivated vaccines have shown promise, whereas peptide vaccines have been less immunogenic. DNA-based vaccines have induced protection in animals and are currently favoured for definitive

clinical trial. Until now, vaccine trials in volunteers with prototype vaccines have been uniformly disappointing. It has also become clear that combination chemotherapy can enhance the response to an HIV vaccine in infected patients and has led to useful clinical remission if not to cure.

> ## Key points
>
> **1** Considerable advances have been made since HIV infection was first observed in 1981, including the identification of the causative virus, the application of HIV antibody testing, the introduction of antiviral agents and the start of vaccine trials. However, no treatment has yet been shown to reverse the disease, which gradually overwhelms the immune system over a period of 10 years or so.
>
> **2** It is transmitted by sexual intercourse, infected blood or blood products, injecting drug use or from infected mother to infant. Approximately 20 million people have died of AIDS and approximately 60 million have been infected with HIV since the pandemic began in 1981.
>
> **3** HIV binding to CD4 and chemokine receptors on T-helper cells leads to fusion of the envelope protein with the T cell membrane.
>
> **4** The decline in T cell function is caused by some or all of the following mechanisms: direct viral lysis, fusion of lymphocytes by the formation of syncitia, immunological destruction of the infected cells, induction of apoptosis and thymic impairment.
>
> **5** Opportunistic infections develop when the count falls below 400 cells mm^{-3} and become severe when it falls below 200 cells mm^{-3}. Much can be done to treat them and progress of the disease can be slowed by antiviral chemotherapy. However, the key prospect for successful intervention is the development of an effective vaccine. Trials are in progress but it is unlikely that this will be swiftly achieved.
>
> **6** In the meantime, public health measures are the only means of slowing the spread of infection in communities. These include safe sexual practices, prompt treatment of other sexually transmitted diseases, preventing drug users sharing needles, and providing safe blood and blood products.

Chapter 12

Immunodeficiency disorders

The immune system and the complex interrelationships of its components have evolved to cope with the enormous variety of pathogens that threaten the host organism. Individuals with congenital or acquired deficiencies of the immune system are much more prone to serious infection and autoimmune complications. These 'experiments of nature' have shed considerable light on the functional significance of the deficient components. It used to be thought that clinical immunodeficiency was confined to a few rare and rapidly fatal disorders but some forms are quite common, e.g. deficiencies of IgA or C2. Every practitioner should be aware of the major kinds of deficiency and ways in which they are diagnosed and managed, as they are often missed altogether or mismanaged even when diagnosed.

Important clues

A diagnosis of immunodeficiency should always be considered when an individual experiences unusually recurrent infections, in unusual locations or with unusual organisms, and it should always form part of the differential diagnosis in children who 'fail to thrive'. There is no hard and fast rule that determines when 'recurrent infections' become suspicious. The organisms involved may be unremarkable but infections with opportunistic organisms, i.e. those that do not usually cause disease, e.g. *Candida* or *Pneumocystis*, should arouse suspicion that immunity is defective. An increased susceptibility to infection can, however, be caused by various non-immunological abnormalities which are considered briefly at the end of this chapter. Figure 12.1 indicates the major sites of involvement of the immune system in the immunodeficiency disorders, which are reviewed in this chapter.

Investigation of suspected immunodeficiency

It is often difficult to decide when children are experiencing more than their fair share of infection, particularly of the upper and lower respiratory tracts. The pattern of infection experienced by the patient often provides a useful clue to the nature of the underlying disorder (Table 12.1) and can simplify the process of investigation.

Initially, investigation is determined by the type of infections, which give clues to the site of the potential defect. Investigation of all patients should include a haemoglobin level, total and differential white cell count, platelet count; careful attention must be paid to the differential white cell count, as a normal total white count can hide severe lymphopenia. Recurrent bacterial infections of the upper and lower respiratory tract suggests humoral immune deficiency and investigations should include serum immunoglobulins (IgG, IgA, IgM), IgG subclasses and specific antibodies against

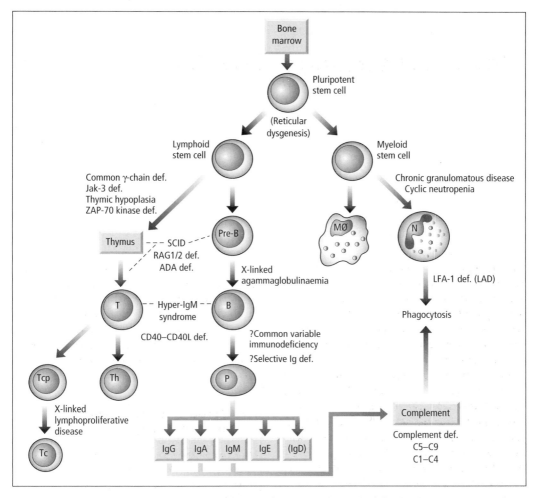

Figure 12.1 Major sites of involvement in primary immunodeficiency disorders. See text for details. ADA, adenosine deaminase; def., deficiency; LAD, leucocyte adhesion deficiency; SCID, severe combined immunodeficiency; Tcp, cytotoxic precursor T cell. See the 'Key to symbols' (p. ix) for the definition of cell types.

Table 12.1 Patterns of infection in selected immunodeficiency disorders.

Deficiency	Example	Pattern of infection
T & B cell	SCID	Viruses, fungi and bacteria
T cell	DiGeorge syndrome	Budding viruses, *Candida*, *Pneumocystis*
B cell	Hypogammaglobulinaemia	Pyogenic bacteria
Spleen	Splenectomy	Pneumococci, meningococci and *Haemophilus influenzae*
Phagocyte	CGD	Catalase-positive organisms, e.g. staphylococci and *Aspergillus*
Phagocyte	LAD	Indolent infection with pyogenic bacteria; poor wound healing
Complement	C3	Pyogenic bacteria
Complement	C5,-6,-7,-8 or-9	*Neisseria*, e.g. gonococci and meningococci

CGD, chronic granulomatous disease; LAD, leucocyte adhesion deficiency; SCID, severe combined immunodeficiency.

vaccination and exposure antigens such as pneumococccal polysaccharides, tetanus, *Haemophilus influenza* type b (Hib), polio types 1–3, measles, mumps and rubella (MMR) and chickenpox (*Varicella zoster* virus). Low levels can be followed up by deliberate test immunization, although it is important that anyone suspected of having an immunodeficiency is *never* given a live vaccine, even if it is attenuated. It is useful to measure isohaemagglutinins, which are naturally occurring IgM antibodies against ABO blood group antigens. Analysis of lymphocyte subsets to measure the absolute numbers and T, B and natural killer (NK) cells and the CD4 and CD8 subsets of T cells is required. As complement deficiency can present with recurrent bacterial infections, particularly recurrent infection with *Neisseria*, measurement of haemolytic complement (classical, alternative and mannan-binding lectin pathways), together with C3 and C4 levels, is required.

Infection with viral or fungal pathogens, or opportunist organisms such as in *Pneumocystis carinii* pneumonia (PCP), suggests a possible T cell defect. As T cells are required to assist B cells to make antibodies, there is often evidence of both T and B cell dysfunction, so investigations for antibody deficiency are required. In addition to these, more detailed studies of T lymphocytes are required, including the analysis of T cell subsets and functional studies in which the T cells are stimulated with mitogens or antigens. These include plant-derived lectins such as phytohaemagglutinin A (PHA) and concanavalin A (conA) which react with sugars on surface molecules, or phorbol esters such as phorbol myristate acetate (PMA) which bind to intracellular enzymes. Antigens are usually mimicked by using mitogenic anti-CD3 monoclonal antibodies, which react with all T cells through the T cell receptor–CD3 complex. All of these agents will cause the T cells to proliferate, and this can be measured by the uptake into the newly formed DNA of tritiated thymidine, which is radioactive. As deficiency of the surface proteins CD40 and CD40 ligand, which are critical for immunoglobulin class switching can also present with PCP, a functional assay of the surface express of CD40L is

required. Deficiency of cytokines and cytokine receptors may lead to infections with mycobacteria and can be identified through measurement of cytokine production and cytokine receptor expression.

Patients with neutrophil disorders present with recurrent bacterial and fungal infections, usually in the form of abscesses. Common organisms are those that produce catalase, an enzyme that degrades the hydrogen peroxide produced by neutrophils, such as *Staphylococcus aureus* and *Aspergillus niger*. Investigation of neutrophil function is complicated. The most serious defects are those that interfere with the neutrophil oxidative burst and are caused by genetic defects in the nicotinamide adenine dinucleotide phosphate (NADPH) oxidase system. This is assessed by the nitroblue tetrazolium reduction test, which is carried out on a microscope slide, or by an equivalent test on a flow cytometer (dihydrorhodamine reduction).

Some primary immune deficiencies do not present with infection, such as hereditary angioedema, which presents with tissue swelling and is brought about by deficiency of the complement regulatory enzyme C1-esterase inhibitor.

Primary or secondary immunodeficiency

Apart from IgA deficiency and complement C2 deficiency, all other primary immunodeficiencies are rare, and the most commonly encountered immune deficiencies will be secondary to other causes, such as malignancy (lymphoma, myeloma), radiation and drug therapy for malignancy or autoimmune disease, infections (HIV, cytomegalovirus, Epstein–Barr virus [EBV], measles, tuberculosis), nutritional deficiency, metabolic problems (diabetes), toxins (cigarettes, alcohol, drugs of addiction), burns (protein loss), renal failure and myotonic dystrophy.

As management will differ, it is important to take a careful history to establish whether immunodeficiency is likely to be a result of a primary or secondary cause.

Severe combined immunodeficiency

Severe combined immunodeficiency (SCID) is the most severe immunological defect of all and is caused by a large number of rare genetic disorders that lead to failure of development of the lymphoid system (Table 12.2). It usually presents during the first few months of life with failure to thrive, persistent oral *Candida* infection, intractable diarrhoea, often caused by persistent viral infection, and PCP. SCID infants may develop overwhelming infection with herpes and measles viruses, and inoculation with live vaccines, e.g. oral polio, bacille Calmette–Guérin (BCG) or smallpox, is invariably fatal in the absence of treatment. Infants often show a red scaly rash, which may be caused by a mild form of graft-versus-host (GVH) disease following the transplacental passage of maternal lymphocytes. Maternal T cells have been identified in the circulation in these cases. SCID is classified clinically on the basis of the presence or absence of B cells and NK cells. The most common cause of SCID (50%) is a result of mutations in the **common γ chain** of the receptors for the cytokines IL-2, IL-4, IL-7, IL-9, IL-15 and IL-21. This is an X-linked disorder and B cell numbers are usually normal. A similar phenotype is seen in **JAK-3 kinase** mutations, which is inherited as an autosomal recessive condition. Some SCID patients lack other formed elements of the blood, e.g. polymorphonuclear leucocytes, because they have

a defect that affects the myeloid stem cells as well (Fig. 12.1), a rare condition known as **reticular dysgenesis**. Immunoglobulin levels are usually also low in SCID and a proportion of cases have a homozygous deficiency of **adenosine deaminase** (ADA), which metabolizes adenosine and deoxyadenosine. Heterozygote carriers for this deficiency can be identified and antenatal diagnosis of the homozygous deficiency is possible. A form of SCID can also develop because of a deficiency of **recombination-activating genes (RAG-1/RAG-2)** (see Chapter 5), resulting in failure of the T cell antigen receptor and immunoglobulin genes to rearrange. Mutations that impair but do not abolish recombination activity give rise to the **Omenn syndrome**, in which T cells are preserved in number but are functionally abnormal. The clinical features resemble SCID but with lymphadenopathy, eosinophilia and a raised serum IgE level in addition. Rare individuals with a SCID-like syndrome fail to express HLA glycoproteins on the surface of their lymphocytes—a condition known as the **bare lymphocyte syndrome**. Other SCID-producing defects include deficiencies of the **CD3** and **CD45** molecular complexes and of the protein **ZAP-70**, involved in signal transduction.

Patients with SCID succumb during the first few years of life unless their lymphoid system is reconstituted by bone marrow transplantation. This requires the identification of a suitable donor, accurate HLA matching of donor and recipient, and graft acceptance by the latter. A further problem is the frequent development of **GVH disease**, the incidence and severity of which can be reduced by 'laundering' the graft to remove T cells using monoclonal antibodies or lectin columns (see Chapter 17). It is now possible to purify the pluripotent stem cells from the donor bone marrow and from umbilical cord blood and infuse these alone, obviating the risk of GVH disease. GVH disease can follow the transfusion of a single unit of stored blood and the T cells contained therein require elimination by irradiation before a blood transfusion is given to any patient who has defective cell-mediated immunity.

Table 12.2 Forms of severe combined immunodeficiency.

Reticular dysgenesis (very rare)
Adenosine deaminase deficiency
RAG deficiency; Omenn's syndrome
Cytokine receptor γ chain deficiency
Jak-3 deficiency
ZAP-70 deficiency
CD3 deficiency
CD45 deficiency
Bare lymphocyte syndrome

RAG, recombination-activating gene.

Thymic hypoplasia (DiGeorge syndrome; 22q11 deletion syndromes)

The thymus, parathyroid glands, and parts of the face, jaw and great blood vessels develop from the third and fourth pharyngeal arches between the sixth and eighth weeks of fetal life. In the **DiGeorge syndrome** their development is arrested, with the result that affected individuals lack a thymus (or have a few small fragments elsewhere in the neck), have hypoplastic parathyroid glands and abnormalities of their great vessels, e.g. transposition or Fallot's tetralogy, and may show facial abnormalities, e.g. low-set ears, small jaw and a short philtrum.

Medical attention is often sought because of congenital heart disease or hypocalcaemia caused by parathormone deficiency, causing neonatal tetany, but the triad of *Candida* infection, PCP and persistent diarrhoea is soon evident. The absence of a thymic shadow on chest X-ray can be a useful pointer if thymic involution has not already occurred because of age or illness. The severity of the T cell defect is variable: most cases have a few T cells detectable in blood, and B cells and immunoglobulin levels are often normal. These individuals are less prone to develop GVH disease following blood transfusion and this is in keeping with their incomplete T cell defect. The immunological abnormality can be corrected by grafts of fetal thymus or the administration of thymic humoral factors. Partial forms of the DiGeorge syndrome are not uncommon and, if the cardiovascular abnormalities permit and the hypocalcaemia can be controlled by the administration of vitamin D and calcium supplements, the infants usually show a progressive increase in T cell numbers and function with age, possibly as a result of extrathymic T cell development. Developmental delay and behavioural abnormalities are usually features in older children. The genes responsible for the DiGeorge syndrome and a number of related congential abnormalities are located at chromosome 22q11.

Table 12.3 T cell deficiencies.

Thymic hypoplasia (DiGeorge)
Purine nucleoside phosphorylase deficiency
Wiskott–Aldrich syndrome
Ataxia telangiectasia
Chronic mucocutaneous candidiasis
Hyper-IgM syndromes (CD154 deficiency, CD40 deficiency, AID)
AIDS (see Chapter 11)

AID: activation-induced cytidine deaminase.

T cell deficiencies

Various T cell defects have been described without evidence of a primary thymic abnormality. Five are referred to here (Table 12.3), in addition to the acquired immunodeficiency syndrome (AIDS) (described in Chapter 11). T cell function can become abnormal for many other reasons, e.g. zinc deficiency (see Table 12.10), when lymphocytotoxins are present (as in various autoimmune diseases) and in many forms of secondary immunodeficiency (see p. 126 and Table 12.9).

Purine nucleoside phosphorylase deficiency

This, like the DiGeorge syndrome, is characterized by low T cell numbers with normal B cells and immunoglobulins but, in contrast, shows progressive deterioration rather than gradual improvement in immune status. These children are particularly susceptible to opportunistic viral infection and live vaccines can prove fatal. Neurological features occur early and are progressive. Purine nucleoside phosphorylase (PNP) is involved in the same purine salvage pathway as ADA and its deficiency is inherited as an autosomal recessive. The toxic metabolite dGTP is preferentially toxic to T cells but eventually B cells are affected as well.

Wiskott–Aldrich syndrome

This X-linked disorder consists of severe eczema, thrombocytopenia with typically small platelets and susceptibility to opportunistic infection, and usually manifests itself during the first few months of life. Most children succumb to infection although intracranial haemorrhage and lymphomas occur eventually in most patients. Affected individuals show a progressive decline in T cell function with profound lymphopenia developing by the age of 6 years. The serum shows decreased IgM, increased IgA and IgE, and normal IgG levels and an absence of antibodies reactive with polysaccharide antigens including blood group isohaemagglutinins. IgG or IgM monoclonal proteins are occasionally present. All the features of this syndrome can be corrected by bone marrow transplantation. In the absence of an available matched donor, splenectomy is useful in reducing the risk of bleeding. Immunoglobulin replacement therapy is valuable in reducing the risk of infection. The defective gene is located on the X chromosome and codes for a protein (**WASP**) involved in signal transduction and interaction with the cytoskeleton. One mutation causes the full syndrome; another gives rise to X-linked thrombocytopenia, in which there is no detectable immune problem.

Ataxia telangiectasia

Cerebellar ataxia is first observed when affected children start to walk in their second year of life, initially with subtle but later progressive clumsiness, although the dilated small blood vessels (telangiectasia), which are most noticeable on the sclerae and the ears, do not usually become apparent until several years later. Repeated respiratory tract infection is usually complicated by bronchiectasis but lymphoma (often of T cell origin) is a common cause of death. T cells (and particularly helper T cells) are reduced in number and function, whereas B cells are normal or increased. IgA is low or absent, IgE is reduced, IgG levels are usually normal and IgM levels are often raised. Autoantibodies to IgA are often present. The condition is caused by a DNA repair defect with increased susceptibility to form chromosomal breaks and translocations and is inherited as an autosomal recessive condition. The mutated protein appears to be a phosphatidylinositol-3-kinase protein. Elevated levels of serum α_1-fetoprotein and carcinoembryonic antigen are also related to abnormal gene control.

Chronic mucocutaneous candidiasis

Chronic mucocutaneous candidiasis (CMCC) is a heterogeneous group of disorders characterized by chronic infection of skin, mouth and nails with *Candida*. Most patients have normal serum immunoglobulins, high levels of anti-*Candida* antibody and impairment of the T cell response to *Candida*. Most CMCC patients with normal specific immune responses to *Candida* respond to the administration of iron and folate and it is likely that iron deficiency is a factor in the development of chronic candidiasis in many of these individuals. Some have associated endocrine abnormalities, e.g. hypoparathyroidism, adrenal insufficiency and hypothyroidism (**APECED**—autoimmune polyendocrinopathy, candidiasis and ectoderaml dystrophy; also known as autoimmune polyendocrine syndrome type 1), and these have been associated with a specific immune defect related to the **AIRE (autoimmune regulator) gene**, as discussed on page 33.

Hyper-IgM syndrome

This X-linked condition is characterized by a profound lack of IgG and IgA but an increased level of polyclonal IgM (which distinguishes it from macroglobulinaemia; see p. 164). These patients often present with *Pneumocystis carinii* and other opportunist infections and are prone to pyogenic infections. They may also develop neutropenia and thrombocytopenia caused by the presence of IgM autoantibodies to neutrophils and platelets. They show lymphoid hyperplasia (but lack germinal centres) and have an increased incidence of lymphoma. Serum IgM levels and the associated lymphoid hyperplasia may decline when immunoglobulin replacement is given. These patients lack a glycoprotein (gp39), CD40-ligand (CD154) normally expressed on the surface of activated T cells with which the B cell CD40 membrane protein interacts during the formation of memory B cells; enabling the switch from IgM to other isotypes characteristic of the response to T cell-dependent antigens. This is an X-linked condition and is treated with bone marrow transplantation. An autosomal form is associated with abnormalities of CD40. Other molecular defects have also been associated with the same phenotype, such as activation-induced cytidine deaminase deficiency.

Mediator defects

Lymphocytes produce a variety of soluble mediators or cytokines and the chemical characterization of some of them, e.g. interleukins and interferon, is well advanced (see Chapter 3). Impaired production of IL-2 is likely to be found whenever there is significant T cell deficiency; specific deficiencies of IL-2 and of the IL-2 receptor have now been described. Several reports point to the existence of patients who fail to produce interferon in response to viral infection and who are prone to develop fulminant hepatitis, herpes encephalitis or persistent EBV infection. Mutations of genes coding for the γ-interferon (IFN-γ) receptor, the IL-12 receptor or IL-12 itself have been identified in patients with increased susceptibility to infection with mycobacteria and *Salmonella*. This demonstrates that cooperation between IL-12 secreting cells (macrophages and dendritic cells) and IFN-γ secreting cells (T cells and NK cells) is required for an effective response to these organisms. Some children experiencing recurrent respiratory tract infection with rhinoviruses have deficient IFN responses and lack IFN in their nasal secretions. Deficient IFN production in leukaemia, systemic lupus and multiple sclerosis is likely to be a secondary phenomenon.

Natural killer cell defects

Natural killer cells, alias large granular lymphocytes (LGL), are particularly effective at lysing virus-infected cells, some tumour cells and cells of bone marrow origin (see Chapter 9) and are activated by all three varieties of IFN and by IL-2. IFN deficiency can be associated with NK deficiency and restoration of the former can correct the latter. Patients with the **Chédiak–Higashi syndrome** are prone to bacterial infection and the development of lymphomas, and their cells show absent NK activity although the oxidative burst is preserved. Their leucocytes and platelets contain abnormally large and misshapen lysosomal granules and it is likely that the granule abnormality is directly linked to their NK deficiency. A similar condition has been described in mutant Beige mice. Impaired NK activity occurs in a subset of patients with late-onset hypogammaglobulinaemia in association with a high incidence of autoimmune disease. NK abnormalities have also been reported in fatal infectious mononucleosis and malignant lymphoproliferative disease, **X-linked lymphoproliferative syndrome (XLPS)**, and it seems likely that this deficiency impairs defences against EBV and so permits the inactivation or transformation of B lymphocytes. These patients, if they do not succumb to overwhelming EBV or lymphoma will develop a pan-hypogammaglobulinaemia. This disorder has been associated with defects in **SLAM-associated protein (SAP)**.

B cell deficiencies: hypogammaglobulinaemia

An increased incidence of infection with pyogenic bacteria occurs with defects of antibody production or complement activation. This is because pus cells, i.e. neutrophil polymorphs, are the chief line of defence against these organisms and are recruited and activated following the interaction of specific antibody and complement. The major varieties of generalized antibody deficiency are described in this section (Table 12.4). Complement deficiencies are described on pp. 124–6.

X-linked hypogammaglobulinaemia

Bruton's disease (XLA)

The classical form of antibody deficiency was described by Bruton in 1952 and is usually referred to as **X-linked agammaglobulinaemia (XLA)** as there is a complete absence of serum immunoglobulins. Affected males usually present with recurrent infection at between 6 months and 2 years of age, as they are protected from earlier infection

Table 12.4 Examples of primary and secondary hypogammaglobulinaemia.

Primary	Secondary
Bruton's disease (XLA)	Myelomatosis
Common variable immunodeficiency	Chronic lymphatic leukaemia
Selective IgA deficiency	Protein-losing enteropathy
IgG subclass deficiencies	Congenital rubella
Hypogammaglobulinaemia with thymoma	
With dwarfism	
Transcobalamin II deficiency	
Transient hypogammaglobulinaemia of infancy	

because of the placental transfer of maternal IgG antibody. *Haemophilus influenzae, Streptococcus pneumoniae* and staphylococci are the most frequent causes, and the respiratory tract and skin the most frequent sites of infection. Septic arthritis may be the first indication of a problem. Episodes of diarrhoea may occur and are often caused by infection with *Giardia lamblia*. A minority of patients develop arthritis, which can be caused by mycoplasma. Some develop a meningoencephalitis resulting from enteroviruses (echovirus); this is the only type of viral infection that affects antibody-deficient patients and the reason for this is poorly understood. Other viral infections are not usually a problem, although paralytic poliomyelitis can follow immunization with the live attenuated vaccine.

The defect blocks pre-B cells differentiating into B cells (see Fig. 12.1) and is caused by the lack of a **B cell-specific tyrosine kinase, btk**. Very few B cells or plasma cells are found in affected individuals, whereas pre-B cells are present in normal numbers in bone marrow and lack surface immunoglobulin in conjunction with the presence of cytoplasmic μ heavy chains. IgM and IgA are usually absent in serum and secretions, and serum IgG levels are low but rarely completely absent. T cell numbers and function are usually normal. Male infants at risk should have their circulating B cell levels measured rather than wait for maternal antibody to decay so that replacement immunoglobulin therapy can be started promptly.

A combination of immunoglobulin replacement therapy, vigorous use of antibacterial agents and measures designed to achieve maximal drainage of infected sites form the basis of the long-term management of generalized antibody deficiencies of all kinds. Immunoglobulin replacement is administered by intravenous or subcutaneous injection, with the aim of restoring trough IgG levels to the normal range. The initiation of immunoglobulin replacement therapy can be as dramatically beneficial as the introduction of insulin therapy to the patient with type I diabetes and, in both situations, follow-up is required for life.

Common variable immunodeficiency

Common variable immunodeficiency (CVID) is more common and less consistent than XLA. It usually presents in later childhood or early adult life and has also been referred to as late-onset hypogammaglobulinaemia. However, the pattern of infection is similar and chiefly affects the lungs, sinuses and gastrointestinal tract. Herpes zoster infection, meningitis, osteomyelitis and skin sepsis also occur. Some patients develop malabsorption resulting from bowel infection with *Giardia* or *Campylobacter*. Gastric atrophy and achlorhydria occur in approximately one-third of patients and is often associated with vitamin B_{12} deficiency, although the typical autoantibodies are not detectable and a diagnosis of classical pernicious anaemia is debatable. There is also an increased incidence of gastric carcinoma and lymphoma.

Nodular lymphoid hyperplasia is often found in the gut. The nodules occur in the small bowel, resemble Peyer's patches and consist mostly of B lymphocytes and are now considered to be preneoplastic. They are usually seen in patients with circulating B lymphocytes and preserved IgM production. Sarcoid-like granulomas are another feature of CVID and are found in the lungs, liver, spleen and skin although no associated microorganisms have been identified. Hepatosplenomegaly is the main clinical feature and can be controlled with steroid therapy. Autoimmune haemolytic anaemia, thrombocytopenia and neutropenia are other complications seen in this group; these usually respond to steroids or may require a cytotoxic agent, e.g. vincristine. Patients with granulomas appear immunologically different from other patients with CVID, as they lack class-switched memory B cells.

CVID is often familial but there is no clear pattern of inheritance. Family members may have selective IgA deficiency, IgG subclass deficiencies or specific antibody deficiency. Some patients have an intrinsic B cell defect, some have an immunoregulatory T cell imbalance and some possess autoantibodies to T or B lymphocytes. In the first instance, the B lymphocytes appear to be immature. In the second instance, B lymphocytes are probably normal but fail to differentiate because of either a lack of helper T cells or overactivity of a suppressor T cell population. Some patients with late-onset disease have low NK activity.

Treatment is as for the X-linked deficiency, i.e. immunoglobulin replacement, antibacterial agents and drainage of infected sites with careful follow-up concerning the other complications to which these patients are prone.

Other forms of hypogammaglobulinaemia (Table 12.4)

Patients with a **thymoma** often have an immunological disorder (**Good's syndrome**). Myasthenia gravis, caused by an autoantibody to the muscarinic acetylcholine receptor on muscle endplates, is the most common, with red cell aplasia and hypogammaglobulinaemia occurring in 10–20% of cases. These patients lack pre-B and B cells. Removal of the tumour can reverse the red cell aplasia but has no effect on the antibody deficiency.

Various kinds of dwarfism are associated with isolated B cell deficiency, one of which is associated growth hormone deficiency. Hypogammaglobulinaemia also occurs in an inherited deficiency of transcobalamin II, which can be reversed by giving large doses of vitamin B_{12}.

Transient hypogammaglobulinaemia of infancy

This condition tends to be underdiagnosed and occurs during the period when maternally derived IgG wanes and the infant's own antibodies appear (IgM followed by IgG and IgA). The trough of antibody level usually occurs between the third and sixth months of life but can be more prolonged and is usually more severe in premature infants. Affected infants often develop troublesome infection; they have normal B cells but a relative lack of T-helper cells. Some have immunodeficient relatives. The antibody deficiency usually resolves by the age of 2 years and immunoglobulin replacement is required until normal levels are attained.

Severe antibody deficiency can occur as a secondary phenomenon in a number of other diseases, e.g. protein-losing enteropathy (classically seen in intestinal lymphangiectasia), myelomatosis, chronic lymphocytic leukaemia and congenital rubella. Immunoglobulin replacement can be of value in addition to measures directed toward the primary abnormality.

Selective immunoglobulin deficiencies

IgG subclass deficiency

As IgG1 accounts for 67% of serum IgG, a deficiency of this subclass will usually be diagnosed as CVID (and some of these patients lack IgA as well). The most common IgG subclass abnormality in adults is deficiency of IgG3, whereas in children it is IgG2. Many normal individuals lack detectable levels of IgG4. Antibodies reactive with the polysaccharide capsules of pyogenic bacteria such as pneumococci and *H. influenzae* are mostly of IgG2 isotype. Serious infections may be associated with IgG2 deficiency even when the total serum IgG level is within the normal range, although some individuals with IgG2 deficiency because of deletion of the γ2 gene are entirely healthy. Recurrent bacterial infection and asthma may complicate IgG3 deficiency but the mechanism is poorly understood. In most cases of IgG subclass deficiency the heavy-chain genes are intact, indicating that the lack of subclass is a result of other genetic factors controlling transcription or translation. Where the patient is symptomatic with recurrent infections and evidence for poor or absent immunization responses, immunoglobulin replacement is effective in preventing infection.

Selective IgA deficiency

IgA deficiency is the most common form of immunodeficiency among white people, occurring in approximately 1 in 600 of the population. Most cases are sporadic but some have family members with varied forms of antibody deficiency. It has been noted in patients treated with phenytoin or penicillamine, although the underlying susceptibility to develop IgA deficiency may be part of the primary disease for which they receive these treatments, e.g. epilepsy or rheumatoid arthritis. There is good evidence of an association between possession of the HLA-A1, -B8, -DR3 haplotype and IgA deficiency. IgA deficiency is also a marked feature of ataxia telangiectasia (see p. 117). Most patients with selective IgA deficiency are asymptomatic, but some patients appear prone to sinopulmonary infection and bowel colonization with *Giardia*, *Salmonella* and other enteric pathogens. IgA deficiency is associated with an increased incidence of autoimmune diseases such as juvenile arthritis, systemic lupus erythematosus, coeliac disease and pernicious anaemia. Atopic disorders (see p. 131) are also more common in IgA-deficient individuals.

Almost all IgA-deficient patients possess circulating B cells bearing surface IgA but these appear immature, often coexpress IgM, and fail to differentiate into IgA-secreting plasma cells. In some cases plasma cells producing the IgA2 subclass are present in the gut with the defect confined to IgA1-producing bone marrow plasma cells; in others,

both subclasses are deficient. In all cases the structural genes for IgA are intact. Circulating T cells that block the differentiation of IgA plasma cells have been identified in some patients with IgA deficiency.

Specific antibody deficiency with normal immunoglobulins

There are well-described patients who have normal levels of serum immunoglobulins and IgG subclasses, but still suffer from recurrent infections typical of antibody deficiency. These patients may be shown to be immunologically unresponsive to bacterial polysaccharide antigens such as pneumococcal capsular polysaccharide. This can be demonstrated by measuring the level of antibodies before and after immunization with pneumococcal polysaccharide vaccine (Pneumovax ®). Treatment is as for CVID.

IgM deficiency

Selective deficiency of this isotype is exceptionally rare. Such patients lack isohaemagglutinins and are particularly susceptible to meningitis and septicaemia with encapsulated organisms, e.g. pneumococci and meningococci. In older adults, isolated IgM deficiency is often an early marker of lymphoma.

Immunoglobulin component deficiencies

Kappa chain, λ chain and secretory component deficiencies have each been described in association with increased susceptibility to infection. In the last case, neither IgA nor secretory component is detectable in saliva or jejunal fluid, whereas the serum IgA level is normal.

Phagocyte defects

Phagocytes, i.e. neutrophil polymorphs and monocytes, have a critical role in defence against many bacterial pathogens. Profound neutropenia is associated with infection, septicaemia and ulceration of the mouth, skin and respiratory tract. Phagocyte function divides into three sequential components:

1 mobility, margination and adherence;
2 phagocytosis; and
3 intracellular killing (see Chapter 7).

The primary phagocyte defects described below illustrate the importance of these different processes (Table 12.5). However, it is important to realize that the presence of infection itself can cause secondary alterations in phagocyte performance. This may be caused by toxic or inhibitory factors produced during infection or result from the recruitment of more mature cells, leaving earlier forms to predominate in the blood (often referred to as a 'left shift' in the segmentation pattern of neutrophil nuclei when viewing the blood film). In some families a cyclical neutropenia (with a periodicity of 21 ± 3 days) can occur and serial studies may be required to identify this problem.

Defects of mobility and phagocytosis

Various abnormalities have been described that affect the ability of phagocytes to migrate to sites of infection. This process involves margination and adherence to endothelial membranes, a directed response to chemotactic stimuli, and adherence at the site of antibody combination and complement fixation. Immune adherence is intimately linked to phagocytosis and it is rare to find defects of phagocytosis alone. However, not all mobility abnormalities are associated with detectable abnormalities of phagocytosis.

Leucocyte adhesion deficiency

These patients usually present with infections of the skin, mouth, respiratory tract and around the rectum but with little evidence of pus formation. Abscesses tend to be 'cold' and their pus 'thin'. Periodontal disease is common. Wound healing is impaired and delayed separation of the umbilical cord is a feature of most cases.

This condition is characterized by a failure of neutrophils and monocytes to migrate to sites of tissue infection (in spite of persisting neutrophilia). Although the clinical manifestations vary considerably between cases, this group of disorders is caused by a defect in the biosynthesis of the β chain (CD18) common to three glycoproteins (of *c*. 150 000 kDa) normally present on the surface of leucocytes. These three **integrins** are known as LFA-1 (CD11a, CD18), Mac-1 or CR3 (CD11b, CD18) and p150/95 or CR4 (CD11c, CD18) and each possess a different α chain (Table 12.6). Neutrophils, monocytes and NK cells possess all three heterodimers, whereas B and T lymphocytes only express LFA-1. Defective synthesis of the β component results in impaired or absent expression of αβ complexes on the cell surface. The condition is usually inherited as an autosomal recessive and several different mutations of the CD18 gene have been described. Patients with complete CD18

Mobility ± phagocytosis	Killing
Leucocyte adhesion deficiency	Chronic granulomatous disease
Schwachman's syndrome	Myeloperoxidase deficiency
Chédiak–Higashi syndrome	G6PD deficiency

G6PD, Glucose-6-phosphate dehydrogenase.

Table 12.5 Primary phagocyte defects.

Integrin receptor	α chain	β chain	Ligands
LFA-1	CD11a	CD18	ICAM-1 and -2
Mac-1 (CR3)	CD11b	CD18	ICAM-1 and iC3b
P150/95 (CR4)	CD11c	CD18	iC3b

Table 12.6 Integrin receptors and their ligands.

deficiency usually die in early life unless recognized quickly, but those with partial defects benefit from prophylactic and acute administration of antibiotics. Bone marrow transplantation has been successful in correcting this condition.

Schwachman's syndrome, in which neutropenia is associated with exocrine pancreatic insufficiency and growth retardation, is another example of a neutrophil mobility defect caused by a defective membrane protein. Cells from patients with the **Chédiak–Higashi syndrome** also show defective mobility but with normal phagocytosis. They contain giant secondary lysosomes which contain the products of fusion of many cytoplasmic granules and the functional abnormalities observed may well be a consequence of the continuous activation that these cells undergo. They fail to kill catalase-positive or catalase-negative organisms and have absent NK activity although the oxidative burst is preserved, suggesting that the granule abnormality is directly linked to the NK deficiency.

Hyper-IgE syndrome (Job's syndrome)

This disorder is characterized by a chronic eczematous dermatitis in association with recurrent skin, lung and bone abscesses, otitis media and sinusitis. The dermatitis and proneness to infection is usually evident within the first 6 weeks of life. Most infections are caused by *Staphylococcus aureus* but *Candida* infections are also common and may take the form of chronic mucocutaneous candidiasis (see p. 117). These patients often have coarse, 'leonine' facial features, osteoporosis and are prone to bone fractures. They have extremely high serum levels of total IgE (usually > 50 000 IU mL^{-1}), raised levels of histamine in blood and urine, and eosinophilia. The condition can be familial but the pattern of inheritance is unclear. The frequent occurrence of skin abscesses, which show little surrounding erythema, gave rise to the earlier description of 'Job's syndrome' but the term **hyper-IgE (HIE) syndrome** is preferred. These patients possess normal numbers of neutrophils which phagocytose and kill normally but respond poorly to chemotactic stimuli. The raised levels of hista-

mine inhibit neutrophil chemotaxis which can be reversed by histamine (H$_2$) antagonists. A chemotactic inhibitory factor of 61 000 kDa is produced by mononuclear cells from patients with HIE syndrome and activation of these cells may cause the bone demineralization observed in these patients. Ciclosporin may be helpful and bone marrow transplantation and intravenous immunoglobulin have been used successfully.

Phagocyte mobility is secondarily impaired in various other disorders. The effect of infection has already been emphasized but impairment also occurs in malnutrition, burns, diabetes, uraemia and following the administration of various drugs and anaesthetic agents.

Defects of intracellular killing

The archetype is the rare but much studied disorder **chronic granulomatous disease** (CGD). Phagocytosis is normal but oxidative killing is absent in both neutrophils and monocytes. It can be either X-linked or autosomal and affected patients develop infection—often taking the form of abscesses—of lungs, lymph nodes, liver and bones. Wound healing is slow and sinus formation may follow attempts at drainage. Other features include splenomegaly and gastrointestinal involvement. The pattern of organ involvement is probably a result of the uptake of neutrophils containing intracellular pathogens by fixed macrophages in bone marrow, liver, lungs and lymph nodes, where chronic granulomas develop and are difficult to eradicate.

The defect arises because of a failure to generate an effective membrane NADPH oxidase to initiate the oxidative burst that normally accompanies phagocytosis (see p. 74). CGD monocytes are also less efficient at antigen processing and presentation. The molecular cause of most cases of membrane oxidase deficiency is defective production of the heavy chain of the cytochrome b involved in the electron transport chain linked to the membrane oxidase. Most of the problem organisms for patients with CGD are **catalase-positive**, i.e. they destroy any excess hydrogen peroxide they produce. Examples include many staphylococci,

Escherichia coli, Serratia marcescens, Salmonella, Aspergillus, Candida and atypical mycobacteria. In contrast, organisms that generate hydrogen peroxide (H_2O_2) and are catalase-negative, e.g. *Haemophilus influenzae* and streptococci, do not cause persistent infection. The reason for this disparity is that H_2O_2 produced in the absence of catalase can be incorporated into the metabolic pathway of the phagocyte to compensate for the lack of endogenous H_2O_2 production so that, in effect, the pathogen commits suicide (Table 12.7).

The outlook for what was previously known as 'fatal granulomatous disease of childhood' has improved with the use of cell-penetrating antibacterial agents, e.g. co-trimoxazole (Septrin®, Bactrim®) and rifampicin, together with prophylactic antifungals such as itraconazole, and an increasing number of patients are now surviving into adulthood. Treatment with recombinant human IFN-γ has produced clinical improvement in some patients with CGD, but the mechanism is unclear. Bone marrow transplantation, preferably early in childhood, using either a matched sibling donor or a matched unrelated donor is curative.

Several other enzyme deficiencies prejudice phagocyte killing, e.g. deficiencies of myeloperoxidase and glucose-6-phosphate dehydrogenase (G6PD). In the former case the enzyme is deficient in neutrophils and monocytes although eosinophil peroxidase is preserved. Deficiency of either enzyme gives a clinical picture resembling CGD although the individuals are less incapacitated.

Complement deficiencies

Heritable deficiencies of each of the nine components of the classical pathway (including the three subunits of C1) as well as properdin, factor D and the inhibitors of C1 (C1 esterase inhibitor) and C3 (H and I) have been identified in humans. Major deficiencies of C3 are associated with severe bacterial infection; deficiencies of components of the membrane attack pathway give increased susceptibility to infection with *Neisseria*, e.g. gonococci and meningococci; whereas deficiencies of early components in the classical pathway are associated with various forms of immune complex disease rather than overt infection (Table 12.8). Deficiency of the C1 esterase inhibitor is the cause of **hereditary angio-oedema** (HAE). Deficiency of the alternative pathway component, properdin, is associated with severe bacterial infection, particularly with neisserial organisms. Factor D deficiency also associates with neisserial infection but is more benign. Genetic abnormalities of factor H have been associated with the development of the **haemolytic–uraemic syndrome**. A relatively common defect (5% of the white population) of complement-mediated opsonization is caused by deficiency of **mannose-binding lectin** (MBL). This protein binds to mannose and *N*-acetylglucosamine on microbial cell walls and activates C3 by a C1q-independent route (see Chapter 6). MBL deficiency may be asymptomatic but if combined with other minor humoral deficiencies may give rise to pyogenic infections in infancy, chronic diarrhoea and failure to thrive. Adults who are homozygous for abnormalities of this protein are also prone to recurrent infection including meningococcal disease.

Each of the deficiencies listed is inherited in autosomal recessive mode except for properdin deficiency, which is X-linked, and HAE, which occurs as an autosomal dominant. C2 deficiency is the most common: approximately 1% of the

	Microbe status		
Neutrophil	H_2O_2	Catalase	Result
Normal	+	+	Oxidative lysis
Normal	+	−	Oxidative lysis
CGD	+	+	Microbial persistence
CGD	+	−	Microbial suicide

Table 12.7 Outcome of interaction between normal or chronic granulomatous disease (CGD) neutrophils and aerobic organisms.

Table 12.8 Clinical associations of primary complement deficiencies.

Component	Clinical picture
C1 esterase inhibitor	Hereditary angioedema
	Immune complex disease
C1q, C1r, C1s	Immune complex disease, e.g. systemic lupus,
C4	vasculitis and glomerulonephritis
C2	
C3, factor I, factor H	Pyogenic infection; haemolytic–uraemic syndrome
C5, C6, C7, C8, C9	Gonococcal and meningococcal infection
Properdin, factor D	Gonococcal and meningococcal infection

population are heterozygous for the deficient gene, which occurs in linkage disequilibrium with HLA-DR2 (see p. 156).

The cleavage products of C3 are pre-eminent in the defence against pyogenic bacteria and the fact that only major deficiencies of C3 associate with severe infection emphasizes the importance of the alternative pathway in achieving C3 conversion when classical pathway components are deficient (see Chapter 6). Components of the membrane attack pathway only seem to be indispensable with regard to neisserial infections. The association of defects in the classical pathway with **immune complex disease** is a consequence of the role of these components in inhibiting the precipitation of immune complexes and facilitating their clearance from the circulation (see pp. 67 and 143). Deficiency of either of the two C3 control proteins—factor H (C3b-binding protein) and factor I (the C3b inactivator)—permits the unchecked activation of C3, leading to secondary C3 deficiency with a pattern of infection very similar to that found in primary C3 deficiency.

Hereditary angio-oedema (HAE)

Although this condition is genetic, symptoms rarely begin before puberty. Presentation is with episodes of subepithelial oedema of the skin, larynx or gastrointestinal tract which last for 2–3 days. Oedema of the gut can present as severe abdominal pain and laryngeal oedema can prove fatal. C1 esterase inhibitor inactivates various serine esterases including plasmin, kallikrein and activated factor XI and factor XII (Hageman factor) as well as the activated forms of C1 ($C\overline{1r}$ and $C\overline{1s}$). In its absence, C1 becomes readily cleaved (especially at extravascular sites where levels of another major enzyme inhibitor—α_2-macroglobulin—are very low) with generation of the activated forms of C4 and C2 and, in particular, a vasoactive peptide derived from C2b by plasmin. This process does not cause effective C3 conversion as it mostly occurs in a fluid phase without the generation of a stable membrane-bound C3 convertase (see Chapter 6). Thus, these patients have low levels of C4 and C2 with normal C3.

The large majority of patients are heterozygous for C1 esterase inhibitor deficiency but their inhibitor levels are usually well below 50% of normal because of increased catabolism. A rarer form consists of heterozygosity for a dysfunctional form of the inhibitor, caused by a point mutation in the active site; these patients have normal or elevated levels of C1 esterase and can only be detected by a functional assay for the inhibitor. Typically, levels of C4 are undetectable during and even between attacks. Patients with HAO also have an increased susceptibility to immune complex disease, probably as a consequence of their secondary deficiencies of C2 and C4. The condition can be treated by giving inhibitors of fibrinolysis, e.g. ε-aminocaproic acid and tranexamic acid, or the administration of attenuated androgenic steroids such as danazol and stanozolol. The latter were thought to increase synthesis of the inhibitor and correct the C2 and C4 deficiency, but this has now been shown not to be correct. Purified C1 esterase inhibitor is now available for replacement therapy by intravenous injection.

Acquired forms of C1 esterase inhibitor deficiency are also associated with lymphoproliferative disease and with autoimmune disease such as systemic lupus erythematosus. This has been variously attributed to absorption of the inhibitor protein by tumour cells, the formation of anti-idiotype complexes or the presence of a monoclonal autoantibody, which inactivates the inhibitor.

The most common cause of angioedema in the older population is the use of the antihypertensive drugs belonging to the class of angiotensin-converting enzyme inhibitors, which prevent the breakdown of bradykinin.

Secondary forms of immunodeficiency

The most common cause of serious immunodeficiency in clinical practice is none of the above but rather the impact of a number of diseases and the therapies used to treat them upon the immune system. Table 12.9 lists some of the more important examples. Depression of T cell responses occurs early on in Hodgkin's disease whereas antibody de-

Table 12.9 Major causes of secondary immunodeficiency.

Leukaemia, e.g. chronic lymphatic leukaemia
Lymphoma, e.g. Hodgkin's disease
Myeloma
Solid tumours
Malnutrition
Burns
Nephrotic syndrome
Protein-losing enteropathy
Uraemia
Down's syndrome
Chronic inflammatory disease
Persistent infection, e.g. malaria or leprosy
Congenital viral infection, e.g. rubella
Immunosuppressive drugs
Ablation of lymphoid tissue by surgery or irradiation
Plasmapheresis

ficiency is usually a progressive feature of chronic lymphocytic leukaemia and myeloma. Other disorders associated with impaired protein intake or protein loss also cause immunodeficiency and secondary impairment develops during the course of most forms of chronic inflammatory disease.

Lymphoid ablation

The surgical removal of tonsils, adenoids, appendix or local lymph nodes has little effect on immunological responsiveness although one should be reluctant to remove lymphoid tissue in individuals who already show signs of immunodeficiency. Removal of the spleen, however, greatly increases the risk of fulminant infection with pneumococci, meningococci and *H. influenzae*. The risk is now known to be lifelong. Polyvalent pneumococcal, Hib and meningococcal vaccines should be given (and, where possible, before splenectomy is performed) in conjunction with lifelong prophylactic antibiotics, usually penicillin V or erythromycin. The immunological changes consist of impaired clearance of intravascular organisms, reduced concentrations of serum complement and IgM, and a disturbance of the normal profile of lymphocyte subpopulations, often with a moderate lymphocytosis.

The use of powerful immunosuppressive drugs, e.g. corticosteroids, cytotoxic agents and antilymphocyte globulin, can also cause profound impairment of the immune system. The suppression of graft rejection in transplant recipients is still a balancing act between the development of serious infective complications resulting from generalized immunosuppression (particularly of T cell responses) on the one hand, and loss of the graft as a result of T cell-mediated rejection on the other. The pattern of infection seen in these individuals is reminiscent of the problems experienced by individuals with primary T cell defects (see Table 12.1).

Non-immunological abnormalities that predispose to infection (Table 12.10)

The skin and other epithelial surfaces of the body provide an important first line of defence against

Table 12.10 Examples of non-immunological abnormalities associated with susceptibility to infection.

Affected site	Disorder
Skin	Burns and trauma
	Eczema
Mucosa	Ciliary dyskinesia
	Cystic fibrosis
Impaired drainage of a duct or hollow viscus	e.g. Bronchiectasis
Cofactor deficiencies	
Zinc	Acrodermatitis enteropathica
Iron	Mucocutaneous candidiasis (see p. 117)
Acid pH	Vaginal candidiasis
Cortisol	Addison's disease
Insulin	Diabetes mellitus
Vitamin B_{12}	Transcobalamin deficiency

infection. Denuded areas of skin, e.g. in severe **eczema** or following **burns**, provide ready access for many organisms. Lysozyme is a bacteriostatic component of mucous secretions, and the acid pH of the skin, gastric juice and vaginal secretions normally inhibit the growth of many microorganisms.

Kartagener's syndrome is a form of ciliary dyskinesia in which an intrinsic defect in ciliary function (absence of the ATPase-containing dynein arms) causes defective mucociliary clearance and pulmonary, nasal and middle ear disease, and impaired sperm motility. In **cystic fibrosis**, ciliary function is normal but impaired clearance results from abnormalities of the mucus component. Impaired drainage of any duct or hollow viscus provokes infection whether it is caused by congenital malformation or the damaging effects of infection itself, e.g. bronchiectasis.

Infection can follow alteration in the level of various other cofactors, e.g. zinc, iron and iron-binding proteins, vitamin B_{12}, cortisol, insulin and interferon. The free iron level may be especially critical. The over-energetic treatment of the anaemia of infection with iron supplementation can exacerbate infection (many bacteria utilize iron), yet some patients with chronic candidiasis respond favourably to iron treatment. The levels of acute phase proteins (e.g. C-reactive protein) adapt to infective stimuli (via interleukin release) but deficiency of acute phase proteins with antienzyme activity can cause tissue destruction without overt infection, e.g. α_1-antitrypsin deficiency and pulmonary emphysema.

Key points

1 Imunodeficiency should be suspected when an individual experiences infections occurring unusually frequently, in unusual locations or with unusual organisms.
2 The pattern of infection often points to the nature of the defect, which may be located in almost any part of the immune system.
3 Severe combined immunodeficiency (SCID) and T cell defects often present in the first few weeks of life, whereas B cell defects do not become apparent for at least 3 months (when the level of maternal immunoglobulin has waned) and sometimes present many years later.
4 The defective genes have been identified in several immunodeficiency disorders, e.g. SCID, Bruton's hypogammaglobulinaemia, immunodeficiency with hyper-IgM and chronic granulomatous disease.
5 The most common forms of immunodeficiency are secondary to other diseases or are a side-effect of therapy, e.g. with immunosuppressive drugs.
6 The prompt diagnosis and treatment of immunodeficiency disorders can have a major and lifelong impact on the affected individual.

Chapter 13

Inappropriate responses to extrinsic and intrinsic antigens

The primary role of the immune system is to protect the host against infection with pathogenic organisms. However, the enormity and intricacy of this task (discussed in Chapter 10) means that survival is often achieved 'at a price', which usually involves appreciable inflammatory damage to host tissues during the course of infection. In addition, the immune response is prone to be activated by extrinsic antigens of a non-microbial nature, and during the course of other diseases it may focus its attention on components of self, i.e. autoantigens. In some otherwise well-documented immunologically mediated diseases the definitive antigens have yet to be identified. This chapter reviews these four categories of immunological disease which together constitute a major part of **immunopathology**.

Responses to microbial antigens

Inflammation is a well-known consequence of infection and its classical signs of **rubor** (erythema), **tumor** (swelling), **calor** (heat) and **dolor** (pain) were described by Celsus around AD 30. However, the subsequent identification of noxious materials produced by pathogens, e.g. diphtheria and cholera toxins, led to the general view that much of the pathology of infectious disease was caused by the evils of the infecting organism whose ill effects the immune response was endeavouring to contain. It is now clear that much of the discom-

fort and disability is often a direct consequence of the activities of the immune response against the pathogen and this is well illustrated by studies performed with lymphocytic choriomeningitis (LCM) virus. If adult mice of a certain strain are inoculated with LCM virus they develop fits and paralysis resulting from an acute encephalitis (experiment 1, Fig. 13.1). If inoculation is performed when the animals are newborn they do not become ill, even when reinoculated as adults, although they remain lifelong carriers of the virus (experiment 2). If adult animals are given a single dose of a cytotoxic drug—cyclophosphamide—shortly after the inoculation of LCM virus they too suffer no ill effects and continue to harbour the virus (experiment 3). Either of these two 'carrier states' can be rapidly terminated by the administration of histocompatible lymphocytes from a normal animal (experiment 4). These findings indicate that the carrier animals lack lymphocytes capable of responding to LCM; the severity of the tissue damage being governed by the vigour of the immune response rather than the continued presence of the virus. Specific responsiveness can be subverted by administering the virus before the animal is immunologically mature or eliminated by the administration of a drug that kills the specifically reactive cells of the immune response as they proliferate in response to the introduction of the virus.

There are many examples of infections in which there is good evidence for a major contribution by

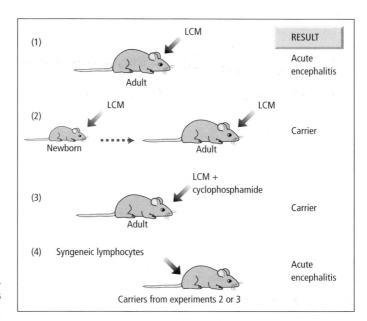

Figure 13.1 Experiments with lymphocytic choriomeningitis (LCM) virus in mice (see text for explanation).

the immune response to the tissue damage that ensues, and some of these are listed in Table 13.1. Massive inflammatory lung damage occurs in acute bacterial **pneumonia** and, even today, this condition carries a mortality rate of approximately 10% even when appropriate antibacterial agents are used. Several of the important organisms concerned, e.g. pneumococci, staphylococci and *Legionella*, possess subtle ways of evading the immune response (see Chapter 10). Much of the tissue destruction (caseation) seen in postprimary **pulmonary tuberculosis** is brought about by the intensity of the cell-mediated immune response to the *Mycobacterium*; the latter presents particular problems to the immune response because of its waxy coat and intracellular location. Infection with *Mycobacterium leprae* is also very difficult for the immune response to eradicate and individuals may show dramatic signs of tissue destruction (tuberculoid leprosy) or the immune response may become overwhelmed (lepromatous leprosy), depending on the type of immune response (see p. 37). Most of the tissue damage seen in secondary and tertiary **syphilis** is immunologically mediated. The severity of infective serum **hepatitis** is largely determined by the intensity of

Table 13.1 Some infectious diseases or their complications in which immunologically mediated tissue damage is a major feature.

Disease	Infectious agent
Acute pneumonia	*Pneumococcus*
	Staphylococcus
	Legionella
Pulmonary tuberculosis	*Mycobacterium tuberculosis*
Tuberculoid leprosy	*M. leprae*
Syphilis	*Treponema pallidum*
Serum hepatitis	Hepatitis B virus
Glomerulonephritis	*Streptococcus*
	Plasmodium malariae
Rheumatic fever	*Streptococcus*

the immune response, and acute infection of the throat with certain strains of β-haemolytic streptococci can be followed by inflammation of the heart and joints (**rheumatic fever**), basal ganglia (**chorea**, i.e. involuntary movements) and kidneys (**glomerulonephritis**).

Table 13.2 includes a list of several organ-based diseases associated with immune responses to microbial antigens. The skin is a frequent battleground for immune responses and **leprosy** and

Table 13.2 Categories of antigens triggering some organ-based diseases.

	1 Microbial antigens	2 Non-microbial antigens	3 Autoantigens	4 Unidentified antigens
Skin	Leprosy Erythema nodosum	Atopic dermatitis Dermatitis herpetiformis	Pemphigus Pemphigoid	Cutaneous vasculitis
Eyes/nose	Scleritis Reiter's syndrome	Allergic conjunctivitis Allergic rhinitis	Lens-induced uveitis Keratoconjunctivitis sicca	Other forms of uveitis Vasculitis
Lungs	Bacterial pneumonia Pulmonary tuberculosis	Allergic asthma Allergic alveolitis	Anti-GMB disease	Pulmonary eosinophilia Sarcoidosis
Gut	Enteric fever Chronic gastritis	Food allergy Coeliac disease	Pernicious anaemia	Crohn's disease Ulcerative colitis
Kidneys	Poststreptococcal nephritis Malarial nephritis	Seasonal nephrotic syndrome	Anti-GBM disease Systemic lupus	Membranous nephritis

GBM, glomerular basement membrane.

erythema nodosum are just two examples; the latter is characterized by tender red nodules which often follow streptococcal infection. **Scleritis** produces a painful red eye, can lead to blindness and may follow infection with bacteria, fungi or viruses. **Reiter's syndrome** consists of inflammation of the anterior part of the uveal tract, conjunctivitis and keratitis, and is a complication of gastrointestinal or urinary tract infection with certain organisms, e.g. *Chlamydia* and *Salmonella*. **Enteric fever** (often called typhoid fever) is caused by the organism *Salmonella typhi*, but many of the pathological changes occurring in the gut, including ulceration, are the direct consequence of the immune response to this organism. It has recently become clear that infection with *Helicobacter pylori* is a common cause of **chronic gastritis** as well as peptic ulceration and, possibly, gastric cancer.

Untoward responses can also occur when vaccines are used. A vaccine against **respiratory syncytial virus** (RSV) was withdrawn when it was discovered that children who received it experienced a greater degree of lung damage (resulting from immune complex formation) when they sub-sequently contracted the natural infection. The first **measles** vaccine to be introduced was a heat-inactivated preparation but this gave rise to an unusually severe and atypical form of measles following natural infection and was withdrawn in favour of the current live attenuated vaccine which does not have this effect.

Types of immune reactions

In the 1960s, Gell and Coombs described a simple system for classifying immunological reactions (see Chapter 14). Four types were identified:

Type I: Immediate hypersensitivity, mediated by mast cells and IgE.

Type II: Antibody mediated, IgG, IgA or IgM antibodies and complement.

Type III: Immune complex mediated.

Type IV: Delayed-type hypersensitivity, mediated by T cells, macrophages and cytokines.

It is important to recognize that these reactions are not mutually exclusive and more than one mechanism will frequently be identifiable in immunopathological disease states.

Responses to non-microbial antigens

The contribution of the immune response to the development of inflammation and the destruction of body tissues is clearly demonstrated when non-microbial antigens (also called **allergens**) are studied. Their ability to induce dramatic responses was first highlighted at the beginning of the twentieth century in two classical descriptions. In the first instance, two French scientists, Portier and Richet, observed that an extract of sea anemone could be safely injected into dogs on a first occasion but induced a severe and fatal reaction when reinjected several weeks later. This adverse reaction took the form of cardiovascular and respiratory collapse and was given the term '**anaphylaxis**' to contrast with the protection induced by prophylaxis. It is now known to be mediated by IgE, mast cells and their mediators (see Chapter 14) and is a typical type I reaction. The second observation was made by Von Pirquet and Schick, who were using hyperimmune horse serum to treat the life-threatening infection diphtheria. They too found that an initial injection was usually uneventful but a fever, rash, joint pains and renal damage often developed approximately 8 days after a subsequent injection of horse serum. This became known as '**serum sickness**' and is now known to be mediated by circulating immune complexes, formed from anti-horse IgG antibodies formed in response to the first injection complexed with complement (see Chapter 14) and is the prototypical type III reaction.

The term '**allergy**' was initially used to describe any form of altered reactivity that followed exposure to antigenic material but currently is most often used to refer to the symptoms and signs that accompany adverse reactions to non-microbial antigens. Table 13.3 lists some of the more common examples of such antigens. There is a marked variation in individual susceptibility to develop allergic responses and many of these responses fall within the general category of **atopic disease**.

It was first recognized in the 1920s that some individuals, and other members of their families, are particularly prone to develop allergic responses to

Table 13.3 Some non-infective materials that can trigger allergic responses.

Plant pollens
Fungal proteins
Animal danders
House dust mite proteins
Insect stings
Food proteins (peanut, shellfish, milk, egg, wheat)
Drugs (antibiotics and anaesthetics) and chemicals (dyes, perfumes)
Metals (chromium, cobalt and nickel)
Vaccines

certain non-microbial antigens. These responses usually express themselves in the skin (**atopic dermatitis**), nose (**allergic rhinitis**), eyes (**allergic conjunctivitis**), lungs (**allergic asthma**) and gut (**food allergy**). The tendency to develop such disorders is known as the **atopic trait** and the underlying abnormality is discussed in Chapter 15. Table 13.2 includes these atopic diseases and some other allergic disorders. Air-borne antigens are a common cause of allergic disease and the size of the antigen-containing particle is a major factor in determining which part of the respiratory tract is involved. Allergic rhinitis is usually associated with particles of more than 15 μm in diameter; allergic asthma is associated with particles of less than 15 μm, as larger particles are trapped by the mechanisms operating in the upper airway, mucus and cilia. These reactions are complex, but IgE is usually involved. However, asthma is multifactorial and involves elements of type III, immune complex, and type IV, T cell mediated, reactions, as well as a neurogenic component from bronchial nerves. The involvement of specific IgE against allergens can be demonstrated by the **skin prick test**, where the antigen is introduced into the skin with a lancet. The allergen binds to IgE on mast cells, causing degranulation and histamine release. This causes the typical wheal and flare to occur within 15 min. The specific IgE can also be detected by analysis of serum, 'RAST' test, but this is more expensive and not as sensitive or specific for some allergens.

Allergic alveolitis occurs in response to particles within the range 1–5 μm. The smallest size of particles is often produced by moulds which form on a variety of biological materials, e.g. hay, barley, sugar cane and cheese (Table 13.4), and those working in close proximity to these materials (e.g. farmers) are prone to develop allergic inflammation of their alveoli. This type of adverse reaction is typified by the presence of IgG antibodies, but there is a component of T cell activation. The reaction has elements of type III and IV reactions. Symptoms occur within 12 h of exposure but are not immediate, unlike the type I allergic diseases, and comprise shortness of breath often accompanied by systemic symptoms of fever and malaise. Because the symptoms settle when exposure ceases, the reactions may sometimes be referred to as Monday morning fever.

Contact dermatitis, although associated with other atopic diseases and often associated with elevated levels of total IgE, up to 10 000 kU mL^{-1}, is a typical type IV reaction with T cells, cytokines and macrophages involved. The elevated IgE is not involved in the reaction. Triggering allergens are usually contact allergens, typically cosmetics, topical drugs, chemicals found in leather and rubber products and metals such as nickel. Testing here is carried out by patch tests, where the substance suspended in petrolatum jelly is left in contact with the skin for 48 h, so that the antigen-presenting Langerhans' cells in the skin can take up the antigen and recruit T cells. The test is read at 5 days, indicating the delay required to recruit and stimulate the T cells. The reaction will show swelling, blistering and on biopsy there is an infiltrate of activated T cells.

Dermatitis herpetiformis and **coeliac disease** are two forms of adverse reaction to the protein gliadin which is present in wheat; the former condition is a blistering skin disease, the latter is characterized by gastrointestinal malabsorption, and both respond to a gliadin-free diet. Here the immunological response is triggered by the interaction of the wheat gliadin with self-proteins, to generate an autoimmune response characterized by the development of IgA antibodies directed against tissue transglutaminase, found extensively in endomysium, hence their detection as anti-endomysial antibodies on sections of monkey oesophagus.

Many kinds of disturbance which have been loosely attributed to 'allergy' have nothing to do with immunological responsiveness and the cardinal features of immune responses (e.g. specificity and memory) should be reviewed (see Chapter 1) when attempting to categorize an adverse reaction as immunological or not. **Favism** is a condition in which haemolytic anaemia and jaundice follow the ingestion of broad beans or various drugs. It was thought to be an immunological phenomenon until a deficiency of glucose-6-phosphate dehydrogenase was identified within the red cell membrane of susceptible individuals. Another example is the adverse response to aspirin and some other drugs and chemicals experienced by a few patients with asthma. In both instances the lack of chemical

Disease	Antigenic material
Farmer's lung	*Micropolyspora faeni* (mouldy hay)
Bird fancier's lung	Avian proteins (bird droppings)
Mushroom worker's lung	Thermophilic actinomycetes (mushroom compost)
Bagassosis	Thermophilic actinomycetes (mouldy sugar cane)
Cheese worker's lung	*Penicillium caseii* (mouldy cheese)
Suberosis	*Penicillium frequentans* (mouldy cork)
Malt worker's disease	*Aspergillus clavatus* (mouldy barley)
Ventilator pneumonitis	Thermophilic actinomycetes (humidifiers/air conditioners)

Table 13.4 Examples of allergic alveolitis.

specificity was always against an immunological explanation. A now classical confusion is that of the inappropriately termed '**total allergy syndrome**' in which some individuals experiencing a variety of symptoms, including dizziness and breathlessness following exposure to many different stimuli, were considered to have an immunological problem. Most of the symptoms described are now known to be psychological in origin.

Responses to autoantigens

A century ago, Ehrlich contemplated the prospect of unbridled autoreactivity and gave it the term '**horror autotoxicus**'. The first intimation of the existence of human autoimmune disease was the identification of a red cell autoantibody (haemolysin) in a haematological complication of syphilis (paroxysmal cold haemoglobinuria). Many diverse forms of autoimmune disease have been studied since then and these disorders form a major part of clinical immunological practice. Autoimmune disease can be predominantly antibody mediated, such as **myasthenia gravis**, where there is an autoantibody that blocks neuromuscular transmission by binding to and removing from the cell surface the acetylcholine receptor on the muscle endplate, or more predominantly T cell mediated, such as **rheumatoid arthritis**. The integration of the humoral and cellular immune systems means that precise distinction is impossible. Autoimmune diseases therefore tend to involve a combination of type II, III and IV mechanisms to varying degrees.

Table 13.2 lists several examples of autoimmune diseases. **Pemphigus** and **pemphigoid** are two blistering skin disorders, which are associated with the presence of autoantibodies that react with epithelial components. In the former, the autoantigen is present in the intercellular substance of the epidermis, whereas in the latter it is located at the basement membrane. **Lens-induced uveitis** is a condition in which inflammation of the uveal tract follows the release of lens protein after traumatic damage to the lens. In **keratoconjunctivitis sicca** (or Sjögren's disease) an autoimmune response impairs the function of the lacrimal and salivary glands resulting in dry eyes and a dry mouth. An autoimmune response to the glomerular basement membrane (GBM) (**anti-GBM disease**), in particular, the α_3 chain of type IV collagen, is characteristic of Goodpasture's syndrome and gives rise to a severe proliferative glomerulonephritis and, in some cases, bleeding from the lungs. The latter is caused by the same autoantibody which cross-reacts with the basement membrane in the lung (see Chapter 14). **Pernicious anaemia** is associated with a form of chronic gastritis and is characterized by the presence of several autoantibodies one of which is specific for intrinsic factor normally produced by the gastric mucosa and which is essential for the absorption of vitamin B_{12}. **Systemic lupus erythematosus** is an autoimmune condition that causes damage to several organs including the kidneys. Many of the antibodies present react with native (double-stranded) DNA and the immune complexes that result deposit in parts of the circulation where the fluid is filtered across membranes, e.g. in the glomerulus (see Chapter 14). It is strongly associated with deficiencies in the complement system, leading to accumulation of abnormal immune complexes.

The cause of autoimmune disease is still one of the unsolved mysteries of immunology. The normal ability of the immune system to discriminate between self and non-self is achieved by:
1 a process whereby self-reactive cells are deleted during development; and
2 the inhibition or regulation of residual self-reactive cells by other cells which suppress them.
Some T lymphocytes escape the censoring process in the thymus by which self-reactive cells are eliminated and **clonal inhibition** is therefore required in addition to **clonal deletion**. B lymphocytes that have survived their self-reactive screening (see p. 17) do not receive a 'go' signal from self-reactive T cells unless the normal immunoregulatory mechanisms have broken down.

Infection as a trigger of autoimmunity

There are often pointers toward microbial or chemical agents that may trigger autoimmune responses and there is considerable individual variation in host susceptibility, which governs the severity and chronicity of these processes (see Chapter 15). The immune response to the protozoan organism, *Trypanosoma cruzi*, which causes **Chagas' disease**, is an interesting example of the way in which autoimmunity can develop during the course of an established infection. Acute infection—in which the parasite can be detected in the blood—is characterized by the presence of fever, muscle pain, enlarged liver, spleen and lymph nodes and, in some cases, inflammatory change in the heart muscle, i.e. myocarditis. Approximately 10–20 years later these patients often present with chronic disease in which cardiac failure and arrhythmias, and impaired motility and dilatation of the gastrointestinal tract are major features. Autoantibodies and T cells from patients with chronic disease show specificity for cardiac and neuronal tissue and their presence is associated with loss of the normal conducting fibres in the heart and the parasympathetic nerve plexuses in the gut. Antigens of *T. cruzi* bind to various host cells spontaneously, and antibodies and T cells reactive with them are able to lyse these host cells. Autoimmune features develop subsequent to this.

There are many other clues to possible microbes that may trigger autoimmune responses, e.g. Coxsackie virus infection and autoimmunity to pancreatic islet cells, and if any infection is at all prolonged it is probably unusual to find no evidence of autoreactivity. It is interesting to speculate that if *Treponema pallidum* had not been identified as the microbial cause of syphilis early on then much of the pathology present in secondary and tertiary syphilis (which includes the development of various kinds of autoreactivity) might well have been regarded as being caused by 'autoimmunity'.

Some of the more important autoimmune diseases and their respective autoantigens are listed in Table 13.5. In some instances, autoantibodies have pathological effects, e.g. the antireceptor antibodies of Graves' disease and myasthenia gravis; in others, tissue damage is largely a result of the activities of T cells. In either case, the presence of autoantibodies in the circulation is of considerable value in the serological investigation of these diseases, which is achieved by using the techniques described in Chapters 5 and 14.

Table 13.5 Some autoimmune diseases and their typical autoantigens.

Organ specific	
Hashimoto's thyroiditis	Thyroid peroxidase, thyroglobulin
Graves' disease (thyrotoxicosis)	Thyroid-stimulating hormone receptor
Pernicious anaemia	Gastric parietal cells (Na^+/K^+ ATPase); intrinsic factor
Addison's disease	Zona glomerulosa of adrenal cortex (including 21-hydroxylase)
Type I (insulin-dependent) diabetes	Islet cells (including glutamic acid decarboxylase, insulin)
Myasthenia gravis	Acetylcholine receptor
Multiple sclerosis	Myelin sheath of nerve fibres (including myelin basic protein)
Pemphigus	Intercellular substance of epidermis (including desmoglein 3)
Pemphigoid	Epidermal basement membrane (BP230 and BP180 antigens)
Goodpasture's disease	Glomerular and alveolar basement membranes (including α_3 chain of type IV collagen)
Primary biliary cirrhosis	Mitochondrial enzymes (M2 antigen)
Systemic	
Systemic lupus erythematosus	Double-stranded (native) DNA, histones, ribonucleoprotein
Mixed connective tissue disease	Ribonucleoprotein
Systemic sclerosis	Nucleoli (including topoisomerase)
Dermatomyositis	Aminoacyl tRNA synthetases
Rheumatoid arthritis	IgG, collagen

Mechanisms of induction of autoimmunity

The various mechanisms that have been proposed fall into two main categories: ways in which unreactive T cells can be bypassed and ways in which autoreactive T cells can be stimulated (Table 13.6). Bypassing the requirement for self-reactive T cells does, however, only provide a means of generating autoantibodies and cannot, of itself, produce autoreactive T cells.

Various agents, e.g. endotoxin and Epstein–Barr virus (EBV), can act as **polyclonal B cell stimulators** without a requirement for T cell help and this is probably why autoantibodies appear transiently during the course of infectious mononucleosis. Some microbes contain sequences that consist of repeating determinants, e.g. lipopolysaccharide, and thus may be able to function as **T-independent B cell antigens**. If there is cross-reactivity between microbial and host antigens then autoimmunity may result. Some forms of monoclonal B cell proliferation also lead to autoreactivity (see Chapter 16).

During the immune response to a foreign antigen (epitope), a second wave of antibodies appears which reacts with the **idiotype** of the initial antibody (see p. 52). The idiotype presents a complementary shape to that of the antigenic epitope and thus one would expect the binding sites of some **anti-idiotype antibodies** to show similarity with the original epitope (Fig. 13.2). If, for example, the antigen is a viral component which binds to host cell components, then a proportion of the

anti-idiotype antibodies may also bind to the virus receptors and appear as 'autoantibodies'. Anti-idiotype antibodies reactive with reovirus antibody have been shown to bind host cells and mimic or inhibit binding of the virus to these cells. This mechanism may help to explain why so many autoantibodies are directed to structures with which viruses combine, e.g. DNA, ribonucleoprotein and various RNA fragments and enzymes, and why so many of the antibodies that develop during infection are not specific for the infecting organism. However, there is little direct evidence for this mechanism operating in human autoimmune disease although several animal models support such a possibility.

A more common form of infection-triggered autoimmunity is the induction of rheumatoid factors. These are antibodies with specificity for the Fc region of IgG, and may be of any class. While they may be seen in high titres in approximately 60–70% of patients with clinical rheumatoid arthritis, they are not specific for this disease and are seen commonly during the course of infections, especially with agents such as EBV, and chronic bacterial infections such as **subacute bacterial endocarditis** (SBE). Once the infection is treated, these antibodies usually disappear. It is thought that they have an important role in the down-regulation of the antipathogen B cell response.

The **carrier effect** (Fig. 13.3) enables autoreactive B cells to receive T cell help when a foreign determinant, e.g. a drug or virus, becomes covalently

Table 13.6 Possible ways of inducing autoimmunity.

Bypassing unreactive T cells
Polyclonal or monoclonal B cell stimulation
T-independent autoantigens
Anti-idiotype reactivity
The carrier effect

Stimulating autoreactive T cells
Molecular mimicry
Impaired immunoregulation
Inappropriate HLA class II expression
Release of sequestered antigen

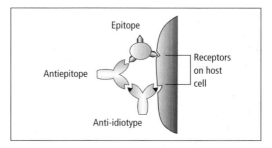

Figure 13.2 How anti-idiotype reactivity can manifest itself as autoimmunity. For example, the epitope could be a viral component and the anti-idiotype might therefore bind to the virus receptor.

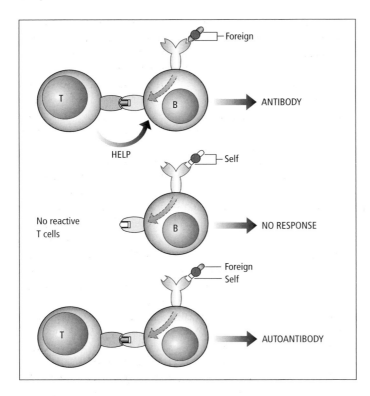

Figure 13.3 The carrier effect by which T cells reactive with foreign determinants can provide help for self-reactive B cells in the presence of covalently linked 'self' and 'foreign' determinants.

linked to a self-determinant. The helper T cells that recognize the foreign determinant can then cooperate with self-reactive B cells to cause them to proliferate and produce autoantibody. Various experimental examples of this phenomenon have been studied and this process is thought to underlie the autoimmune haemolytic anaemia that develops following the administration of the drug α-methyldopa or during infection with *Mycoplasma pneumoniae*. These foreign materials become intimately associated with the red cell membrane.

Molecular mimicry describes the situation whereby a pathogenic organism contains a chemical determinant that exactly mimics a component of self. For example, rheumatic fever is a condition in which cardiac inflammation follows streptococcal infection and molecular mimicry has been invoked to explain the presence of antibodies cross-reactive with cardiac muscle, which normally react with the M proteins of streptococci. Sequence similarities between the M proteins and

human host proteins can be identified. Indeed, it is possible that mimicry has a functional value for pathogenic microorganisms as they evade the destructive effect of the immune response by taking advantage of the immunological tolerance of the host to its self-determinants. Sequence homology between a ribosomal protein of *Trypanosoma cruzi* and the human β_1-adrenergic receptor may be relevant to the development of autoimmune myocardial injury in Chagas' disease. Molecular mimicry may be restricted to the B cell compartment with non-homologous microbial determinants stimulating helper T cells (as in the 'carrier effect' described above), or it could involve the stimulation of cross-reactive T cells as well. A reason why autoreactive T cells may be stimulated initially by cross-reactive foreign antigens, but not by the autoantigens themselves, may depend on the way in which the antigens are presented, i.e. their immunogenicity. There is evidence that the immune system maintains **self-ignorance** to many potential autoantigens because they are not presented by activated 'professional' antigen-presenting cells (i.e. dendritic cells and macrophages) which express HLA class II and co-stimulatory adhesion molecules (see Chapter 4). By contrast, foreign antigens are normally presented in this way and, once activated by them, T cells may react against cross-reactive autoantigens.

The fact that some individuals and their families are inordinately prone to a variety of autoimmune disorders suggests that **impaired immunoregulation** may underlie their susceptibility. The exact identity and role of 'suppressor' T cells in humans are ill defined but various studies suggest that failure to control autoreactive helper T cells is of major importance in some autoimmune disorders. In particular, it may be critical in determining whether an autoimmune response is chronic or short lived. CD4$^+$CD25$^+$ regulatory T cells have been shown to have an important regulatory role and, as discussed on page 34, impaired development of T$_{Reg}$ cells resulting from mutations in a gene for a transcription factor called Foxp3 is associated with a disease called **IPEX** (immune dysregulation, polyendocrinopathy, enteropathy, X-linked syndrome) in which patients develop endocrine autoimmunity and allergies. Studies in mice demonstrate that red cell autoantibodies can be readily induced by injecting the red cells of another species. The autoimmune response declines promptly in normal animals because of the presence of regulatory cells, in contrast to animals prone to develop spontaneous autoimmune disease, e.g. the NZB/NZW hybrid mice. The increased prevalence of autoimmune phenomena in various forms of immunodeficiency also lends support to this possibility. As discussed in Chapter 3, some T cells can inhibit others via the cytokines they secrete. Many autoimmune diseases involve inflammatory Th1 cells and these may respond unchecked if there is inadequate activation of Th2 cells which are a source of the Th1-inhibitory cytokines: IL-4, IL-10 and transforming growth factor β (TGF-β).

Class II glycoproteins of the HLA system (see Chapter 2) are normally only expressed on antigen-presenting cells, e.g. macrophages and dendritic cells, and B lymphocytes. There is some expression by other cell types including endothelium and cells lining the bronchi and small intestine. **Class II expression** has, however, been described on cells from tissues in which autoimmune disease has become established, e.g. thyrocytes in thyroiditis, pancreatic islets in type I diabetes and liver cells in biliary cirrhosis. It has been proposed that this stimulates autoreactive helper T cells to induce autoreactive cytotoxic T cells and B lymphocytes and ongoing autoimmune destruction. This could, conceivably, have survival value in enabling the host to eliminate persistent viruses within host cells, albeit at the cost of self tissue damage. The antigen-presenting capacity of cells such as thyrocytes is further supported by their ability to express the intercellular adhesion molecule-1 (ICAM-1) and to generate IL-1 as a second signal for helper T cell stimulation. However, class II expression is a feature of most infective foci and sites of inflammatory damage, and is possibly a secondary rather than a primary phenomenon; it may even have a role in inducing suppression as the immune response gets under way.

Self-components that do not make contact with the cells of the immune system during development will not be regarded as 'self'. If material containing such components is released during adult life from a site in which it has been sequestered then a vigorous immune response will ensue and will be regarded as autoimmune. Lens protein and sperm antigens have been placed in this category to explain the development of lens-induced uveitis and mumps orchitis, respectively, although it is by no means clear how many other kinds of autoimmune disease can be explained by the **release of sequestered antigen**. However, reactivity against released components of cells undergoing apoptosis may account for the autoimmunity to such ubiquitous cellular constituents as DNA, nucleosomes and ribonucleoproteins in connective tissue diseases such as systemic lupus.

A similar phenomenon may occur at the level of individual epitopes which are not normally presented to the immune system and can be regarded as cryptic self-determinants. The immune system is tolerant of dominant determinants of the same autoantigens, but not to the cryptic epitopes to which a response can occur if they are inadvertently presented in an immunogenic form.

In most situations, it is likely that autoimmune disease arises because of combinations of the processes listed in Table 13.6, e.g. molecular mimicry is unlikely to wreak havoc in the absence of other assistance such as class II expression, and immunoregulatory impairment will become apparent when other forces, such as the development of cross-reactive idiotypes, stimulate the production of autoreactive specificities. Transient autoimmune phenomena are extremely common in infectious disease and after the administration of some drugs and chemical agents. What is not clear is why some patients present with severe and intractable autoimmune disturbances, which can be resistant to the most powerful immunosuppressive drugs.

Autoreactive T cells have been identified and isolated from patients with autoimmune disease and studies using such cell lines are providing valuable information concerning ways in which the activity of these cells is regulated. The fact that they can be obtained from animals that have recovered from an autoimmune disease suggests that their active suppression is a normal state of affairs.

The subdued but specific ability of the immune system to recognize self-components is undoubtedly an important attribute, e.g. recognition of self-HLA glycoproteins and recognition of self-idiotypes, and is in keeping with the specialization of the immune system from innate properties of intercellular recognition. Thus, autoreactivity may have greater physiological importance than was at first thought and should only be considered as untoward when expressed as the destructive lesions of autoimmune disease.

Responses to unidentified antigens

Although much is known about the nature and identity of antigens triggering human immune responses there is still a long list of serious, and often chronic, diseases that are immunologically mediated but for which the key antigens have yet to be identified. A few examples are included in Table 13.2. There are many forms of inflammation that affect blood vessels, i.e. **vasculitis**, and many of them produce changes in the skin as well as other organs. One example is polyarteritis nodosa and, although a very small proportion of cases have been found to be caused by infection with hepatitis B virus, the cause of the remainder is obscure. Henoch–Schönlein purpura is another variant in which the predominant immunoglobulin involved is IgA, suggesting that the immune response originates in the gastrointestinal tract. The nature of the stimulus in most forms of **uveitis** is still unknown. This condition usually affects *either* the anterior (iris and ciliary body) or posterior (choroid) part of the uveal tract and can show a histological appearance typical of *either* an immune complex-mediated or cell-mediated form of tissue damage (see Chapter 14); it is likely, therefore, that several causal agents may be responsible.

Nasal polyps cause obstruction of the nasal airway and can be a sequela to long-standing allergic rhinitis. They are seen particularly in patients with asthma who are highly sensitive to aspirin, a conditon known as **Samter's triad**. **Pulmonary eosinophilia** is characterized by infiltration of the lung with eosinophils and a raised blood eosinophil count. Worldwide, the most common form is that of tropical eosinophilia, which is a sequela to infection with helminths, but the mechanism responsible for cases arising in other parts of the world is unclear. **Sarcoidosis** has a similar histological appearance to tuberculosis but without the presence of recognizable mycobacteria (see Chapter 14). **Crohn's disease** is another condition characterized by chronic granulomatous inflammation and usually affects the gastrointestinal tract. Similar studies have been conducted in the search for a microbial cause but with less success, thus far, than in sarcoidosis. Currently, attention has focused on a bovine mycobacterium, which causes Jonne's disease in cattle. Furthermore, there is evidence that Crohn's disease is associated with mutations in a cytoplasmic protein called NOD2, which normally limits the stimulation of antigen-presenting cells by microbial components that bind to Toll-like receptor 2; reduced inhibition by NOD2 therefore confers increased sensitivity to the Th1 activating inflammatory effects of gut flora. There is evidence of acute inflammation in **ulcerative colitis** but the definitive trigger has eluded detailed study so far. **Membranous nephritis** is a form of glomerulonephritis characterized by marked signs of immune complex deposition in the kidney (when examined by immunohistochemical techniques). It is still far from clear why certain individuals develop this condition, which responds only poorly to conventional therapy.

Despite the many puzzles that remain, a number of previously mysterious diseases have had their microbial causes identified in recent years, e.g. *Borrelia burgdorferi* as the cause of Lyme disease (affecting skin, joints and the brain); *Escherichia coli* 0157 as a cause of haemolytic–uraemic syndrome; *Helicobacter pylori* as a cause of gastrointestinal disease (see above); hepatitis C, D and E viruses as causes of previously obscure cases of liver inflammation; and parvovirus B19 as the cause of a characteristic rash, arthropathy and anaemia (see Chapter 10, Table 10.2). Those conditions that remain 'orphans', i.e. without an identified trigger for the immune response that ensues, are likely to be resolved in the near future by using molecular microbiological techniques to study the 'footprints' of infection (rather than relying on *in vitro* culture) and modern epidemiological techniques to identify risk factors.

Classification of immunological disorders

Use of the term 'idiopathic' (i.e. cause unknown) is becoming less common in modern textbooks of medicine as causative agents are identified in an increasing number of diseases of infective origin. As time goes by, it is likely that many of the conditions that currently fall within categories 3 and 4

(Table 13.2) will transfer to categories 1 and 2. The striking manifestations of autoimmunity that can be observed during conditions that are incontrovertibly triggered by infection suggest that autoimmunity is rarely, if ever, likely to be the *primary* cause of disease but, rather, reflects the complex nature of the interactions between host and parasite. It is possible that autoimmune phenomena may have survival value for the host or they may demonstrate yet another technique by which parasites are able to divert the aggressive intentions of the immune response.

The upshot of this gradual reclassification of immunological disorders brings us back to the view that all four kinds of response represent 'altered reactivity' (the original definition of allergy) to environmental antigens—be they of microbial or non-microbial origin.

Key points

1 In addition to coping with the complexity of microbial antigens, the immune system is also prone to be activated by antigens of a non-microbial nature, as well as by autoantigens, and also shows evidence of activation in diseases in which the triggering antigens have yet to be identified.

2 Experiments in animals have clearly demonstrated that the severity of the tissue damage and illness experienced in infectious diseases is often caused by the vigour of the immune response rather than by toxic factors released from microbes.

3 Allergic disease is common and usually occurs in response to air-borne or ingested antigens.

4 Immune responses to autoantigens have been described in many diseases but unrecognized infection is likely to be the triggering event in most examples. Several mechanisms have been proposed to explain this sequence which may, in some instances, represent another mechanism of evasion by the triggering pathogen.

Chapter 14

Mechanisms of immunological tissue damage

Whatever the primary cause of a particular immunopathological disorder may be, the mechanisms by which host tissues become damaged belong to four main categories, as originally described by Gell and Coombs:

1 IgE-mediated (immediate) hypersensitivity.

2 IgG, IgA or IgM mediated (cell or membrane reactive).

3 Immune complex mediated.

4 Cell mediated (delayed-type hypersensitivity, DTH).

This classification grew out of the contrasting features of 'immediate' and 'delayed' forms of allergic reaction—often referred to as hypersensitivity. In Table 14.1 the physiological role of each mechanism is contrasted with pathological examples of each kind of tissue damage. Figure 14.1 illustrates these processes diagrammatically. It is important to be aware that clinical disease is often mediated by more than one mechanism.

Immediate hypersensitivity (type I)

Immediate hypersensitivity refers to the events that follow the combination of antigen with IgE molecules specific for the antigen, which are bound to IgE receptors on the surface of mast cells. This involves the release of various mediators, e.g. histamine, leukotrienes (LTC$_4$, LTD$_4$, LTE$_4$), chemotactic factors (eosinophil and neutrophil chemotactic factors of anaphylaxis, ECF-A and NCF-A) and platelet-activating factor (PAF), which induce smooth muscle contraction and increase capillary permeability (reviewed in Chapter 8). The histamine is stored in the mast cell granules and is released immediately upon triggering of the IgE receptor. The leukotrienes are synthesized *de novo*, with their biological effect peaking 4–6 h after the onset of the reaction. This gives rise to a **biphasic reaction**, with immediate and delayed components; this is clinically important. Histamine and leukotrienes have very similar effects, leading to vasodilatation and increased vascular permeability. The physiological value of this process has its origins in antiparasite immunity in which increased vascular permeability promotes the extravascular recruitment of immunological components, e.g. IgG, neutrophils, eosinophils and monocytes, which then act in concert to inflict damage on the parasite by various forms of lysis. Smooth muscle contraction assists the process and, if it occurs in the gut, can lead to expulsion of the parasite.

Acute **anaphylaxis** is the severe systemic form of immediate hypersensitivity and manifests itself as pallor, nausea, hypotension, itching, wheezing, cyanosis, abdominal pain, urticaria and loss of consciousness, all of which can develop over a remarkably short period of time, e.g. 5–10 min. In a susceptible individual, it can follow inoculation of venom by a stinging insect, parenteral or enteral administration of an antibiotic or ingestion of

Table 14.1 The four main categories of tissue damage with examples divided into those known to be triggered by foreign antigens (termed extrinsic) and those deemed to be autoimmune.

Mechanism	Physiology	Pathology	
		Extrinsic	**Autoimmune**
Type I: immediate, IgE-mediated	Extravascular recruitment of immunological components Parasite expulsion	Anaphylaxis Allergic asthma Allergic rhinitis	? Chronic urticaria
Type II: IgG, IgA, or IgM-mediated	Lysis of pathogens by extracellular or intracellular events	Incompatible blood transfusion Haemolytic disease of the newborn Hyperacute graft rejection	Haemolytic anaemia Thrombocytopenia Pemphigoid Goodpasture's disease Myasthenia gravis* Thyrotoxicosis*
Type IIII: immune complex mediated	Neutralization of pathogen-derived factors, e.g. toxins Transport of antigen to germinal centres	*Local:* Arthus reaction Dermatitis herpetiformis Allergic alveolitis *Systemic:* Serum sickness vasculitis	*Local:* Rheumatoid arthritis *Systemic:* Systemic lupus Widespread vasculitis
Type IV: cell mediated	Defence against intracellular parasites	Tuberculosis Leprosy Contact dermatitis Graft rejection	Thyroiditis Adrenalitis Pernicious anaemia Diabetes

* The receptor antibodies present in these two conditions have inhibitory or stimulatory effects on the respective receptors rather than complement-mediated lysis.

foods. The most common triggers are peanuts, shellfish, penicillins, bees and wasps, and latex. Otherwise, pathological effects usually arise as a consequence of IgE produced in response to inhaled or ingested antigens, e.g. pollens, animal danders and foods. The responses express themselves as extrinsic asthma in the lungs, allergic rhinitis in the nose and allergic conjunctivitis in the eyes. Non-anaphylactic reactions to food include abdominal discomfort, nausea, vomiting and diarrhoea. The atopic triad is eczema, asthma and rhinoconjunctivitis, and these disorders tend to appear in this order through childhood, with one waning as the next peaks.

Autoreactivity mediated by IgE is not well docu-mented but autoreactive IgE responses have been suggested to underlie some cases of chronic urticaria.

The diagnosis of IgE-mediated disease is by the demonstration of antigen-specific IgE, either by skin prick testing, using prepared solutions of the antigen to demonstrate an immediate wheal and flare response, or by the demonstration in the blood of specific IgE by an enzyme-linked immunoassay or by a radioimmunoassay. The blood tests are colloquially known as RAST tests, standing for radioallergosorbent test, a name that has stuck despite the fact that the assays are no longer carried out in this way.

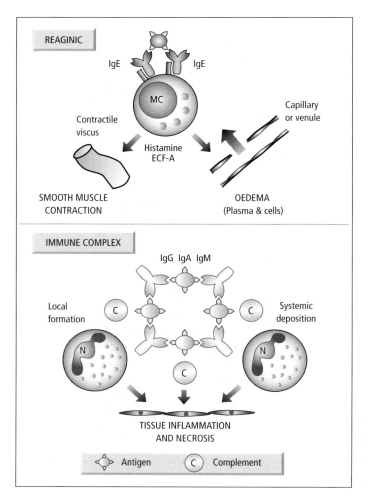

Figure 14.1 Mechanisms of immunological tissue damage. APC, antigen-presenting cell; ECF-A, eosinophil chemotactic factor of anaphylaxis; IFN-γ, γ-interferon IL-2, interleukin-2; Mø, macrophage; MC, mast cell; N, neutropril; Tc, cytotoxic T cell; Tcp, cytotoxic precursor T cell; Th, helper T cell.

IgG, IgA or IgM cell- or membrane-reactive mechanism (type II)

Cell- or membrane-reactive tissue damage occurs when specific autoreactive or cross-reactive antibody (of classes IgG, IgA or IgM) combines with antigen on the surface of a cell or basement membrane and which is then able to activate complement and polymorphonuclear leucocytes. Its physiological role is the lysis of pathogens by these extracellular or intracellular processes. Their activity can prove disastrous, however, following an incompatible blood transfusion and during the antibody-mediated 'hyperacute' rejection of tissue grafts. Similar processes are involved in haemolytic disease of the newborn in which maternal antibody reacts with paternal blood group antigens (usually of Rhesus specificity) present on fetal cells.

This mechanism plays a major part in various autoimmune disorders, e.g. autoimmune haemolytic anaemia, idiopathic thrombocytopenic purpura, the bullous skin diseases (e.g. pemphigus and pemphigoid) and Goodpasture's disease (characterized by antiglomerular basement membrane antibodies).

In some autoimmune disorders, antibodies are present which combine with receptors on cell surfaces rather than other target antigens and have

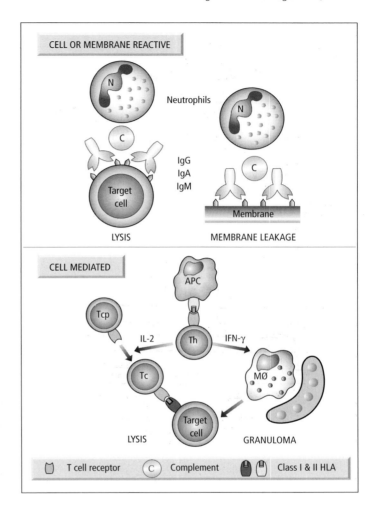

Figure 14.1 *Continued.*

effects mediated via receptor stimulation or blocking rather than causing lytic damage, e.g. anti-acetylcholine receptor antibodies in myasthenia gravis and antithyroid-stimulating hormone receptor antibodies in thyrotoxicosis.

Diagnosis of type II reactions depends on demonstration of the presence of the autoreactive antibodies in the circulation, together with evidence of the physiological damage. For example, in haemolytic anaemia, the blood film will show evidence of fragmented red cells, the levels of haptoglobin, which bind free circulating haemoglobin, will be reduced, and there will be an increase in immature red cells in the circulation (reticulocytes). The Coombs' test will demonstrate the presence of antibody and complement on the surface of the red cells. Many circulating antibodies can be detected by overlaying them onto tissue sections and then using fluorescently labelled antibodies against human IgG or IgM to detect the binding of the autoantibody (immunofluorescence) or by a solid phase immunoassay, when a purified antigen is available (see Fig. 5.12).

Immune complex mechanism (type III)

Immune complex-mediated tissue damage is probably the most common form of all and occurs when

143

soluble antigen combines with soluble antibody. In other words, this form of tissue damage is not confined to the surfaces of cells and can occur locally in a particular tissue or systemically via the circulation. Normally soluble immune complexes are rapidly inactivated by binding to complement receptors on red cells which then carry the complexes on their surface to the spleen where the complexes are stripped off the surface by phagocytic cells in the red pulp and processed for presentation to T and B cells in the germinal centres of the white pulp. The cleaned up red cells then recirculate to adsorb more complexes. Abnormalities of the complement system and the red cell receptors increase the risk of developing immune complex disease, typically seen in systemic lupus erythematosus. As with the previous mechanism, its inflammatory effects follow the activation of complement and phagocytic cells by immunoglobulins of classes IgG, IgA or IgM. The damage will be determined by the location of the complexes and the degree of complement activation that occurs at the site of trapping.

If local concentrations of antigen become great then an excess of immune complexes will form, leading to local tissue damage. This was originally described in the skin as the **Arthus phenomenon** following the repeated injection of heterologous serum. Another example is farmer's lung in which the repeated inhalation of a provoking antigen gives rise to an allergic alveolitis. If excessive amounts of antigen occur in the circulation then immune complexes may deposit systemically. This was first described in the form of **serum sickness** in which a rash, fever, arthritis and glomerulonephritis followed the injection of antidiphtheria horse serum. Similar reactions can follow the administration of drugs and during or following various infections. Immune complex-mediated damage is the basis of poststreptococcal glomerulonephritis, dermatitis herpetiformis, Henoch–Schönlein purpura (IgA complexes) and other forms of **widespread vasculitis**. Serum sickness-like features occurring in the early phase of viral hepatitis are also caused by immune complex formation. This mechanism of damage is also seen in various autoimmune disorders, e.g. locally in joints in rheumatoid arthritis and in many organs, especially the kidney and skin, in systemic lupus erythematosus.

The diagnosis of immune complex disease is difficult and is usually dependent on demonstrating the presence of immune complexes in the affected tissue. During an acute response, levels of the complement components C3 and C4 may fall to very low levels.

Cell-mediated mechanisms— delayed type hypersensitivity (type IV)

The cell-mediated mechanism is independent of antibody and occurs when T lymphocytes are recruited and activated. The process is dependent upon uptake of antigen by specialized antigen-presenting cells (APCs), such as Langerhans' cells in the skin, dendritic cells and macrophages. T cells are recruited by the local activation of APCs and are in turn activated, releasing locally damaging cytokines, recruiting further inflammatory cells and T cells. Effector cytotoxic T cells will be generated, leading to further damage through target cell lysis. Physiologically, cytotoxic T cells are of particular importance in protection against intracellular parasites, e.g. mycobacteria and budding viruses. This mechanism of tissue damage is prominent in postprimary tuberculosis, leprosy and contact dermatitis and is the more usual means by which foreign grafts are rejected.

The cell-mediated mechanism is one of the slowest to develop and is often referred to as delayed hypersensitivity. The classical cutaneous reaction is usually evident within 24–48 h but granuloma formation (in which macrophages fuse to form multinucleate giant cells; see Fig. 14.2d) takes at least 14 days. Jones–Mote or cutaneous basophil hypersensitivity is a variant in which the cellular infiltrate contains many basophils and takes 7–10 days to develop, usually in response to soluble antigen. However, basophils or mast cells can be found in classical cell-mediated reactions if the necessary methods of fixation and staining are employed (see p. 77). The organ-specific group of autoimmune diseases, e.g. thyroiditis, adrenalitis, pernicious anaemia and type 1 diabetes, are all characterized by lymphocytic infiltration and lysis of hormone-producing cells, and T cell clones have been derived from such patients which are reactive with organ-specific targets. This is a reminder that clinical disease may involve more than one mechanism, with clinical effects from antibody being combined with tissue damage by effector T cells and activated macrophages.

Type IV reactions may be diagnosed by patch testing, where the putative chemical agent triggering the reaction is placed in contact with the skin for 48 h and then removed. After a further 24–72 h, a local eczematous reaction may be seen. Other tests based on this principle include tests for immunity to tuberculosis, such as the Heaf and Mantoux tests.

Antibody-dependent cell cytotoxicity

Each of the four mechanisms described above require *either* specific antibody *or* T cells for their generation. There is another form of tissue damage which requires the cooperation of both antibody and lymphocyte-like cells, i.e. antibody-dependent cell cytotoxicity (ADCC). Various studies have demonstrated that combinations of IgG antibody and lymphocytes, IgG antibody and monocytes, or IgE antibody and monocytes are able to lyse target cells for which the antibody has specificity. Other work shows that eosinophils can also lyse target cells in the presence of IgG or IgE antibody. Some of these events have been alluded to in the preceding discussion concerning the physiological role of the IgE mechanism. However, it is not yet clear how important this group of mechanisms is in human immunopathology. Large granular lymphocytes are also able to lyse target cells and do not require the presence of specific antibody. As discussed in Chapter 9, these cells overlap with lymphocyte-like cells that mediate ADCC and natural killer cells.

These different mechanisms have been contrasted with each other for simplicity but it is not uncommon for more than one mechanism to coexist in a particular disease, e.g. injections of immunogenic material can give rise to anaphylactic and serum sickness-like reactions and both antibody- and cell-mediated mechanisms have been identified in autoimmune thyroid disease. Attention has also focused on the role of immune complex formation in the lung in allergic asthma (in addition to the IgE-mediated mechanism) and this helps to explain the longer time course of some asthmatic responses to antigen (see below). Unravelling the respective importance of these different processes in particular diseases is one of the challenges of clinical immunology.

Clinical examples

Lung disease

The mechanisms already discussed and their clinical effects are usefully contrasted by taking examples of immunologically mediated tissue damage occurring in the lung (Fig. 14.2).

Extrinsic allergic asthma in its immediate form typifies the IgE-mediated type I mechanism as exacerbations of this condition are induced when inhaled antigen makes contact with specific IgE on the surface of mucosal and submucosal mast cells, causing their degranulation and release of inflammatory mediators. These mediators cause contraction of bronchial smooth muscle and a degree of bronchial oedema (Fig. 14.2a). Both processes cause narrowing of the airways and intermittent airway obstruction is the hallmark of this condition in contrast to chronic obstructive pulmonary disease (COPD) and emphysema in which airway obstruction persists. However, chronic antigen exposure leads to other inflammatory processes developing which are not IgE-mediated, including the release of proinflammatory cytokines and chemokines by activated eosinophils and neural activation involving neurons producing substance P. Type IV reactions involving activated T cells and immune complex reactions may also occur, making asthma an immunologically complex disease to understand. Chronic asthma may then develop many similarities to COPD at this stage, with excess fibrosis occurring in the airways.

Maximal reduction in airflow occurs within 10–20 min of bronchial challenge with the rele-

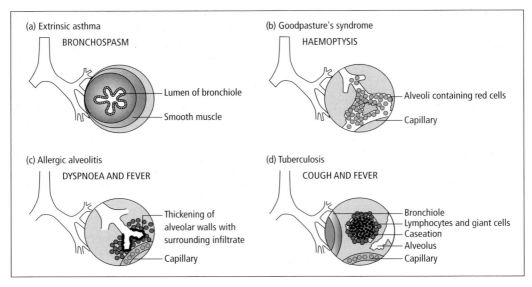

(a) Extrinsic asthma
BRONCHOSPASM
— Lumen of bronchiole
— Smooth muscle

(b) Goodpasture's syndrome
HAEMOPTYSIS
— Alveoli containing red cells
— Capillary

(c) Allergic alveolitis
DYSPNOEA AND FEVER
— Thickening of alveolar walls with surrounding infiltrate
— Capillary

(d) Tuberculosis
COUGH AND FEVER
— Bronchiole
— Lymphocytes and giant cells
— Caseation
— Alveolus
— Capillary

Figure 14.2 Examples of the four main types of immunological tissue damage occurring in the lung.

vant antigen. A similar latency of response is observed when prick tests are performed in the skin of susceptible subjects. This is in keeping with the earlier description of **immediate hypersensitivity** for the IgE mechanism. However, a significant proportion of patients with extrinsic asthma show a second and more prolonged phase of airway obstruction several hours after inhalation of antigen, demonstrating the biphasic response.

A pulmonary example of the cell- or membrane-reactive mechanism is **Goodpasture's syndrome** (Fig. 14.2b) in which autoantibodies react with an antigen present in both glomerular and pulmonary basement membranes, giving rise to acute proliferative glomerulonephritis and parenchymal lung damage with bleeding from the lungs (haemoptysis). Damage to the basement membrane follows attachment of IgG antibody and activation of complement and phagocytic cells, culminating in the leakage of blood across it. Little is known about the cause of this condition although epidemiological evidence points to exposure to petrochemicals which, in susceptible subjects of HLA-DR2 phenotype (see Table 15.4), may be followed by the development of antibase-ment membrane antibodies. These recognize type IV collagen, which is present in both the pulmonary and renal basement membrane.

Immune complex-mediated damage is exemplified by **extrinsic allergic alveolitis** in which IgG antibody is produced with specificity for inhaled antigen (Fig. 14.2c). The classical example is farmer's lung in which the antigen is a component of spores found in mouldy hay (see Table 13.4). IgG antibody complexes with antigen across the alveolar capillary membrane, followed by complement fixation and activation of neutrophils. Clinically, this is manifest as breathlessness (dyspnoea), cough and fever occurring several hours after challenge and a similar latency is observed when skin tests are performed with the appropriate material. This led to the designation of **intermediate hypersensitivity** in contrast to the more rapid immediate form. The dyspnoea, which follows acute exposure, is caused by a decrease in gas transfer across the alveolar capillary membrane with reduction in the oxygen content of arterial blood. Wheezing or airway obstruction is not a feature of this condition. The proportions of inspired air to perfused blood present in different parts of the lung vary largely because of the effects of gravity on the circulation. In the upright position, the ventilation : perfusion ratio is high in the upper lobes of the lung and low in the lower lobes. Thus, the changes of extrinsic allergic alveolitis are more commonly seen in the upper lobes whereas those of the intrinsic form are more commonly found in the lower zones.

Intrinsic (**cryptogenic**) **alveolitis** arises as a consequence of the deposition of blood-borne immune complexes in the pulmonary circulation, where they cause complement and phagocyte activation within the alveolar capillary membrane. This condition has a more insidious onset without evidence of acute exacerbation but produces similar effects on gas transfer. It often occurs in association with other autoimmune diseases, e.g. rheumatoid arthritis and systemic lupus erythematosus.

Pulmonary tuberculosis and **sarcoidosis** are examples of cell-mediated pulmonary damage. The former follows the inhalation of *Mycobacterium tuberculosis* and usually occurs in the upper lobes. Primary exposure to *M. tuberculosis* causes a small peripheral focus of infection (the Ghon focus) but with associated enlargement of the lymph nodes at the hilum of the lung. The primary focus usually heals without symptoms developing and it is only following subsequent (in this context usually referred to as 'postprimary') infection that severe damage to parenchymal pulmonary tissue develops in the upper zones of the lung (Fig. 14.2d). These changes follow activation of various subpopulations of T lymphocytes and the recruitment of macrophages as they respond vigorously to the reintroduced mycobacteria. The involvement and recruitment of both lymphocytes and macrophages is probably why the tempo of this mechanism is the slowest of all and is often referred to as **delayed hypersensitivity**. An equivalent reaction takes place in the skin when sensitized subjects receive an intradermal injection of a mycobacterial extract as in the Heaf, Mantoux or Tine tests. A positive response is characterized by erythema, induration and itching occurring maximally 24–48 h after challenge. The intensity of the inflammatory response is such that, in the

centre of a lesion, lung tissue is replaced by cheese-like 'caseous' material often with the formation of cavities, which eventually become sealed off by fibrosis and calcification. It was only following the introduction of effective antituberculous drugs that this condition (previously called 'consumption') lost much of its notoriety. The efficacy of some of the more successful agents, e.g. rifampicin, is caused in part by an immunosuppressive effect.

Sarcoidosis is a mysterious disease in which granulomas occur in many sites, but most usually the lungs and the hilar lymph nodes. The pathology appears similar to mycobacterial infection, except that caseous necrosis does not occur, and no pathogen has ever been isolated.

Skin disease

The skin and kidneys are also involved in immunopathological disorders and Fig. 14.3 contrasts examples of membrane-reactive and immune complex damage in these two organs. The bullous or blistering skin diseases and various forms of glomerulonephritis demonstrate how relatively subtle variations in the mechanism and locus of an immunopathological disorder can produce major differences in clinical effects.

Pemphigus and **pemphigoid** are both caused by circulating autoantibody reactive with cutaneous antigens. In the former, the antigen forms part of the intercellular substance (ICS) of the epidermis and the interaction of IgG autoantibody with it gives a typical 'chicken wire' pattern of staining on immunofluorescent examination of the skin (Fig. 14.3a). Complement fixation and disruption of the ICS leads to intraepidermal blister formation. In pemphigoid, the antigen is a component of the epidermal basement membrane and immunofluorescent examination for IgG shows linear staining of this structure (Fig. 14.3b). Subepidermal blister formation follows complement activation at that site. **Dermatitis herpetiformis** is a bullous disorder in which IgA-containing immune complexes deposit in the papillary capillaries (Fig. 14.3d). The disease is strongly associated with gluten-sensitive enteropathy, coeliac disease, and it is thought that the antigen is derived from

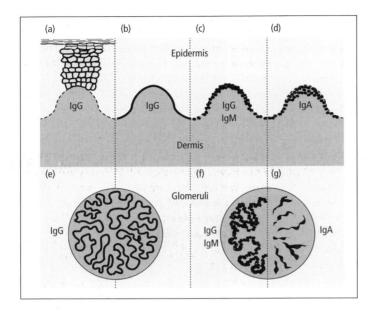

Figure 14.3 Examples of immunological tissue damage in skin (a–d) and kidney (e–g). (a) Pemphigus; (b) pemphigoid; (c) systemic lupus; (d) dermatitis herpetiformis; (e) Goodpasture's disease; (f) systemic lupus; (g) IgA nephropathy.

wheat gluten, as the skin disease will disappear on a gluten-free diet. The complexes activate the alternative complement pathway in the dermal papillae and cause subepidermal blister formation. In **systemic lupus erythematosus** (SLE) IgG-containing immune complexes are found beneath the basement membrane of the epidermis (Fig. 14.3c) and although this may be associated with an erythematous rash this does not cause blisters to form.

Contact hypersensitivity to chemicals gives an excellent example of delayed hypersensitivity. This can occur to any chemical in contact with the skin. The antigen is taken up by dermal antigen-presenting Langerhans' cells to trigger the reaction. The most common clinical example is allergy to the metal nickel, present in cheap jewellery, jean studs and coins, and this presents with a weeping eczematous reaction at the site of contact. Similar reactions may be seen to cosmetics, hair dyes and topical antibiotics such as neomycin.

Kidney disease

In **Goodpasture's disease**, autoantibody to the glomerular basement membrane (GBM) can be de-

tected by the presence of diffuse linear staining of the GBM on immunofluorescent examination (Fig. 14.3e). It usually causes an acute proliferative glomerulonephritis with reduced urine production (oliguria), blood in the urine (haematuria) and failure of the clearance function of the kidney (uraemia). Renal failure occurs rapidly if the disease is not diagnosed promptly. Complement activation and infiltration by neutrophil polymorphs are pronounced features of this condition. Immune complex-mediated damage to the glomerulus takes many forms. Diffuse granular deposition of immune complexes containing most classes of immunoglobulin occurs in **SLE** (Fig. 14.3f) and thickening of the basement membrane as well as some degree of proliferative change is usually found in association with marked protein loss in the urine (proteinuria) and uraemia. In **IgA nephropathy** (Berger's disease), IgA-containing complexes preferentially localize in the mesangium of the glomerulus with relative sparing of the basement membrane, giving a radial pattern of deposition (Fig. 14.3g). The clinical features may range from haematuria and proteinuria to no clinical disturbance whatsoever. In some forms of immune complex deposition in the kidney, e.g.

membranous glomerulonephritis, complexes localize in a subendothelial position where they are least able to recruit neutrophil polymorphs but give rise to considerable thickening of the basement membrane and marked proteinuria.

These examples have been selected to illustrate different patterns of immunologically mediated tissue damage in selected organs. More detailed descriptions of these and other disorders will be found in postgraduate texts.

Key points

1 The mechanisms of immunologically mediated tissue damage are classified into four main types: type I: IgE-mediated immediate hypersensitivity; type II: antibody mediated; type III: immune complex mediated; type IV: T cell-mediated delayed-type hypersensitivity. More than one mechanism may operate in a single disease.

2 Immediate hypersensitivity involves IgE, mast cells and their mediators (including histamine, leukotrienes and chemotactic factors), which give rise to oedema and smooth muscle contraction. Clinical examples include acute anaphylaxis and allergic asthma.

3 The cell- or membrane-reactive mechanism involves IgG, IgA or IgM molecules which, after complexing with antigens on the surface of cells or basement membranes, activate complement and phagocytes resulting in lysis or inflammatory change. Clinical examples include various forms of haemolytic disease, thyroid disease, myasthenia gravis, pemphigoid and Goodpasture's disease.

4 The immune complex mechanism involves the combination of soluble antigens with soluble immunoglobulins in the circulation or extracellular fluid followed by deposition of the complexes and activation of complement and phagocytic cells. Clinical examples include the Arthus phenomenon, allergic alveolitis, serum sickness in response to reinjection of foreign protein and SLE.

5 Delayed-type hypersensitivity involves T cells and macrophages.. Clinical examples include tuberculosis, sarcoidosis, contact dermatitis and graft rejection.

6 Immunoglobulins may also work in concert with various kinds of lymphocyte and monocyte to mediate antibody-dependent cell cytotoxicity although its relative importance in many diseases is not yet clear.

Chapter 15

Susceptibility to immunological disease

The number of diseases in which immunological processes have been shown to play an important part has steadily increased in recent years and doctors working in all medical specialties need to be aware of the manifestations of immunological disorders. Selected examples are listed by specialty in Table 15.1.

It is still far from clear why some individuals are prone to develop certain kinds of immunological disease whereas others are spared. There is often evidence in favour of a genetic predisposition which, in conjunction with a particular kind of environmental insult, e.g. infection or chemical challenge, produces the critical interaction leading to disease expression. Well-studied examples include allergic asthma, dermatitis herpetiformis, type 1 diabetes and rheumatoid arthritis.

In this chapter, the nature of individual susceptibility is reviewed under three headings: atopic disorders, immune complex disease, and HLA and disease.

Atopic disorders

Atopic disorders form a significant part of human immunopathology in the Western world, occurring in at least 5% of individuals. The **atopic trait** can be defined as the spontaneous tendency for an individual to produce high levels of IgE reacting with one or more common antigens in association with antigen-provoked disorders in which an IgE-mediated mechanism can be identified. Table 15.2 lists some of the more important conditions (also mentioned in Chapter 13) in which there is good evidence for the involvement of IgE antibody, mast cells and their mediators. The physiological role of the IgE mechanism (described in Chapter 14) is concerned with defence against protozoan and metazoan parasites most of which, e.g. plasmodia, schistosomes and trypanosomes are now rarely experienced in the Western world. Parasite killing by IgE plus monocytes, eosinophils, platelets or mast cells, or IgG plus eosinophils (the last recruited following ECF-A release by IgE-sensitized mast cells) have each been identified in recent years. The itching, scratching, hypersecretion, sneezing, coughing and contraction of smooth muscle which follows mast cell degranulation is also likely to be of considerable value in effecting the physical removal of parasites and their vectors.

Improvements in public health and hygiene have led to a major decrease in infections (particularly of the respiratory tract) but the introduction of novel environments associated with central heating, double glazing, modern diets (including formula feeding of infants), high pollen exposure and the keeping of pets, has led to frequent contact with antigens by inhalation or ingestion. Genetic factors are important in determining susceptibility to atopic disease and the identity of the genes involved and the perturbations that they cause are the subject of current research. Antibody-mediated

Table 15.1 Selected examples of immunologically mediated disease. (Modified from Reeves G. *Lancet* 1983;**ii**:721 with permission.)

Medical specialty	Disease
Cardiology	Rheumatic carditis, cardiomyopathy, postcardiotomy/postinfarction syndromes (Dressler's syndrome)
Respiratory medicine	Extrinsic and intrinsic alveolitis, extrinsic asthma Goodpasture's syndrome (anti-GBM disease)
Dermatology	Bullous skin disorders, angioedema, contact dermatitis
Endocrinology	Addison's disease, type 1 diabetes, thyroiditis
Ear, nose and throat	Allergic rhinitis, secretory otitis media
Gut and liver	Coeliac disease, ulcerative colitis, acute and chronic hepatitis, primary biliary cirrhosis
Haematology	Autoimmune haemolytic anaemia, neutropenia and thrombocytopenia, pernicious anaemia
Infectious and tropical diseases	Tuberculosis (granuloma), Chagas' disease (myocarditis), malaria (anaemia, nephrotic syndrome)
Obstetrics and gynaecology	Rhesus disease, miscarriage (antiphospholipid syndrome), infertility
Ophthalmology	Allergic/vernal conjunctivitis, uveitis, keratoconjunctivitis sicca (Sjögren's syndrome)
Nephrology	Glomerulonephritis, e.g. poststreptococcal, shunt, bacterial endocarditis, Goodpasture's disease, mesangiocapillary, serum sickness, systemic lupus erythematosus
Neurology	Polymyositis, polyneuritis, multiple sclerosis, myasthenia gravis, postinfective/postimmunization encephalitis
Paediatrics	Atopic eczema, milk and food allergy, juvenile chronic arthritis, Henoch–Schönlein purpura
Rheumatology	Rheumatoid arthritis, systemic lupus erythematosus, dermatomyositis, widespread vasculitis

GBM, glomerular basement membrane.

Table 15.2 Atopic disorders.

Extrinsic allergic asthma
Allergic rhinosinusitis
Allergic conjunctivitis
Atopic dermatitis
Allergic gastroenteropathy
Seasonal nephrotic syndrome

responses (orchestrated by Th2 cells; see p. 37) are most evident during fetal life but Th1-directed cell-mediated responses tend to predominate after birth. This switch is sluggish in children with the atopic genotype and the 'hygiene hypothesis' proposes that reduced microbial exposure in early life promotes the persistence of Th2-directed responses to environmental antigens. This does not explain why only some children with Th2-polarized responses develop atopic disease or the reason for its variable organ distribution. Confusingly, early antigen exposure such as to pet dander may have both a triggering and protective effect. Children with older siblings are less likely to develop atopic disease than those with no siblings.

Various other factors have been proposed as explanations for the atopic trait. IgA is the usual protective antibody at mucosal surfaces and several studies have shown an increased prevalence of IgA deficiency in atopic individuals and their relatives. A variant of the gene for the β subunit of the high-affinity Fc receptor for IgE (Fc$_\varepsilon$RI), present on chromosome 11, is strongly associated with the atopic trait when the gene variant is inherited maternally, and variants of a gene that regulates IgE levels show associations with severe asthma. Polymorphisms of the α chain of the interleukin-4 (IL-4) receptor and the IL-9 gene have been associated with atopic asthma in some families. A polymorphism for the gene coding for the receptor for bacterial lipopolysaccharide has also been shown to associate with the severity of atopy. This may operate by subduing IL-12 production by antigen-presenting cells that bear this receptor so that Th2 responses predominate. Atopic disease is clearly a polygenic disorder.

Immune complex disease

It is interesting to speculate why some individuals should be particularly prone to the development of widespread immune complex disease following otherwise straightforward infections. Recently, attention has focused on the role of complement components (particularly C4, C2 and factor B) in maintaining immune complexes in soluble form in body fluids. Some individuals prone to conditions in which immune complex-mediated damage is a feature, possess genetic variants of these proteins which are functionally less efficient (see p. 70) and this is probably the major reason why complexes precipitate so readily in these patients and cause an inappropriate degree of tissue damage.

Table 15.3 lists various factors that govern the deposition of immune complexes within the circulation. Overloading of the normal pathways by which immune complexes are cleared is most likely to occur when there is an excessive quantity or persistence of antigenic material which has sufficient epitope density to form immune complexes of a sufficient size to precipitate (see Fig. 5.9). The isotype (i.e. class and subclass) of the antibodies in-

Table 15.3 Factors governing the deposition of circulating immune complexes (IC).

Antigen quantity and persistence
Antibody isotype and affinity
Solubilization capacity of serum (C1, C4, C2)
Removal of complexes (erythrocyte complement receptors)
Local factors
Site of immune complex formation
Turbulence
Capillary permeability
Filtration effects

volved, as well as their affinity of binding, determine their biological effects, and the efficiency of both classical and alternative complement pathways governs how readily immune complexes are solubilized and thus how well they are transported to cells of the mononuclear phagocyte series which are able to ingest and process them. Approximately 1% of the population are heterozygotes for C2 deficiency, and deficiencies of C1q, C1r, C4 and C2 are each associated with a susceptibility to develop immune complex disease (see Chapter 12). Patients with systemic lupus erythematosus (SLE) have also been shown to have reduced receptors for complement on their red cells, thus reducing the rate at which abnormal complexes can be cleared.

The sites at which circulating immune complexes are deposited are determined partly by their site of formation, e.g. the release of large quantities of antigen from heart valve endothelium in bacterial endocarditis and its combination with circulating antibody give rise to considerable deposition downstream in the kidneys (and other organs that are major recipients of the arterial supply). Turbulence of blood flow and local increases in vascular permeability also affect localization. Immune complexes are often deposited at the various sites at which plasma colloid is filtered to produce other body fluids, e.g. renal glomeruli, choroid plexus, synovium, epidermal basement membrane and uveal tract. An aggregation/concentration effect occurs as soluble complexes pass across these semipermeable membranes and this is why the localization of circulating immune complexes may appear to be confined to a single location and in a subepithelial position, e.g. as in membranous glomerulonephritis.

The formation of soluble immune complexes has an important physiological role and it is only when their formation or clearance become grossly disturbed that the manifestations of 'immune complex disease' become of clinical concern.

HLA and disease

Initially, HLA typing was mainly performed to determine the degree of compatibility between donors and recipients prior to organ transplantation (see Chapter 17). However, it was soon realized that the presence of certain HLA types (often called 'antigens' because they have been defined by using antibodies specific for them) was positively associated with particular diseases (Table 15.4). For many years, serological typing (using a technique known as microlymphocytotoxicity) was only applicable to the HLA-A and HLA-B series of antigens (see p. 173) and thus the first disease associations described were with variants at these loci, e.g. ankylosing spondylitis (B27) and haemochromatosis (A3). Many other A and B locus associations were described but when serological typing became possible for D locus antigens, i.e. DR typing, it was realized that many HLA-associated diseases, e.g. type 1 diabetes, coeliac disease and rheumatoid arthritis, were more strongly associated with DR variants. The diseases listed in Table 15.4 are only a selection of those that have been described in the literature.

B locus associations are often with diseases that are not of an immunological nature, whereas most of the conditions that are closely related to D locus

variations are diseases in which immunological processes play an important part and this may give a clue to the underlying mechanism of association (see below). Some disorders, e.g. type 1 diabetes and coeliac disease, show association with more than one DR antigen and, in the former case, individuals heterozygous for the two antigens, i.e. who are DR3/DR4, are at greater risk than those homozygous for either DR3 or DR4, suggesting the presence of two different susceptibility genes or the formation of a novel class II heterodimer (see p. 21).

In view of the critical requirement for these polymorphic HLA glycoproteins to present antigenic peptides to helper T cells when an immune response is triggered, one would expect variations between HLA types to be associated with marked differences in the outcome of infectious diseases. A study performed in West Africa has shown a strong association between HLA-B53 and resistance to severe malaria, which is probably mediated by a heightened immune response to an antigen expressed during the liver stage of malarial infection. There is a need for more work on the relationship

Table 15.4 Some examples of associations between HLA types and disease. (After Svejgaard *et al. Immunological Reviews* 1983;**70**:193–218.)

Disease	HLA type	Frequency of patients (%)	Controls	Relative risk	Aetiological fraction
Idiopathic haemochromatosis	A3	76	28.2	8.2	0.67
Congenital adrenal hyperplasia	B47	9	0.6	15.4	0.08
Ankylosing spondylitis	B27	90	9.4	87.4	0.89
Dermatitis herpetiformis	DR3	85	26.3	15.4	0.80
Coeliac disease	DR3	79	26.3	10.8	0.72
Sicca syndrome	DR3	78	26.3	9.7	0.70
Graves' disease	DR3	56	26.3	3.7	0.42
Type 1 diabetes	DR3	56	28.2	3.3	0.39
Type 1 diabetes	DR4	75	32.2	6.4	0.63
Systemic lupus	DR3	70	28.2	5.8	0.58
Membranous nephropathy	DR3	75	20.0	12.0	0.69
Multiple sclerosis	DR2	59	25.8	4.1	0.45
Narcolepsy	DR2	100	21.5	135.0	1.0
Goodpasture's syndrome	DR2	88	32.0	15.9	0.82
Rheumatoid arthritis	DR4	50	19.4	4.2	0.38
Hashimoto's thyroiditis	DR5	19	6.9	3.2	0.13
Pernicious anaemia	DR5	25	5.8	5.4	0.20

between HLA genotypes and the response to infectious agents as, until now, most studies have been concerned with non-infective disorders prevalent in Western environments.

Measuring the strength of associations

There are various ways of estimating the strength of these associations (Table 15.4). A convenient way to display data obtained for a series of patients and controls with respect to the presence or absence of a particular antigen is in the form of a 2×2 table (Table 15.5). The **relative risk** (RR) is then the cross or odds ratio, i.e. $(a \times d)/(b \times c)$. This value indicates how many times more frequently the disease develops in individuals positive for this antigen compared with individuals who lack it. Another estimate is to compute the **aetiological fraction** (AF), i.e. how much a disease is directly caused by the disease-associated factor under investigation. This value can only be used when the relative risk value is greater than 1 (i.e. for those individuals who have an increased risk) and is determined by the following calculation:

$$AF = \left(\frac{RR - 1}{RR} \right) \left(\frac{a}{a + b} \right)$$

Those associations having a greater relative risk usually also possess a greater aetiological fraction but this is not universally so, for, where a particular gene has a very low frequency in the healthy population and is present in only a minority of patients with the disease, the aetiological fraction will be disproportionately low. An example of this is the

possession of B47 which confers a relative risk of congenital adrenal hyperplasia of 15.4, which in Table 15.4 can be seen to be the same as for the association between HLA-DR3 and dermatitis herpetiformis, whereas the aetiological fractions for these two associations are 0.08 and 0.80, respectively.

The strongest HLA–disease association discovered so far is that between DR2 and narcolepsy, giving a relative risk of 135 and an aetiological fraction of 1.0. The magnitude of the latter strongly suggests that HLA-DR2 is intimately involved in the disease process and may be linked to a receptor or neurotransmitter defect.

Phenotypes, genotypes and haplotypes

In the absence of a significant degree of consanguinity, each individual is likely to possess a different set of HLA genes on paternal and maternal chromosomes. The total set is known as the **phenotype**, which can be rewritten as the **genotype** when sufficient other members of the family have been studied to identify which genes belong to which chromosomes (Fig. 15.1). The collection of particular antigens that are under the control of genes borne on a single chromosome is known as the **haplotype** (e.g. a, b, c or d in Fig. 15.1). HLA haplotypes can be written in even more detail, e.g. the haplotype A1/B8/Cw7/DR3 usually possesses the following alleles at the intervening complement loci: C2C, C4AQO, C4BB1 and BfS so that this becomes (reading from left to right along the short arm of chromosome 6, as depicted in Fig. 2.10) DR3–C4BB1–C4AQO–BfS–C2C–B8–Cw7–A1. This is termed the **extended haplotype**. Even though each of these loci is very polymorphic, and the loci on each chromosome bear one of many possible alleles, certain alleles at one locus, e.g. HLA-A, are found much more often with certain alleles at other loci, e.g. HLA-B. These non-random arrangements are a common occurrence within particular populations and this phenomenon is known as **linkage disequilibrium**. Indeed, with the advent of typing for HLA-DP and -DQ, it has been found that the DQ2 and DQ8 alleles that are in linkage disequilibrium with DR3 and DR4,

Table 15.5 A 2×2 table to display data concerning a possible association between the presence of an HLA antigen and the presence or absence of a disease.

	Number of individuals	
	HLA antigen positive	HLA antigen negative
Patients	a	b
Controls	c	d

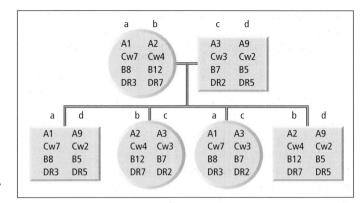

Figure 15.1 The inheritance of HLA haplotypes.

respectively, show strong associations with type 1 diabetes.

Until recently, HLA typing was usually performed to determine variations at the HLA-A, -B, -C and -DR loci. These data, obtained using serological techniques, are now augmented by DNA techniques that enable the genes associated with particular specificities to be identified.

Genotype nomenclature

The nomenclature used to describe these more detailed genotypes contains information about the locus (and for class II, which α or β chain) before an asterisk, followed by numerals assigned to the specificity and gene number.

For class I: locus/*/specificity/gene number, e.g. A*1102 is the second gene belonging to specificity 11 of the A locus.

For class II: locus/chain/*/specificity/gene number, e.g. DQA1*0401 is the first gene belonging to specificity 4 of the first DQ α chain locus, whereas DRB3*0201 is the first gene belonging to specificity 2 of the third DR β chain locus.

Mechanisms of association

Several proposals have been made to explain the mechanism of association between HLA types and disease (Table 15.6). Genes controlling specific immune responses were originally characterized in the murine major histocompatibility complex (MHC) and described as **immune response (Ir)**

Table 15.6 Mechanisms of association of disease with HLA.

Effects of class II polymorphism on antigen presentation
Effects of class I polymorphism on target recognition by cytotoxic T cells
Complement or phagocyte polymorphisms
Molecular mimicry
Receptor interaction

genes. Similar phenomena have been documented in humans, e.g. the immune response to ragweed antigen (associated with HLA-Dw2), insulin (associated with HLA-DR7) and streptococcal extracts (associated with HLA-Dw6), and other work favoured the existence of specific immune suppression (Is) genes. It is now clear that the Ir (or Is) genes are the HLA class II genes themselves by virtue of the differential ability of their αβ heterodimers on the surface of antigen-presenting cells to present antigen (of self or exogenous origin) to T cells. This proposal is supported by the finding that the presence of an arginine residue at position 52 of the DQ α chain and the absence of an aspartic acid residue at position 57 of the DQ β chain are strongly correlated with susceptibility to type 1 diabetes in white people (with a relative risk of over 40 for homozygotes). The presence of these structural features in the HLA-DQ8 molecule facilitates the binding of a particular peptide derived from insulin, which may then be presented to insulin-specific autoreactive T cells. Class I associations—of an immunological kind—are likely to be mediated by variation in the way cytotoxic T cells recognize their targets.

The human MHC also contains four loci coding for important complement (C4 and C2) components and several of the extended haplotypes known to associate with some of the DR-related diseases contain genes that code for functionally inadequate or absent complement proteins. Individuals bearing certain haplotypes, typically 'null alleles' are less able to clear immune complexes from the circulation (see Chapter 6) and show significant differences in phagocyte function. It seems likely that variations in the quality of effector systems such as complement and phagocytic cells, i.e. **complement** or **phagocyte polymorphisms**, could be important in determining the outcome of virus infections which may damage host tissues whether an autoimmune response follows or not.

Others have argued that these disease associations occur because of chemical similarity, often called **molecular mimicry**, between the chemistry of these self-proteins and chemical determinants present on invading microorganisms (see p. 136). Much attention has been paid to the relationship between the possession of HLA-B27 and various reactive arthritides, e.g. those that follow infection with organisms belonging to species of *Salmonella*, *Shigella* and *Yersinia*.

Evidence is also accumulating that HLA proteins may intimately associate with hormone and virus receptors on the surface of cells, i.e. **receptor interaction**, and the extremely strong association between DR2 and narcolepsy may be an example of this.

Contributions from other gene loci

Genes coding for structural variations in IgG molecules (the Gm system) and the acute phase protein α_1-antitrypsin (the Pi system) are both present on chromosome 14. These allotypic variations influence susceptibility to a number of diseases and Gm and Pi alleles have been shown to have an interactive effect with HLA alleles in various disorders, e.g. multiple sclerosis, myasthenia gravis and coeliac disease.

Approximately 20 genetic loci contribute to susceptibility to type 1 diabetes, although the HLA association is greatest, accounting for almost half of the genetic risk.

Developments in DNA technology involving the use of HLA gene probes and endonuclease restriction enzymes have enabled many polymorphisms to be identified within the HLA complex. This approach enables disease susceptibility or resistance genes to be mapped with greater accuracy and disease associations to be identified even when there is no evidence of association with HLA polymorphisms.

Other strong candidate genes associated with type 1 diabetes include those for insulin, IL-12 and CTLA-4. Insulin is an important autoantigen and gene polymorphisms that influence its expression in the thymus may affect the induction of insulin-specific T cell tolerance (see Chapter 3), whereas polymorphisms in IL-12 (see p. 39) and CTLA-4 (see p. 35) may influence the activation and control of autoreactive T cells.

Finally, it has long been known that many autoimmune diseases are more common in females than males, indicating the importance of sex-related genetic effects on the immune system.

Key points

1 Doctors working in all medical specialties are confronted by immunologically mediated diseases but the reasons why some individuals are susceptible to particular examples of them are incompletely understood.

2 Atopic diseases occur in at least 5% of individuals in developed countries and include allergic asthma, allergic rhinitis and atopic dermatitis. The atopic trait is associated with the predominance of Th2-mediated responses and the 'hygiene hypothesis' proposes that reduced microbial exposure in early life enhances such responses to environmental antigens. Genetic factors are also important and genes coding for variants in receptors for IgE or for bacterial lipopolysaccharide positively associate with atopy.

3 A number of disorders are caused by the inappropriate deposition of immune complexes. Various factors govern the formation and clearance of immune complexes and the complement system has a critical role in ensuring their solubilization and transport to cells of the mononuclear phagocyte system. Deficiency of certain complement components such as C2 and C4 is often associated with immune complex disease.

4 The HLA type of an individual is a contributory factor toward the susceptibility of many immunological disorders. Most of the studies performed so far have focused on chronic diseases in developed countries but work in West Africa demonstrates that the HLA phenotype has a major influence on the outcome of malarial infection. The most likely explanation for these associations is the effect that polymorphism of class I and II HLA glycoproteins has on T cell cytotoxicity and antigen presentation, respectively. Polymorphism of genes for components of complement and phagocyte function may also play a part.

Chapter 16

Lymphoproliferative disease

The study of lymphoid tissue used to be a difficult task in view of the lack of clear and constant structural features and readily distinguishable cell types. Lymphocytes numerically overshadow the other cell types present in lymph nodes and recirculate through the lymphatic system. The delineation of the follicle-containing cortex from the medulla, and the identification of specialized postcapillary venules (PCV) at their junction, started the process of understanding the relative roles and cellular constituents of these compartments and their cell traffic patterns (see Fig. 4.5). The development of reagents (e.g. monoclonal antibodies) specific for T and B lymphocytes and their subpopulations and the identification of various kinds of antigen-presenting dendritic cell, in conjunction with *in vivo* studies of lymphocyte traffic patterns, have led to an appreciation of the complex dynamics of lymphoid tissue and the way these processes are perturbed in disease.

Lymphocytosis and lymphadenopathy

The common clinical problems are those associated with an excessive number of lymphocytes in the blood (**lymphocytosis**), enlarged lymph nodes (**lymphadenopathy**) or lymphocytic infiltration of other tissues. These can have many causes, including infection, autoimmune disease

and neoplastic disorders. **Leukaemias** are characterized by the presence of abnormal white cells in blood and bone marrow. In **lymphomas** the normal structure of lymphoid tissues is replaced by abnormal cells of lymphoid origin and in some conditions, e.g. chronic lymphocytic leukaemia, both features coexist. Some forms of lymphoproliferative disease, e.g. **myeloma** and **macroglobulinaemia**, are associated with the production of excessive quantities of immunoglobulin products of individual clones of lymphocyte-derived cells and are collectively known as monoclonal gammopathies.

The distinction between the characteristics of peripheral blood lymphocytes and lymphoid tissues (i) in the normal resting state, (ii) during antigenic stimulation, and (iii) in established lymphoproliferative disease has been greatly facilitated by the use of markers for normal, activated and transformed cell types. These markers include cytogenetic abnormalities; enzyme activities and polymorphisms; immunoglobulin isotypes (e.g. κ vs. λ light chains); cell surface glycoproteins (e.g. HLA and various receptors); and the ability to detect rearrangements in the genes coding for immunoglobulins and the T cell receptor proteins. This powerful armoury not only makes it possible to distinguish the cell type responsible for lymphocyte excess or infiltration, but also enables the distinction to be made between proliferations that are **monoclonal**, i.e. derived from a single progenitor cell, and those that are **polyclonal**, i.e. derived from a variety of cells.

The three main categories of lymphoproliferative disease—leukaemias, lymphomas and monoclonal gammopathies—are reviewed below. In each case, the abnormal proliferation of lymphoid or myeloid cells relates to a physiological counterpart and the particular stage of differentiation involved is indicated in Fig. 16.1.

Viruses and oncogenes

The pathogenesis of lymphoproliferative diseases is poorly understood but the identification of several lymphotropic viruses, e.g. Epstein–Barr virus (EBV), human T cell leukaemia virus-1 (HTLV-I) and human immunodeficiency virus (HIV), in association with various kinds of lymphoma and leukaemia, suggests that infection with a virus belonging to this group may be a critical requirement. However, the large majority of EBV infec-

tions, for example, are self-limiting, because of an effective T cell response and it is probably only when this is deficient, e.g. in chronic malarial infection or in patients with acquired immunodeficiency syndrome (AIDS) or other forms of immunodeficiency, that B cell proliferation leads to overt lymphoma.

Cell-transforming or oncogenic RNA viruses contain **oncogenes** (V-onc) which, following the production of DNA transcripts (via reverse transcriptase), are able to alter the proliferative behaviour of the host cell because they code for growth factors, growth factor receptors or their second messengers, e.g. tyrosine kinases. The genome within human cells also contains similar sequences (C-onc) which are normally present in latent form (proto-oncogenes). These become activated in particular circumstances, e.g. during embryogenesis or clonal stimulation of lymphocytes. Several of the **chromosomal translocations** found in lymphoproliferative disease are known to affect

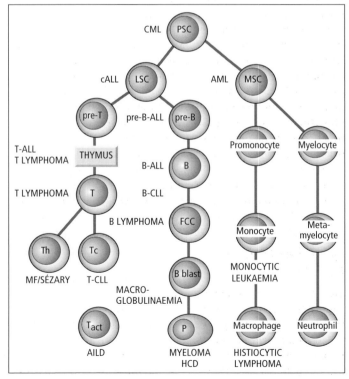

Figure 16.1 Differentiation pathways of lymphoid and myeloid cells, indicating the cell stages from which lymphoproliferative diseases arise. AILD, angio-immunoblastic lymphadenopathy with dysproteinaemia; ALL, acute lymphoblastic leukaemia; AML, acute myeloid leukaemia; cALL, common acute lymphoblastic leukaemia; CLL, chronic lymphocytic leukaemia; CML, chronic myeloid leukaemia; FCC, follicle centre cell; HCD, heavy chain disease; LSC, lymphoid stem cell; MF, mycosis fungoides; MSC, myeloid stem cell; P, plasma cell; PSC, pluripotent stem cell; T$_{act}$, activated T cell.

the expression of host oncogenes, e.g. the transfer of material between chromosomes 8 and 14 in Burkitt's lymphoma, and between chromosomes 9 and 22 which gives rise to the Philadelphia chromosome in chronic myeloid leukaemia. The relationship between infection with oncogenic viruses and the expression of host oncogenes is an area of active investigation.

Epstein–Barr virus and infectious mononucleosis

This common condition is usually self-limiting but has implications for various lymphoproliferative diseases. It occurs when primary infection with **EBV** is delayed beyond childhood. The virus is spread by saliva and replicates in B lymphocytes. The transformation and proliferation of infected B cells is brought under control by T cells of cytotoxic phenotype which recognize EBV-determined antigens on the B cell surface. These immunological events coincide with the development of fever, sore throat, lymphadenopathy, splenomegaly and the appearance of **atypical mononuclear cells** (activated T cells) in the peripheral blood. A variety of virus-specific antibodies can be detected against early antigen (EA), viral capsid antigen (VCA) and EB nuclear antigen (EBNA) as well as the typical heterophile antibody of the Paul–Bunnell test, and some autoantibodies, e.g. against red cells and smooth muscle, occur transiently. After recovery, latently infected B cells are released into the circulation throughout life and are constantly eliminated by cytotoxic T cells.

The **Duncan** or **X-linked lymphoproliferative (XLP) syndrome** is a familial condition in which a defective T cell response fails to control primary EBV infection, leading to uncontrolled B cell proliferation and the development of lymphoma. The molecular defect has now been identified as a deficiency of **SLAM-associated protein (SAP)**. EBV infection also has a role in the pathogenesis of Burkitt's lymphoma, Hodgkin's disease and non-Hodgkin's lymphomas (as well as nasopharyngeal carcinoma and smooth muscle tumours) but the nature of any genetic susceptibility is still unclear. The development of a vaccine against EBV is the subject of current research.

Leukaemias

Leukaemia can develop slowly over a period of years or may present abruptly with clinical evidence of bone marrow involvement, e.g. anaemia, bleeding or infection. Leukaemia is designated 'acute' when more than 50% of bone marrow cells are lymphoblasts or myeloblasts.

Acute lymphoblastic leukaemia (ALL)

This condition mostly affects children and is classified into five distinct types. Three types arise from B cell precursors; have leukaemic cells that are positive for B cell lineage markers; and show rearrangements of their immunoglobulin genes. They are known as **early B cell precursor ALL** (previously designated 'null'), **common ALL** and **pre-B-ALL** (Table 16.1). Common ALL cells are also positive for CD10 (previously referred to as the common ALL antigen; CALLA) whereas pre-B-ALL is distinguished by the presence of cytoplasmic immunoglobulin. The cells of each of these B cell precursor types of ALL contain a nuclear enzyme—terminal deoxynucleotide transferase (TdT) (Table 16.1). By contrast, **B-ALL** cells are negative for TdT and CD10 but possess surface immunoglobulin. Approximately 15% of ALL are designated **T-ALL**. They arise from early thymocytes and their leukaemic cells possess T cell lineage markers and nuclear TdT. Multiple gene abnormalities have been associated with ALL, including *HOX* genes and *BCR-ABL*.

Children with common ALL do well (over a 5-year span) on a regimen of repeated courses of combination chemotherapy. T-ALL and B-ALL are more resistant to cytotoxic agents and have a greater tendency to relapse. Bone marrow transplantation in first or second remission can enhance survival.

Acute myeloblastic leukaemia (AML)

This occurs at all ages but is the most common form of leukaemia in adults. It arises following the

Table 16.1 Cell markers in acute leukaemia.

	B cell lineage						T lineage	Myeloid
	nTdT	CD10	CD19 cCD22	cIg	sIg	Class II	CD7 cCD3	CD13 CD33
Early B cell precursor ALL	+	−	+	−	−	+	−	−
Common ALL	+	+	+	−	−	+	−	−
Pre-B-ALL	+	+/−	+	+	−	+	−	−
B-ALL	−	−	+	−	+	+	−	−
T-ALL	+	−	−	−	−	−	+	−
AML	−	−	−	−	−	−	−	+

nTdT, nuclear terminal deoxynucleotidyl transferase; CD10 was previously known as the common ALL antigen (CALLA); CD19 and cytoplasmic CD22 are B-lineage markers; cIg, cytoplasmic immunoglobulin (μ chains); sIg, surface immunoglobulin; Class II, HLA class II glycoprotein; CD7 and cytoplasmic CD3 are T-lineage markers; CD13 and CD33 are myeloid lineage markers.

clonal proliferation of the **myeloid stem cell** (Fig. 16.1), normally the precursor of both mono-cytes and neutrophils. In AML the blasts usually show some evidence of differentiation to granulo-cytes, in contrast to ALL in which the blast cells show no differentiation at all. AML cells are posi-tive for myeloid cell markers (e.g. CD13 and CD33), myeloperoxidase and non-specific esterase but are negative for TdT and the markers that characterize T and B cell precursors, including CD10.

Combination chemotherapy is used in AML but remission is more difficult to achieve and marrow failure is more difficult to reverse. Bone marrow transplantation is giving encouraging results in younger patients with AML in first remission al-though this option largely depends on the avail-ability of a suitable donor.

Chronic lymphocytic leukaemia (CLL)

This is a disease of the elderly; it develops insidi-ously, and can remain stable for many years. The circulating lymphocyte count may be 100 times normal and often without symptoms or physical signs. Younger patients have a more active course. Infection complicating secondary antibody defi-ciency and bone marrow failure are later sequelae

to which patients usually succumb. CLL does not transform into acute leukaemia but can develop into lymphoma.

In the majority of cases the cell phenotype is that of the mature B cell, i.e. positive for surface im-munoglobulin (sIg) and HLA-DR, and is designated **B-CLL**. The B cells usually express CD5 and mono-clonal sIg. This phenotype relates to an early em-bryonic B cell in normal development, which produces low-affinity polyreactive antibodies. In approximately 10%, a monoclonal immunoglobu-lin is secreted of the same isotype as that detected on the surface of the CLL cells. Autoimmune haemolytic anaemia and thrombocytopenia occur in a minority. Rare cases are of T cell phenotype and can be CD4⁺ or CD8⁺ (**T-CLL**). Cutaneous in-volvement is common and there is considerable overlap with Sézary's syndrome, mycosis fun-goides and T cell lymphomas (see p. 163). The dis-ease has been associated with many disease loci, including the *ATM* gene, which is mutated in ataxia telangiectasia.

CLL is treated with prednisolone and/or an alkylating agent when there is evidence of bone marrow failure, involvement of lymph nodes or spleen, or autoimmune haemolytic anaemia or thrombocytopenia. Intravenous immunoglobulin is an important adjunct in those patients with sec-ondary hypogammaglobulinaemia.

Chronic myeloid leukaemia (CML)

CML is a disease of middle life but usually presents with symptoms and signs of leukaemic infiltration, e.g. splenomegaly. The blood shows a marked increase in leucocytes (at least fivefold and often much higher). The abnormal cells derive from the **pluripotential stem cell** (see Fig. 16.1) and show a cytogenetic abnormality—the **Philadelphia chromosome**—resulting from translocation of part of the long arm of chromosome 22 to the long arm of chromosome 9 with reciprocal translocation of part of chromosome 9 containing the *ABL* oncogene to chromosome 22. Most patients develop a blast crisis in which the cell type transforms to give a picture resembling AML or ALL, underlining the common origin of the two cell types concerned.

Most patients with CML respond to treatment with an alkylating agent and splenic irradiation or splenectomy, where necessary. Bone marrow transplantation is being increasingly used in younger patients who have an HLA-matched sibling and this offers the prospect of long-standing remission.

Lymphomas

In these forms of lymphoproliferative disease normal lymphoid tissue is replaced by abnormal cells of lymphoid origin.

Hodgkin's disease

Hodgkin's disease typically presents in young adults with painless enlargement of regional lymph nodes. Histologically, it is characterized by the presence of large multinucleate cells of irregular shape known as **Reed–Sternberg cells**, which are surrounded by a mixed cellular infiltrate consisting of T and B lymphocytes, macrophages, neutrophils, eosinophils and plasma cells. Systemic symptoms such as fever, anorexia and weight loss are often present, particularly when lymph node involvement has progressed to other sites.

Reed–Sternberg cells are positive for HLA class II glycoproteins, IgG Fc receptors and the granulocyte marker CD15 but are not phagocytic. They also express the IL-2 receptor (CD25) typical of activated T cells, and the transferrin receptor. It is likely that the Reed–Sternberg cell arises from an early lymphoid cell. Hodgkin's tissue is often positive for the EBV genome and epidemiological data support a role for EBV in the pathogenesis of this condition.

Hodgkin's disease is classified histologically into four subtypes: lymphocyte predominant, nodular sclerosis, mixed cellularity and lymphocyte depleted. Nodular sclerosis is distinct from the other three histological subtypes and shows a nodular pattern surrounded by collagen bands. Once this pattern is established it remains constant throughout the course of the disease. The subtype of Hodgkin's disease is important in predicting survival: those with lymphocyte predominant disease have the best survival; mixed cellularity and nodular sclerosis have an intermediate prognosis; and those with lymphocyte depletion have the worst.

Treatment is dependent on the stage of the disease. If it is localized, radiotherapy is the treatment of choice but if further advanced, multiple agent systemic chemotherapy is used. Approximately three-quarters of patients treated for Hodgkin's disease survive for at least 5 years. Autologous bone marrow transplants are used for patients who relapse.

Non-Hodgkin's lymphomas

The increase in knowledge of the biology of the lymphocyte has led to a greater understanding of the most common tumours of the immune system—the non-Hodgkin's lymphomas (NHL). This has given rise to more informative classifications of these neoplasms. The Kiel classification was used initially but has now been superseded by the REAL (revised European American Lymphoma) classification and a WHO classification. This groups NHL by cell type (T, B, Hodgkin's) and as precursor or mature cell derived. The more recent classifications include not only the histological features but also immunophenotypic and genotypic features, linked to clinical outcomes.

There is an increased incidence of NHL in patients with impaired T cell immunity resulting from therapeutic immunosuppression (given for autoimmune disease or to suppress graft rejection), HIV infection or inherited deficiencies. EBV can be detected in most lymphomas occurring in graft recipients. LMP-1 is an oncogenic protein expressed by EVB, with similarities to tumour necrosis factor (TNF) receptor proteins, which mimics T cell activating signals to B cells. A chromosomal translocation between chromosomes 14 and 18 is present in approximately 80% of B cell lymphomas. It gives rise to overexpression of the *BCL*-2 oncogene, which prevents apoptosis (programmed cell death).

Diffuse large B cell lymphoma is the most common non-Hodgkin's lymphoma and represents between 30% and 40% of lymphomas. Although aggressive it will respond well to chemotherapy. The cells are usually CD20 positive and the cells may exhibit cytogenetic abnormalities with translocations [t(14;18); t(3;14); t(8;14)]. The tumours often contain abundant polyclonal T cells. The next most common lymphoma is the **follicular lymphoma**, an indolent tumour. Most tumours of this type have the t(14;18) translocation and overexpression of *BCL-2*; they have a mature B cell phenotype and are CD10, CD19, CD20 and CD22 positive. The normal counterpart of the malignant cell is the reactive germinal centre cell. Response to therapy is good. Monoclonal antibodies against CD20 are used in this type of tumour along with conventional chemotherapy. **Maltomas** are tumours arising from cells in the mucosal associated lymphoid tissue. These tumours present outside lymph nodes in, for example, the stomach (associated with *Helicobacter pylori* infection), thyroid gland (associated with autoimmune thyroiditis) and salivary glands (in Sjögren's syndrome). Treatment of the *Helicobacter* infection will cure the gastric maltoma.

Malignancies of small lymphocytes are relatively common. They form a spectrum of disease ranging from cases with extensive marrow involvement, a peripheral blood lymphocytosis and inconspicuous lymphadenopathy to those whose clinical picture is dominated by lymph node involvement. The former picture is that of **chronic lympho-cytic leukaemia** and the latter is termed **lymphocytic lymphoma**. The malignant cell appears identical in both processes and is a CD5$^+$ B cell, belonging to a separate pathway of B cell differentiation in the majority of cases. Thirty per cent of cases have trisomy 12. Plasmacytoid differentiation of the B cells leads to **Waldenström's macroglobulinaemia**, in which the B cells produce large quantities of monoclonal IgM. The main complications of this disease are caused by the increase in plasma viscosity, a **hyperviscosity syndrome**, from the high molecular weight IgM and the presence of **cryoglobulins**, abnormal monoclonal immunoglobulins which precipitate in the blood vessels in the cooler parts of the body such as the hands, feet, nose and ears, causing blockage of the blood vessels (see below). Lymphocytic lymphoma/B-CLL is an indolent but incurable disease and many patients live for long periods, dying with the disease rather than as a result of it.

Burkitt's lymphoma is a B cell tumour usually seen in children and originally described in Africa in areas endemic for malaria; it also occurs as a consequence of immunosuppression in HIV infection. It is strongly associated with infection with EBV. It is a rapidly growing tumour with characteristic translocations involving chromosome 8, leading to overexpression of the *c-myc* oncogene [t(8;14); t(2;8); t(8;22)]. Malignant lymphocytes may be seen in the peripheral blood. The cells are of a mature B cell phenotype, CD10, CD19, CD20 and CD22 positive, and CD5 negative.

T cell lymphomas are much less common. **Mycosis fungoides** is a cutaneous T lymphocytic lymphoma which can spread to other organs and **Sézary's syndrome** is a related condition in which the skin changes are more diffuse and abnormal lymphocytes, **Sézary cells**, are found in the circulation. In both instances the abnormal cells are usually of T helper cell phenotype. More aggressive T (or null) cell lymphomas include the systemic **anaplastic large-cell lymphoma**, which is characterized by the expression of the surface marker Ki-1 (CD30), although this may also be seen in Hodgkin's disease. Cells show a typical cytogenetic abnormality, t(2;5)(p23;q35), and have an aberrant phenotype, losing many characteristic T cell surface antigens such as CD3 and CD45RO, but express some cytotoxic T cell-specific antigens such as granzyme B and perforin. **Adult T cell lymphoma/leukaemia** is seen in Japan and the Caribbean and is caused by infection with the retrovirus **HTLV-1**. Infection may occur through sexual relations, blood transfusion and transplacentally.

Non-Hodgkin's lymphoma is usually treated with radiotherapy if localized and with single or combination chemotherapy if the disease is more extensive or aggressive. Monoclonal antibodies against CD20 (rituximab) and other surface antigens are now increasingly used to target therapy at the malignant cells. Intensive chemotherapy followed by transplantation with autologous bone marrow purged of lymphoma cells is used in patients who fail on standard chemotherapy or relapse while in remission.

Angioimmunoblastic T cell lymphoma

This condition is characterized by generalized lymphadenopathy, hepatosplenomegaly, skin rashes, fever and a polyclonal increase in serum IgG (and often IgA and IgM). Lymphoblastoid cells may be present in peripheral blood. The diagnosis is made on the histological changes observed in lymphoid tissue, i.e. a mixed cellular infiltrate containing immunoblasts, lymphocytes, plasma cells, eosinophils and histiocytes, marked proliferation of small blood vessels and deposition of an amorphous acidophilic material between the infiltrating cells. Anecdotal reports suggest that this condition may be triggered by various drugs, e.g. phenytoin or penicillin, or other antigens. A variety of autoantibodies are present and there is usually a haemolytic anaemia with a T cell lymphopenia and anergy on delayed hypersensitivity testing. Some cases spontaneously remit or respond to steroid treatment but 5–10% of patients develop an immunoblastic lymphoma. The cellular infiltrate and blood vessel proliferation are probably caused by cytokine release from the abnormal cells which are usually of T cell origin.

Monoclonal gammopathies

This is a group of disorders in which evidence of monoclonal proliferation is readily obtained because the abnormal cells derive from terminal stages of the B cell maturation pathway (see Fig. 16.1) and secrete large quantities of a chemically homogeneous immunoglobulin product. In **macroglobulinaemia**, the abnormal cell is a **B lymphoblast** which is found in lymph nodes, spleen and marrow and the secreted product is of class **IgM**. In **myeloma**, the abnormal cells resemble **plasma cells** and produce lesions in marrow-containing bones without involvement of secondary lymphoid organs and the secreted immunoglobulins are of classes **IgG, IgA, IgD** or **IgE**. The organ distribution of the abnormal cells in macroglobulinaemia is in keeping with the presence of IgM-producing plasma cells in the medulla of lymph nodes and the red pulp of the spleen, but the localization to the bone marrow of monoclonal plasma cells producing immunoglobulins of other isotypes is more difficult to explain unless these are cells that differentiate directly from pre-B cells in bone marrow or represent cells that have switched from IgM production and seeded secondarily in bone marrow.

Macroglobulinaemia

Virtually all the symptoms of this condition are caused by the presence of a **monoclonal IgM** of κ or λ type secreted by a population of cells infiltrating lymph nodes, spleen, liver and bone marrow which give the appearance of a slowly growing lymphoplasmacytoid lymphoma. The pentameric nature of secreted IgM (1 million Da molecular weight) leads to symptoms of blood **hyperviscosity** when levels exceed 30 g L^{-1} and causes circulatory problems in the retina, central nervous system and extremities. Interaction of monoclonal IgM with the surfaces of platelets, red cells and neutrophils may cause bleeding, anaemia and infection, and in some cases the abnormal protein behaves as a **cryoglobulin**, i.e. a protein that precipitates at a cool temperature, giving rise to cold-induced peripheral vasospasm, i.e. **Raynaud's phenomenon**, as well as vascular inflammation in the small vessels of the skin, leading to necrotic lesions.

In contrast to myeloma, lytic bone lesions and the production of plentiful free light chains are not features of this condition and thus bone pain, hypercalcaemia and renal failure are rarely seen. In contrast, rare cases of monoclonal monomeric (7S) IgM usually have the clinical features of myeloma (Table 16.2). Macroglobulinaemia is usually treated with prednisolone and a cytotoxic agent and by plasmapheresis when hyperviscosity or cryoglobulinaemia is a problem.

Myeloma

This is a malignant proliferation of plasma cells secreting a single immunoglobulin isotype of class **IgG, IgA, IgD, IgE or 7S monomeric IgM** and containing light chains of κ or λ type. In approximately 20% of cases the plasma cells secrete light chains in the absence of a heavy chain (Table 16.2). The abnormal plasma cells accumulate in bone marrow, replacing the normal marrow elements, and cause **bone pain** and, in some cases, pathological fracture (Table 16.3). Decalcification of the

Table 16.2 Incidence of monoclonal isotypes in myeloma.

IgG	55%
IgA	20%
IgM*	0.5%
IgD	1.5%
IgE	0.01%
Light chain only	20%

* This refers to monomeric 7S IgM. Monoclonal pentameric 19S IgM occurs in macroglobulinaemia.

Table 16.3 Clinical features of myeloma at presentation.

Anaemia	>90%
Bone lesions	80%
Infection	50%
Hypercalcaemia	45%
Renal failure	45%

surrounding bone and **hypercalcaemia** are caused by the release of osteoclast-activating factors. These factors include IL-1, IL-6 and TNF, but IL-6 is the most potent and also mediates the effects of the other two. Levels of C-reactive protein (see p. 102) are also raised and can be used to monitor disease activity.

IL-6 is the major cytokine controlling the differentiation of plasma blast cells into mature plasma cells and is an important growth factor for myeloma cells *in vitro*. Human herpesvirus 8 (previously associated with Kaposi's sarcoma; see p. 107) has recently been identified in bone marrow dendritic cells of patients with myeloma and these cells were also found to transcribe IL-6. Monoclonal antibodies to IL-6 inhibit myeloma cell proliferation but it is not possible to achieve this *in vivo* because the levels of IL-6 are usually too high. However, corticosteroids such as dexamethasone, oestrogens and inhibitors of IL-1 and TNF also inhibit IL-6 and are currently under investigation for the treatment of myelomatosis. γ-Interferon may also have a role in inhibiting IL-6-induced proliferation.

There is an increased incidence of **infection** resulting from the development of secondary hypogammaglobulinaemia, neutropenia or interaction of the monoclonal immunoglobulin (if of isotypes IgG1 or IgG3) with phagocytic cells. Patients often show a bleeding tendency because of interaction of the myeloma protein with platelets or coagulation factors. **Hyperviscosity** of the blood is less likely with increased levels of monomeric immunoglobulins but occurs when these approach 100 g L^{-1} and is particularly marked with IgA and IgG3 proteins which have a spontaneous tendency to aggregate. Some myeloma proteins also behave as **cryoglobulins** (see p. 167), giving rise to cold sensitivity phenomena.

Plasma cells normally synthesize an excess of **light chains** compared to their level of heavy chain production. Large quantities of monoclonal free light chains are produced in myeloma and this material, being of low molecular weight, passes readily into the urine. This feature has become known as **Bence Jones protein** after the author of its first description in 1847. These excessive

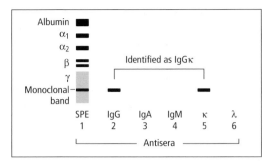

Figure 16.2 Serum protein electrophoresis (SPE) with immunofixation. Patient's serum is electrophoresed in six lanes on an agar gel. Strips soaked in antisera specific for IgG, IgA, IgM, κ or λ light chains are placed over lanes 2 to 6, respectively. These antisera form immune complexes with any M proteins present and 'fix' them in the gel by precipitation (see p. 61). Unfixed serum proteins are then washed out of the gel and the fixed M proteins are visualized by a protein stain. The total serum proteins electrophoresed are stained in lane 1. In the example shown, the monoclonal band seen in the SPE γ region (lane 1) is identified as an IgGκ paraprotein (lanes 2 and 5) by immunofixation.

Table 16.4 Causes of monoclonal gammopathy.

Myeloma
Macroglobulinaemia
Non-Hodgkin's lymphoma
Chronic lymphocytic leukaemia
Primary cold agglutinin disease
Benign monoclonal gammopathy
Chronic infections
Connective tissue disease

amounts of light chain can, however, be toxic to renal tubules, and other factors, e.g. hypercalcaemia, hyperuricaemia, amyloidosis and dehydration, also contribute toward the development of **myeloma kidney**, a cause of renal failure.

A **compact M (monoclonal) band** is usually present on zone electrophoresis of serum (see p. 51) but this can have causes other than a monoclonal gammopathy. Monoclonal immunoglobulins are identified by **immunofixation** (Fig. 16.2) and a diagnosis of myeloma cannot be excluded until this has been performed on serum and urine. Some patients will only show a monoclonal immunoglobulin in serum, whereas others with 'Bence Jones only' myeloma will only show the presence of light chains in urine unless there is impaired filtration resulting from renal failure. In more severely affected cases the immunoglobulins belonging to other classes are reduced, probably related to marrow infiltration and suppression of normal plasma cells.

Abnormal plasma cells are usually apparent on conventional examination of a bone marrow sample obtained by aspiration or trephine biopsy. Most patients show radiological evidence of bone destruction. Examination of bone marrow cells by immunofluorescence (see p. 61; Fig. 5.12) is also useful in confirming the diagnosis of a monoclonal proliferation and in identifying the isotype.

The treatment of myeloma has been unsatisfactory, with only a modest increase in survival following courses of melphalan (a cytotoxic drug) and prednisolone. However, the more aggressive use of combination therapy (e.g. vincristine, doxorubicin and steroids followed by high-dose melphalan) has improved the outlook in recent trials and the application of bone marrow transplantation (allogeneic or autologous stem cells), interferon and inhibitors of IL-6 have been shown to be successful.

Monoclonal gammopathy of uncertain significance

Monoclonal immunoglobulins also occur in other conditions (Table 16.4) and some patients have monoclonal proteins that are either transient or persistent but of undetermined significance and not associated with malignant disease. This condition has been called **monoclonal gammopathy of uncertain significance (MGUS)** but the diagnosis is difficult to establish prospectively. However, patients who have a level of monoclonal immunoglobulin less than $20\,g\,L^{-1}$, have few (<5%) plasma cells in bone marrow, do not show suppression of other immunoglobulin classes, do not have an excess of urinary light chains and lack bone lesions, show a much more benign course, and may remain well for many years. However, careful follow-up has revealed that approximately 20% of such patients develop myeloma, macroglobulinaemia or amyloidosis within a 10-year period.

Heavy chain diseases

Rare patients have been identified who show excessive production of free heavy chains, e.g. the α chain of IgA, the γ chain of IgG, the μ chain of IgM or the δ chain of IgD. α **chain disease** is the most common of this group. It is associated with severe diarrhoea, malabsorption, abdominal pain and weight loss and is also called immunoproliferative small intestinal disease (IPSID). The small gut shows diffuse infiltration with lymphoplasmacytoid cells secreting α chain dimers, which usually show deletion of the variable (V_H) region. Free α chains can be detected in serum by the technique of **immunoselection** in which the sample is electrophoresed through agarose-containing antisera reactive with κ and λ chains in order to precipitate all the intact immunoglobulin molecules, thus leaving any free heavy chains to react with an anti-α chain reagent in a second zone.

The incomplete nature of the abnormal immunoglobulin in this condition makes it difficult to be certain that this is a monoclonal abnormality. Some cases have remitted following oral treatment with antibiotics but most cases transform into an immunoblastic lymphoma of B cell type. γ chain disease behaves like a malignant lymphoma and γ chain fragments (often of the $γ_3$ subclass) can be detected in serum. μ chain disease resembles chronic lymphocytic leukaemia with pentameric μ chain fragments present in serum and κ light chains in the urine, suggesting a monoclonal proliferation. A case of δ chain disease resembled myeloma but with free δ chains in the serum.

Cryoglobulinaemia

The serum of some patients contains proteins that spontaneously precipitate or form gel-like polymers at temperatures below 37°C and are termed **cryoglobulins**. Approximately 25% of cases are **type I** resulting from the presence of **monoclonal** immunoglobulins which have an intrinsic tendency to cryoprecipitate (Table 16.5). **Type II** cryoglobulins are of mixed type (**monoclonal–polyclonal**) and contain a monoclonal protein (most often of class IgM) with rheumatoid factor-like activity, i.e. it has specificity for IgG and forms complexes with it. These also tend to precipitate in the cold. This type of cryoglobulinaemia is associated with various kinds of lymphoproliferative disease including macroglobulinaemia. Overall, approximately 10% of monoclonal IgM proteins have cryoglobulin activity: half of them spontaneously (type I) and half as a complex with IgG

Table 16.5 Types of cryoglobulinaemia.

Type	Cases (%)	Composition	Serum level (g L⁻¹)	Diseases
I	25	Monoclonal Ig IgM, IgG or IgA	1–30	Macroglobulinaemia Myeloma Lymphoma
II	25	Monoclonal–polyclonal Ig IgM–IgG IgG–IgG IgA–IgG	1–5	Macroglobulinaemia Lymphoma CLL MEC–HCV infection
III	50	Polyclonal–polyclonal Ig IgM–IgG	0.1–1	Systemic lupus Sjögren's disease Rheumatoid arthritis Vasculitis Chronic infection

CLL, chronic lymphocytic leukaemia; HCV, hepatitis C virus; MEC, mixed essential cryoglobulinaemia.

Table 16.6 Types of amyloidosis and their fibril proteins.

Clinical type	Amyloid protein	Precursor protein
Lymphoproliferative Myeloma Macroglobulinaemia Heavy chain disease Primary amyloidosis	Amino-terminal (variable region) of light chains (AL)	Light chains
Reactive systemic Chronic inflammation Chronic infection Malignant disease	Protein A (AA)	Serum amyloid A apolipoprotein (SAA)
Following chronic haemodialysis	β_2-microglobulin (Aβ_2M)	β_2-microglobulin (β_2M)
Heredofamilial amyloidosis	AA or pre-albumin	SAA or pre-albumin

(type II). Some of the latter give rise to a clinical picture consisting of purpura, arthralgia, lymphadenopathy and hepatosplenomegaly in the absence of other primary disease—a condition known as **mixed essential cryoglobulinaemia** (MEC). This is strongly associated with chronic hepatitis C virus infection, and typically complement C4 is also reduced or absent.

The remaining 50% of patients with cryoglobulinaemia (**type III**) are of mixed polyclonal type (**polyclonal–polyclonal**) in which polyclonal IgM rheumatoid factor-like antibodies complex with IgG and precipitate in the cold. These patients usually have an obvious immune complex disease (e.g. systemic lupus or rheumatoid arthritis) or chronic infection (e.g. bacterial endocarditis). In each case the symptoms can be alleviated by plasmapheresis and/or the use of prednisolone and cytotoxic agents, although treatment is directed against the primary disorder where possible.

Amyloidosis

Virchoff gave the term **amyloid** or 'starch-like' to the material that stains with iodine which he observed in tissue following chronic inflammation. These days this material is detected by the use of dyes such as Congo red or thioflavine T; by its birefringence under polarized light; or by its fibrillary structure on electron microscopy. The amyloid fibrils that deposit in tissues are, in fact, all derived from protein precursors (Table 16.6) and are formed following enzymatic action which promotes their polymerization in β-conformation. Amyloid deposits also contain a non-fibrillary glycoprotein—amyloid P component—which is derived from a serum protein designated SAP.

Light chain-associated or lymphoproliferative amyloidosis occurs in several related conditions, including myeloma, and follows the excessive production of monoclonal free light chains. It can affect various tissues including the heart, kidneys and peripheral nerves, and is an important cause of myeloma kidney (see p. 166). The main component of the amyloid fibrils is a protein, designated AL, which consists of light chains or fragments thereof which include the V_L domain. Another form of amyloid protein occurs in association with chronic stimulation of the immune system and is called amyloid A protein (AA). It has a circulating serum precursor (SAA), which is an acute phase protein (see p. 103). This reactive form of amyloidosis affects the liver, spleen and kidneys causing enlargement and functional impairment. β_2-Microglobulin and pre-albumin are also able to form amyloid fibrils when their metabolism is disturbed as in chronic haemodialysis and various forms of familial amyloidosis, respectively.

Key points

1 Abnormal proliferation of the cells of the immune system takes many forms, e.g. leukaemia, lymphoma, myeloma, macroglobulinaemia and heavy chain diseases. Cryoglobulinaemia and amyloidosis are also associated with the abnormal production of proteins involved in the immune response.

2 The characterization of proteins present on the surface and in the cytoplasm of lymphocytes and myeloid cells is the chief means of diagnosing and identifying the abnormal cell in the six main types of acute leukaemia, which vary in their management and prognosis.

3 Epstein–Barr virus is a potent stimulus for B cell proliferation, and infection with it usually results in the self-limiting condition, infectious mononucleosis. However, this virus is also implicated in the pathogenesis of Hodgkin's disease, non-Hodgkin's lymphoma and Burkitt's lymphoma, and the development of these conditions is likely to be associated with as yet unidentified forms of genetic or acquired susceptibility.

The origin of the disease-defining cell in Hodgkin's disease — the Reed–Sternberg cell — is still debated but most of the evidence suggests a lymphoid source. More than 90% of non-Hodgkin's lymphomas are derived from the B cell lineage.

4 The monoclonal gammopathies are caused by the uncontrolled proliferation of a single clone of plasma cells (in myelomatosis) or B lymphoblasts (in macroglobulinaemia). In macroglobulinaemia, the excess production of pentameric IgM is associated with hyperviscosity and cryoglobulinaemia. In myeloma, the monoclonal immunoglobulin can be of class IgG, IgA, IgD, IgE or monomeric IgM. Decalcification, hypercalcaemia and bone pain is mediated by the release of IL-6 from the marrow cells (including dendritic cells that have recently been shown to contain a human herpesvirus). Agents that inhibit IL-6 are under investigation for the treatment of myelomatosis.

5 Amyloidosis is caused by the deposition of amyloid fibrils in body tissues. It arises when various kinds of proteins are overproduced in certain chronic diseases and polymerize following enzymatic action.

Chapter 17

Transplantation

Histocompatibility systems

Vertebrates possess the ability to reject most cells or tissues obtained from sources other than those of their own genetic type and some invertebrates also display incompatibility reactions, e.g. genetically distinct corals growing on a reef. The speed and vigour with which tissues are rejected are related to their mutual degree of foreignness and the terms used to describe these differences are summarized in Fig. 17.1. Most of these inherited chemical differences belong to the **major histocompatibility complex** (MHC) designated **H-2** in the mouse and **human leucocyte antigen (HLA)** in humans (described in more detail in Chapter 2). Other minor systems have a weaker influence on tissue compatibility. The genes of the MHC code for two kinds of cell surface glycoprotein: **class I** are present on all nucleated cells, whereas **class II** glycoproteins are normally only present on cells involved in immune recognition, e.g. dendritic cells, macrophages and B cells, and activated T cells (see p. 22).

It has been estimated that at least 10% of peripheral T cells can express reactivity to alloantigens. This seemingly inappropriate ability to react to foreign tissue specificities does, however, have important physiological significance—implicit in the phenomenon of **dual recognition** (see p. 21 and Figs 2.8 and 4.7).

In essence, T lymphocytes—unlike B lymphocytes—recognize antigenic determinants conjointly with self-HLA glycoproteins. T helper cells recognize antigen in association with class II glycoprotein on the surface of specialized antigen-presenting cells, whereas cytotoxic T cells recognize antigen in association with class I glycoprotein on the surface of any nucleated cell. This ensures that each subpopulation of T lymphocytes is guided to react with antigen in a functionally relevant situation. Studies with T cells specific for peptide antigens have demonstrated that such cells often show preferential binding for certain *allogeneic* histocompatibility glycoproteins, reinforcing the view that T cells see foreign tissues as 'self + *x*' (see p. 24).

The rejection process

The specificity and tempo of allograft rejection has already been illustrated in Fig. 1.4. Skin allografts continue to look normal for approximately 5 days after grafting but perivascular infiltration with lymphocytes develops around day 7, followed by vascular obstruction and leakage with oedema and necrosis of the graft epithelium. Necrosis is usually complete by day 14 when the graft takes on a black and shrunken appearance. This process is accelerated if the recipient's lymphocytes have direct vascular access to the graft, e.g. as in a renal transplant.

RELATIONSHIP	NOUNS	ADJECTIVES
Autograft	Syngeneic
Isograft	Syngeneic
Allograft	Allogeneic
Xenograft	Xenogeneic

Figure 17.1 Terms used to describe immunological relationships.

Afferent limb

For grafts that do not involve the construction of a vascular anastomosis, the process of recognition or 'sensitization' usually requires intact lymphatic access, and grafts placed in specially constructed skin flaps or epithelial pouches or within the central nervous system may avoid rejection indefinitely: these locations have been referred to as **privileged sites**. The critical stimulus for the rejection of human tissues placed in unprivileged locations is the expression of HLA class II molecules on the surface of antigen-presenting cells of the tissue graft (Fig. 17.2). HLA class I differences alone may not be sufficient to *induce* an allograft response. The necessity for HLA class II differences to be present and that these should be expressed on intact cells is illustrated by the use of **mixed lymphocyte culture** (MLC) as an *in vitro* correlate of the afferent limb of the allograft response (Fig. 17.3). MLC relies on the ability of mixtures of

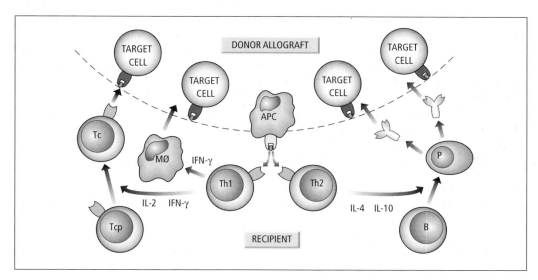

Figure 17.2 The induction of allograft rejection. Class II HLA-bearing fragments of donor tissue proteins on antigen-presenting cells (APC) of donor origin are very effective stimulators of recipient helper T cells. Th1 cells release IL-2 and IFN-γ which enable cytotoxic T cells to differentiate from their precursors and lyse class I HLA–donor peptide-bearing target cells in the graft. IFN-γ also activates macrophages (MØ) which mediate non-specific inflammatory effects. Th2 cells release IL-4 and IL-10 which enable plasma cells (P) to differentiate from B cells and secrete immunoglobulin molecules with specificity for donor antigens. These immunoglobulins, working in conjunction with complement, neutrophil polymorphs or other Fc receptor-bearing cells can then mediate lysis of donor cells. Alloantigens can also be processed by recipient APC but this indirect route is a less efficient way of inducing rejection.

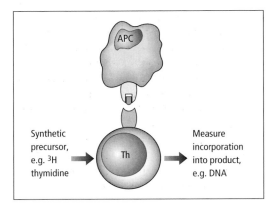

Figure 17.3 The mixed lymphocyte culture (MLC). When allogeneic mononuclear cells purified from peripheral blood are set up in culture with mononuclear cells of self origin, the class II-bearing cells act as antigen-presenting cells (APC) for peptides derived from donor tissue proteins, and activate a proportion of the T helper cell population, i.e. the MLC mirrors the initial steps of allograft rejection as depicted in Fig. 17.2. This is quantified by adding a radiolabelled precursor of DNA, RNA or protein which becomes incorporated into these products as the cells increase synthesis and proceed to cell division.

mononuclear cells from non-identical individuals to stimulate each other in culture even when identical at HLA-A and HLA-B loci and this led to the identification of the HLA-D class II locus. Variations at HLA class II loci are now more usually characterized by serology or DNA typing.

As discussed in Chapter 3 (see p. 31 and Fig. 3.4), T cell education during development in the thymus involves positive selection of those T cells whose antigen receptors (TCR) interact weakly with HLA molecules bearing 'self' peptides derived from processing of the body's own proteins; thus, these T cells are not activated by autoantigenic peptides (Fig. 17.4a), but bind strongly to foreign antigenic peptides associated with self-HLA molecules and react against them (Fig. 17.4b). A major advance in recent years has been the realization that much of the immunogenicity of grafted tissues is caused by the presence of donor antigen-presenting cells—originally referred to as **passenger leucocytes** but now known to be **dendritic cells** (p. 10)—which express (as **alloantigens**) allogeneic HLA class II molecules bearing peptides derived from donor tissue proteins that undergo **direct recognition** by the recipient's T cells. **Peptide-dominant** direct

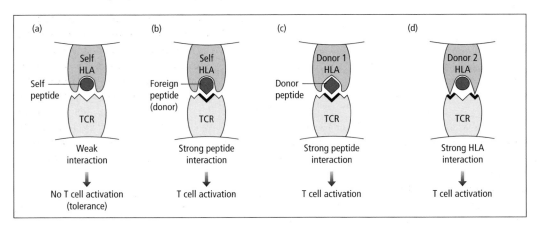

Figure 17.4 Alloantigen recognition by T cells. (a) In the thymus, T cells are positively selected whose T cell antigen receptors (TCR) interact weakly with HLA molecules bearing self-peptides. (b) These selected TCR interact strongly with foreign peptides bound to self-HLA molecules—the foreign peptides could include alloantigenic peptides derived from allogeneic donor tissue grafts. (c) Donor antigen presenting cells (APC) in allogeneic grafts can also present alloantigenic peptides that are recognized by the recipient's T cells. (d) The donor's allogeneic HLA molecules themselves may also bind strongly to the TCR of the recipient's T cells. In these diagrams the strength of TCR interaction is indicated by the darkly shaded areas of the TCR combining site.

recognition involves strong interaction between the recipient's TCR and the donor's HLA-bound allogeneic tissue peptides, termed **minor histocompatibility antigens**, which are seen by the recipient as foreign antigenic peptides because they differ from the recipient's own tissue peptides (Fig. 17.4c). **HLA-dominant** direct recognition involves strong binding of the recipient's TCR to the allogeneic HLA proteins themselves, regardless of the associated antigen peptides (Fig. 17.4d). Indirect recognition involves processing and presentation of donor alloantigenic peptides (i.e. minor histocompatibility antigens) by the recipient's antigen-presenting cells, as occurs for any foreign antigenic peptide (Fig. 17.4b). Very few donor dendritic cells are required to elicit an allograft response by direct recognition and if they are removed prior to grafting so that induction of the allograft response has to occur via indirect recognition then the response is very much weaker and less immunosuppressive therapy is required to prevent rejection. The relative immunogenicity of different allogeneic tissues follows the descending sequence of bone marrow, skin, pancreatic islets, gut, heart, kidney and liver, and largely relates to the quantity of HLA class II-bearing cells within them.

Efferent limb

Once T helper cells become activated then the normal cooperative events (including the release of interleukins) enable cytotoxic T cells to differentiate from cytotoxic precursors (Tcp) with specificity for class I-bearing allogeneic cells, and B cells to differentiate into plasma cells secreting antibody of allogeneic specificity. Graft rejection is also associated with the activation of macrophages, which are induced by γ-interferon (IFN-γ).

The response to an allograft transferred a second time—the 'second set' reaction—is more vigorous because of an expanded population of effector T cells which can operate without T helper cell stimulation. Specific antibody may also contribute to the more rapid rejection process. The balance between T cell and antibody-mediated effects varies according to the circumstance, e.g. the **acute rejection** of renal allografts is predominantly T cell-mediated, whereas **chronic rejection** can be caused by either, or by a combination of both. In contrast, the dramatic events of **hyperacute rejection**, in which the kidney develops vascular stasis with platelet aggregation, neutrophil adherence and loss of function, are caused by the presence of complement-fixing antibody in the recipient's circulation. This is usually avoided by a pretransplant cross-matching procedure in which the recipient's serum is examined for the presence of antibody cytotoxic to donor cells.

Ways of modifying the rejection process

Patients with end-stage organ failure are terminally ill or severely disabled and, when the kidneys are involved, face the prospect of regular dialysis for the rest of their lives. The realization that patients in this category can be restored to a healthy and useful life following organ transplantation has stimulated the search for ways of ameliorating the normal allograft response (Table 17.1).

HLA typing and matching

Typing of kidney donors and their recipients at the major class I loci—**HLA-A** and **HLA-B**—demonstrated that the degree of mismatch affected graft survival although the extreme polymorphism of these two loci means that it is relatively unusual to obtain a complete match between the four possible specificities of both donor and recipient. Incompatibility at the HLA-C locus seems to have little effect on graft survival. The introduction of **HLA-DR** typing by serological means indicated

Table 17.1 Factors that promote graft survival.

HLA typing and matching
Source and preparation of the graft
Selection and preparation of the recipient
Monitoring the allograft response
Non-specific immunosuppression
Specific immunosuppression (including the blood
    transfusion effect)

that matching for the rather smaller number of specificities at this class II locus had an even greater effect on graft survival in keeping with the pre-eminent role of class II glycoproteins in invoking the allograft response. However, the deleterious effect of mismatched grafts has diminished following the addition of ciclosporin to modern immunosuppressive regimens and the urgent need of individual patients and the difficulties of finding perfect matches means that mismatched grafts are often used in renal transplantation. This is less feasible in bone marrow transplantation where the requirements are more stringent (see below).

The procedures by which the limited supply of cadaveric organs is matched to the recipients' characteristics has reached an advanced state of organization in many countries through national and international transplant agencies.

Source and preparation of the graft

Most renal allografts are obtained from unrelated cadaveric donors and are often transported considerable distances in order to provide a satisfactory match between donor and recipient. The period of time during which the kidney is not perfused with an oxygenated blood supply (ischaemia time) is critical and should not exceed 45 min at 37°C or 24 h at 4°C. For liver transplantation the cold ischaemia time is reduced to approximately 8 h.

Living related donors are sometimes used in renal transplantation and in this situation it is possible to match entire haplotypes (see Fig. 15.1). Living donors are the normal source of bone marrow for transplantation and can donate on successive occasions.

The pretreatment of grafts with antibodies specific for class II-bearing dendritic cells linked to cytotoxic agents may render the graft considerably less immunogenic. Purging of bone marrow to remove T lymphocytes is now widely used as a means of reducing the incidence and severity of graft-versus-host disease and is discussed further on p. 178.

Selection and preparation of the recipient

Many patients awaiting renal transplantation develop cytotoxic antibodies reactive with lymphocytes or endothelium following previous transfusion, grafting, pregnancy or infection. This state of presensitization to allogeneic tissue can lead to hyperacute rejection of a renal allograft and it is now routine procedure to perform a cytotoxic cross-match between the recipient's serum and the donor's lymphocytes. However, only antibodies with HLA-A and -B specificity cause hyperacute rejection. Antibodies reactive with products of class II loci are much less damaging and other autoreactive antibodies may even facilitate graft survival. Soon after renal transplantation began it was noticed that the strict avoidance of blood transfusion to prevent presensitization *increased* the chances of graft rejection and a protocol of pregraft exposure to allogeneic blood was introduced in most renal transplant centres (see p. 177).

Monitoring the allograft response

Allograft rejection conjures up a dramatic picture of immunological events, which should be eminently suitable to monitoring by the examination of peripheral blood for changes in antibody or lymphocyte characteristics. Many attempts, involving a wide range of antibody and lymphocyte assays, have failed to provide a clinically useful means of distinguishing rejection episodes from other events such as infection, or one that gives sufficient warning to be able to modify the outcome by therapeutic intervention. This is because the specific cells and antibodies of interest are mostly preoccupied within the graft and thus not available for peripheral sampling.

Fine needle aspiration biopsy enables samples (10 μL) of renal grafts to be removed on alternate days without significant damage to the graft. The nature of the cellular infiltrate is a useful guide to the development of rejection and its severity: the presence of T and B cell blasts occurs early in the rejection process and infiltration with monocytes indicates severe and possibly irreversible change. A significant improvement in the survival of cardiac allografts—for which HLA matching is not attempted—followed the introduction of serial myocardial biopsy in order to observe the early histological changes of rejection. Otherwise, one is left with the non-immunological observation of graft function, using physical, biochemical, isotopic or electrocardiographic techniques and these changes can be very non-specific.

Non-specific immunosuppression

The potency of the antiallograft response is such that none of the factors cited thus far is sufficient to achieve graft survival without the administration of drugs, which suppress the immune system non-specifically. It is only following the exchange of grafts between identical twins (i.e. isografts) or when transferring tissue within the same individual (i.e. autografts) that immunosuppressive measures are unnecessary. In allotransplantation most rejection episodes occur during the first 3 months but a reduced level of immunosuppressive treatment is required indefinitely in most cases.

In the early days of renal transplantation, immunosuppression was usually achieved using the antiproliferative drug, **azathioprine** (in a dosage of *c.* 2.5 mg kg^{-1}day^{-1}), in conjunction with the powerful anti-inflammatory corticosteroid, **prednisolone** (initially in a dosage of 30–100 mg kg^{-1}day^{-1} and gradually reduced toward a maintenance dosage of 10 mg kg^{-1}day^{-1}). The introduction of **ciclosporin**—a fungal metabolite—in the early 1980s had a major impact on graft survival and the combination of low-dose ciclosporin with azathioprine and prednisolone is still used in many centres.

Azathioprine inhibits DNA and RNA synthesis and blocks IL-2 production by lymphocytes. It can cause bone marrow aplasia and frequent monitoring of the white cell count is required. Corticosteroids probably have an effect on T cell function in addition to their anti-inflammatory effect on phagocytic cells. They have many side-effects (Table 17.2) but these are less of a problem with the lower dosage used in modern triple therapy. Ciclosporin binds to a calcium-dependent intracellu-

Table 17.2 Side-effects of non-specific immunosuppression.

Infection
Viral, e.g. CMV, HSV, varicella-zoster virus
Fungal, e.g. *Aspergillus*, *Candida*, *Pneumocystis*
Bacterial, e.g. tuberculosis, *Listeria*, *Nocardia*

Malignancy
Lymphomas (herpesviruses)
Skin tumours (papillomaviruses)
Kaposi's sarcoma (HHV-8)

Antiproliferative effects	
Marrow suppression	Infertility*
Ulceration of	Hair loss*
gastrointestinal tract	Cystitis*

Teratogenesis	
Steroid effects	
Cushingoid appearance	Osteoporosis
Hypertension	Avascular bone
Diabetes	necrosis
Peptic ulceration	Cataracts
Stunted growth	Myopathy

Ciclosporin	
Nephrotoxicity	Hypercholesterolaemia
Hirsutism	Hypertension
Gum hypertrophy	Hepatotoxicity

Antilymphocyte globulin
Serum sickness, fever

CMV, cytomegalovirus; HHV-8 human herpesvirus 8; HSV, herpes simplex virus.
* Seen particularly with cyclophosphamide.

lar protein, cyclophilin, and inhibits the production of IL-2 by helper T cells. It does, however, have several important side-effects including nephrotoxicity, hirsutism, gum hypertrophy, hypercholesterolaemia, hypertension and hepatotoxicity, most of which are dose-related.

Several other immunosuppressive drugs have been introduced recently, e.g. tacrolimus, sirolimus (rapamycin) and mycopholate mofetil. Tacrolimus resembles ciclosporin in its effect on the proteins involved in IL-2 production although its chemical structure is very different. It has similar side-effects to ciclosporin with the exception of hirsutism and gum hypertrophy. Sirolimus resembles tacrolimus in structure but acts distal to IL-2 production. Mycophenolate mofetil is gradually replacing azathioprine in immunosuppressive regimens as it is more effective in preventing acute rejection and is less toxic than azathioprine. It is a more specific and potent inhibitor of T and B cell proliferation because of its inhibition of purine biosynthesis.

Antilymphocyte (ALG) or **antithymocyte globulin (ATG)** has been in use for many years but lacks a standardized bioassay to quantify its potency and preparations raised in other species such as rabbit and horse can induce serum sickness. It is mostly used to treat acute rejection episodes that have failed to respond to a high dose of corticosteroid. Murine antibodies against CD3 (OKT3) have been shown to be as potent as ALG, but easier to standardize. Various monoclonal antibodies to lymphocyte surface proteins have been evaluated, e.g. anti-CD3, anti-CD4 and anti-CD8, anti-CD25 (IL-2 receptor) and anti-LFA-1, and molecular techniques have been developed to incorporate their hypervariable regions into immunoglobulin molecules of human sequence to form **humanized antibodies** that will not provoke a host response. However, serious infection has been a problem in some patients treated with these preparations and this emphasizes the overall limitation of non-specific immunosuppression. Monoclonal antibodies reactive with the IL-2 receptor (anti-CD25) have been shown to reduce the incidence of acute rejection episodes without significant side-effects.

Opportunistic infection is still a major cause of death in most transplantation programmes and emphasizes the need for more sophisticated forms of immunosuppression. The small but significant increase in the incidence of lymphomas and skin tumours is caused by impaired immunity to oncogenic viruses. The subject of secondary immunodeficiency is discussed in more detail in Chapter 12.

Specific immunosuppression

The prospect of inducing antigen-specific immunosuppression at will in the adult animal has been the goal of transplantation immunology since the 1950s when Medawar *et al.* were able to induce a similar state in neonatal mice (Fig. 17.5). Experiment 1 demonstrates the normal rejection of a strain A skin graft by a mouse of the allogeneic B strain. Experiment 2 shows that if cells from strain A mice are inoculated into newborn mice of strain B then the latter animals accept skin grafts derived from strain A throughout their adult life,

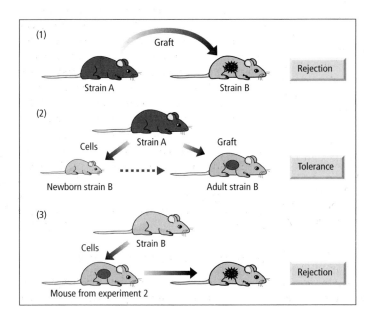

Figure 17.5 The induction of immunological tolerance in the mouse. Normally, skin grafts from strain A are rejected by the allogeneic strain B animal (experiment 1). However, if an animal of strain B is injected with cells from strain A when newborn it becomes tolerant to skin grafts from strain A for the rest of its life (experiment 2). This state of immunological tolerance can be broken by transferring lymphocytes from a strain B animal (that has not been pretreated) to a tolerant mouse. This is followed by prompt rejection of the strain A graft (experiment 3). These experiments were first performed by Billingham *et al.* (Billingham, Brent, Medawar *Nature* 1956;**172**:603–6).

having become specifically tolerant of this histocompatibility type. That the tolerant animals are immunologically normal apart from their specific unresponsiveness to allografts from strain A is demonstrated in experiment 3 in which the natural tendency to reject the strain A graft the animal already bears is restored by the infusion of cells from a strain B animal that has not been pretreated with strain A cells when newborn. This kind of immunological tolerance is attainable in the mouse because of its immunological immaturity at birth and does not apply to most other mammals, including humans.

Many other attempts have been made to induce **immunological tolerance** in adult animals, often with considerable success, but the means by which graft acceptance has been achieved have not usually been clinically applicable or acceptable. It has been known for many years that the administration of graft-specific antibody can promote graft acceptance although there is always a risk of hyperacute rejection. This phenomenon of antibody-mediated **enhancement** has been studied extensively and, at one stage, received limited clinical application for renal transplantation. In experiments where prolonged graft acceptance has been achieved by this means it is clear that the initial phase of induction (or passive enhancement) achieved by antibody is replaced by a maintenance phase (of active enhancement) in which other mechanisms operate. Enhancement can also be actively induced by the administration of allogeneic cells or cell extracts prior to transplantation. These effects have usually been achieved across relatively minor transplantation barriers and only succeed in some donor–recipient combinations. When successful, the animals bearing enhanced grafts tend to show a progressive unresponsiveness to the donor strain. Some clinical examples have been recorded in which graft recipients have gradually 'adapted' to their allografts and been able to have most or all of their immunosuppressive drugs withdrawn.

Experimental studies have shown that the initial antibody-mediated phase of enhancement consists of the depletion of allogeneic class II-bearing cells from the graft. This may be achieved by a direct cytotoxic effect or may involve opsonization by phagocytic cells. Other experimental models support the proposal that the maintenance phase of enhancement is a result of the progressive development of **T-suppressor cells**. A third explanation concerns the development of **autoanti-idiotype antibodies** (idiotypes and anti-idiotypes are described on p. 52). Experimentally, it has been possible to demonstrate that the injection of T lymphocytes bearing idiotypes specific for allogeneic specificities can induce anti-idiotype antibodies which will suppress allograft responses. However, it is usually necessary to inject idiotype-bearing cells or molecules in the presence of powerful adjuvants—a procedure that is not applicable to clinical transplantation. It is possible that suppressor cells, which act to enhance graft acceptance, may achieve this by expressing anti-idiotype activity (see below).

The blood transfusion effect

The realization that blood transfusion prior to allografting paradoxically increased graft survival led to the inclusion of this procedure in renal transplantation programmes. The efficacy of donor-specific transfusions in living related kidney transplantation could well be a result of a specific effect akin to tolerance or enhancement. The fact that single, random transfusions had a beneficial effect in approximately 25% of patients receiving unrelated cadaveric grafts was more difficult to explain, although the appearance of suppressor cells with anti-idiotype specificity has been documented in animal models. Minor histocompatibility determinants may be important in the transfusion effect, which may follow the release of specific or non-specific factors from suppressor cells induced by transfusion. However, the magnitude of the transfusion effect has waned following the introduction of ciclosporin and many centres have abandoned the policy of pretransplant transfusion.

Recurrent and transferred disease

Quite a few diseases leading to end-stage organ failure have an immunological pathogenesis and in these (as well as other conditions) it is possible that the original disease will recur in the transplanted organ. This problem is well documented in renal transplantation and the frequency of recurrence in dense deposit disease and focal glomerulosclerosis negates the value of transplantation. IgA nephropathy, Goodpasture's disease and Henoch–Schönlein purpura also recur but with less severity.

The transplantation of pancreatic islets is under investigation as a means of reversing type 1 (insulin-dependent) diabetes. However, specific destruction of the insulin-producing β cells can occur soon after allografting, emphasizing the role of the immune system in this disease. Cardiac allografts often fail because of atherosclerosis, which may resemble the patient's original disease, and individuals who receive a graft for congestive cardiomyopathy are prone to develop a lymphoma. It is not unusual for leukaemia to recur in some patients treated with bone marrow transplantation (BMT) but, rarely, the cells of the recurrent leukaemia have been shown to be of donor origin, suggesting transfection of an oncogene (see Chapter 16). Several examples of the transfer of atopic or autoimmune disease by BMT have also been recorded.

The transfer of infection and malignancy are other possible hazards of organ grafting. In one case, a carcinoma developed following transfer of a kidney from a donor who was later found to have malignant disease. Fortunately, the tumour was rejected with the graft when immunosuppressive therapy was terminated.

Bone marrow transplantation

An advantage of BMT is that live donors are used and can be sources of marrow on successive occasions. A problem that is almost unique to BMT is that allograft reactions can occur in both directions, i.e. **graft-versus-host (GVH)** and **host-versus-graft (HVG)**. This means that tissue matching has to be closer than is required for organ transplantation and involves mixed lymphocyte culture as well as serological or DNA typing at class

I and II loci. The permutations of the polymorphisms at these various loci are such that it is very unusual to find a satisfactory match from an unrelated donor and most marrow grafts are performed between siblings or parents and their offspring. The ideal situation, of course, is to have an identical twin. Marrow is aspirated from the iliac crests under local or general anaesthetic and is administered intravenously after passage through a wire mesh filter. The usual dose is approximately 10^8 marrow cells kg^{-1} body weight.

Graft acceptance is achieved by giving **conditioning treatment** to the recipient. This usually takes the form of cyclophosphamide with total body irradiation; total lymphoid irradiation; ALG or ATG given in addition. The risks of intensive irradiation are considered unacceptable in children, who usually receive a course of busulfan. This treatment means that the recipient shows severe deficiency of all blood cells (pancytopenia) for 2–4 weeks until engraftment takes place. Intensive support is required during this period in the form of red cell, white cell and platelet transfusions, intravenous feeding, antibacterial agents and a protected pathogen-free environment. The immune responsiveness of the recipient is severely depleted during the first 6 months and infection is a considerable hazard. Interstitial pneumonia resulting from *Pneumocystis carinii* or cytomegalovirus is a common problem and varicella-zoster virus infections also occur. B cell function may take several years to recover, and in some cases never recovers. Intravenous immunoglobulin will then be required as replacement therapy.

Graft-versus-host disease

This complication might be expected to occur in all bone marrow transfers that are not syngeneic but is only obvious in 35–45% of cases although it seriously affects the outcome. It is characterized by a diffuse rash, fever, abdominal pain and diarrhoea with disturbed liver function and, almost always, superadded infection. Its incidence is proportional to the degree of mismatch between donor and recipient and in recent years it has become customary to pretreat the donor marrow with T cell-specific reagents in order to reduce the risk of GVH; a technique known as **purging** or **laundering**. Clearly, it is important to spare stem cells although how the subsequent differentiation of recipient-specific T cells from them is regulated is not clear. Possibly, such cells are brought under control by processes that survive the conditioning regimen and are comparable to the way in which T cell differentiation normally occurs in the thymus.

The introduction of ciclosporin in the management of BMT has further reduced the incidence of GVH because of its preferential effect on helper T cells. However, in recent years it has become clear that there is a reciprocal relationship between the development of GVH and HVG responses in that a lower frequency of GVH is associated with a higher incidence of graft rejection. The persisting problem of bone marrow graft rejection has led to trials of monoclonal antibodies specific for T cell subsets given to the recipients and this has increased the incidence of engraftment, e.g. when reagents specific for both CD4 and CD8 cells are combined. There is also evidence to suggest that the responsiveness of T cells within the graft may be beneficial in patients who receive BMT for leukaemia, i.e. an antileukaemia effect, although the existence of leukaemia-specific antigens is still a matter of debate.

Indications for BMT

The indications for BMT are the major immunodeficiencies, storage diseases and other inborn errors of metabolism, osteopetrosis, marrow aplasia and leukaemia (Table 17.3). BMT can be very successful in immunodeficiency and aplasia and the use of BMT to provide enzyme replacement for inborn errors is showing some promising results. BMT has given encouraging results in patients with acute myeloid leukaemia in their first remission, for without such intervention most patients die from their leukaemia. However, the success rate with chemotherapy for acute lymphoblastic leukaemia is so much better that BMT is usually retained for a subsequent relapse although patients who are prone to relapse can be identified and offered BMT early on. BMT is receiving increasing application in

Table 17.3 Indications for bone marrow transplantation.

Immunodeficiency
Severe combined immunodeficiency (SCID)
Chronic granulomatous disease (CGD)
Leucocyte adhesion deficiency (LAD)
Wiskott–Aldrich syndrome

Storage/metabolic defects
Mucopolysaccharidoses, e.g. Hurler's disease
Lipidoses, e.g. Gaucher's disease

Marrow deficiency
Aplasia
Agranulocytosis

Leukaemia
Acute myeloid
Chronic myeloid
Acute lymphoblastic

Lymphoma
Hodgkin's disease
Non-Hodgkin's lymphoma

Myelomatosis

Haemoglobinopathies
Sickle-cell anaemia
Thalassaemia

Osteopetrosis

chronic myeloid leukaemia where elective intervention during the chronic phase is favoured before progression to blast crisis and this often produces cytogenetic remission with disappearance of the Philadelphia chromosome (see p. 162). It is also increasingly used in non-Hodgkin's lymphoma to treat relapse

Autologous transplantation

Some centres are adopting a more aggressive approach to certain haematological and solid tumours, in which the patient's marrow is stored before the patient is treated with intensive irradiation and/or chemotherapy, after which their marrow is returned. This also creates the opportunity to treat the marrow with antitumour antibodies and this approach has given encouraging results in acute lymphoblastic leukaemia. A more recent development is **peripheral stem cell transfusion** in which stem cells are harvested from peripheral blood during the recovery phase of chemotherapy-induced neutropenia. The inclusion of granulocyte colony-stimulating factor (G-CSF) in the regimen enhances the yield of stem cells and the infusion of stem cells from peripheral blood as opposed to bone marrow reduces the hazard of contamination with malignant cells. Stem cells can be enriched by selection for CD34$^+$ cells, as this marker is expressed by pluripotent stem cells. This form of stem cell replacement may also be useful for allogeneic transplants although the normal donor would also need to be given G-CSF. Stem cell banks are being established using umbilical cord blood.

Key points

1 The critical stimulus for the rejection of foreign grafts is the recognition of class II HLA glycoproteins on the surface of allogeneic antigen-presenting cells (APC) by helper T cells. Recipient APC can also process and present allogeneic class I HLA proteins but this indirect route of sensitization is less effective.

2 Rejection is mediated primarily by cytotoxic T cells specific for allogeneic class I HLA proteins on graft cells. These cells differentiate from cytotoxic precursors under the influence of IL-2 released by Th1 cells. Macrophages are activated by IFN-γ and plasma cells differentiate from B cells under the influence of IL-4 and IL-10. Both of these processes can augment destruction of the graft.

3 Graft survival can be promoted by:
- Close matching of HLA types between donor and recipient
- Ensuring that the donor tissue is optimally prepared
- Treating the recipient with an optimal immunosuppressive regimen
- Prompt detection and management of rejection episodes

4 All forms of non-specific immunosuppression have side-effects—some of which are serious—and it is hoped that a readily applicable form of antigen-specific immunosuppression will soon be available for clinical use.

5 The requirements for successful bone marrow transplantation (BMT) are even more stringent as incompatibility can be manifest as host-versus-graft or graft-versus-host reactions. BMT has been successfully used to correct various forms of immunodeficiency and metabolic defect and is being increasingly applied to the management of leukaemia, lymphoma, myelomatosis, haemoglobinopathies and marrow failure.

Chapter 18

Immunological therapy

The approach to immunotherapy

As discussed in the previous chapter, the clinician needs to manipulate the immune system to ensure a good clinical outcome in transplantation. However, immunotherapy is much broader than this. It is often forgotten that every day millions of people undergo immunotherapy in the form of active and passive immunization, making this the most widely practiced immunotherapy. It is also the oldest, being practiced by Edward Jenner in the late eighteenth century, to protect against the deadly smallpox by inoculating the related cowpox virus. As discussed in Chapter 1, this practice developed because it was observed that milkmaids exposed to cowpox did not develop severe illness with smallpox.

Other aspect of immunological therapy include modulation of allergic disease by desensitization therapy, modulation of inflammatory disease by drugs and by biological agents such as monoclonal antibodies against tumour necrosis factor (TNF), suppression of the immune system in autoimmune diseases, manipulation of the bone marrow with colony-stimulating factors, replacement of missing factors by transfusion, treatment of immunodeficiency by bone marrow or stem cell transplants or by direct gene manipulation (gene therapy). The development of chimaeric and humanized monoclonal antibodies has at last allowed monoclonal antibody technology to be used directly in the treatment of cancer, e.g. the use of anti-CD20 (rituximab) in the treatment of lymphoma. This is a very exciting area of medicine. Overall, modern applications and developments in immunotherapy take advantage of the basic and clinical understanding of the immune system, which is described in the preceding chapters of this book.

Passive immunotherapy

Passive immunotherapy refers to the transfer of immunity, usually antibody, to a naïve recipient. This has the advantage of providing instant protection, but as there is no direct stimulation of the recipient's immune system by antigen, there is no long-lasting memory. This is how a newborn infant is protected for the first 6 months of life, while it makes its own antibody; transplacental passage of IgG, but not IgM or IgA, takes place through an active transport process (see p. 54), with the highest level of transfer taking place in the last trimester (Fig. 18.1). If there is a delay in development of the child's immunity, then a physiological trough develops at approximately 6 months of age. This, if prolonged, may lead to an increase in infections: **transient hypogammaglobulinaemia of infancy**. Premature infants will be more at risk as there will have been less transplacental transfer.

Passive transfer of antibody will therefore provide protection for no more than 6 months.

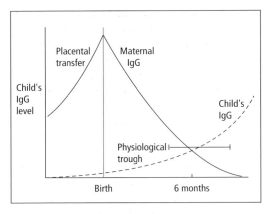

Figure 18.1 Changes in maternal and neonatal IgG levels before and after birth. Transplacental transfer of IgG takes place in the last 3 months of pregnancy and, after birth, maternal antibody disappears gradually over the first 6 months of life.

Table 18.1 Time scale of key development in immunization.

1721	Variolation (smallpox)
1796	Vaccination (cowpox)
1885	Rabies vaccine
1925	Diphtheria toxoid; tetanus toxoid
1931	Viral culture in chick embryo developed to allow production of viruses for vaccines
1937	Yellow fever vaccine
1949	Viral tissue culture
1954	Inactivated poliovirus vaccine (Salk)
1956	Attenuated live poliovirus vaccine (Sabin)
1960	Measles vaccine
1966	Rubella vaccine
1975	Hepatitis B vaccine
1980	Smallpox eradicated as a result of WHO immunization campaign
1988	Hib conjugate vaccine introduced
1995	Hepatitis A vaccine (replaces passive immunotherapy for protection)

It has been used in conjunction with active immunotherapy to provide immediate protection while awaiting the recipient's response to the active component, although the simultaneous administration of antibody with antigen may reduce the recipient memory response. Typical uses of passive immunization include protection against **tetanus** and **rabies** after exposure, usually in conjunction with a course of active immunization, and prophylaxis for hepatitis A prior to travel (although this has now been replaced by an effective vaccine). A monoclonal antibody, **palivizumab**, is licensed for prevention of respiratory syncitial virus infection in infants at high risk.

Passive immunotherapy is also the mainstay of the management of antibody-deficient patients (see Chapter 12). In order to prevent infection, patients with **X-linked agammaglobulinaemia** and **common variable immunodeficiency** (see p. 119) receive pooled **normal human IgG** either intravenously or subcutaneously in a regimen that maintains their trough IgG levels within the normal range. The IgG is purified from pooled human plasma, obtained from carefully screened donors, to avoid the transmission of blood-borne viruses such as hepatitis B, hepatitis C and HIV. There is concern over the transmission of **prions** by plasma and currently donated plasma is sourced from countries where there is no or little evidence of **variant Creutzfeldt–Jakob disease (vCJD)**.

Patients with **hereditary angio-oedema** and α_1**-antitrypsin deficiency** also receive passive immunotherapy with the purified missing components, C1-esterase inhibitor and α_1-antitrypsin, respectively, as either treatment for acute exacerbations or as prophylaxis.

Passive therapy with cells is used only rarely, but occasionally granulocyte transfusions are used from matched donors to provide phagocytic activity, e.g. in patients with severe neutropenia after bone marrow transplantation or with neutrophil defects and severe infections.

Active immunotherapy

The most desirable form of immunotherapy is one that produces a long-lasting change in the immune system with the generation of specific immunological memory, as discussed in Chapter 1. This represents the most widely used immunotherapy. Immunization provides the mainstay of protection against infectious disease, and developed from Edward Jenner's pioneering work. Table 18.1 shows the historical development of immunization.

Principles of active immunization

The aim of active immunization is to produce both a humoral and cellular response. In most cases, the aim is to produce antibody that will **opsonize** bacteria and facilitate **phagocytosis, bind complement**, leading to direct bacterial lysis, bind to and **neutralize bacterial toxins**, prevent uptake of viruses into cells by **blocking surface receptors**, and enhance phagocytosis of viral particles, preventing dissemination. To enable an optimum antibody response, stimulation of antigen-specific T helper cells is required. Some vaccines also lead to the development of specific cytotoxic T cells. Normally, however, the effectiveness of a vaccine is measured by the production of specific protective antibodies.

The induction of the immune response is achieved by the subcutaneous or intramuscular administration of the antigen. The form in which the antigen is administered is carefully chosen to optimize the protective response. As Jenner was aware, administration of smallpox itself ('**variolation**') is too dangerous, as disease usually results even though protection for the survivors is absolute. Use of cowpox ('**vaccination**') is safer, as disease does not occur but there is cross-protection against smallpox. Vaccines are therefore developed using either related non-pathogenic organisms or organisms modified to reduce or abolish their capacity to produce disease, a process of **attenuation**. Administration of live organisms is to be preferred as the replication of the organism in the recipient increases the stimulation of the immune system and mimics the natural disease more closely. However, there are risks in using live vaccines. For example, patients with an undiagnosed immune deficiency will be unable to clear even an attenuated organism. This has been seen with antibody-deficient patients given the attenuated live polio vaccine. In such patients the attenuated virus continues to replicate and the mutation, which attenuated the organism, can then spontaneously revert to the wild-type virus and lead to paralytic disease. As a result of this risk, oral polio vaccine is now being withdrawn in the UK and a killed vaccine substituted.

In other cases, it is not the infection itself that causes the disease but a toxin released by the bacteria, e.g. tetanus and diphtheria toxins. Administration of the toxin as a vaccine would be too dangerous, so the toxin is modified to prevent it causing disease, while retaining sufficient immunogenicity to stimulate an immune response against the unmodified toxin. The toxin can be modified by controlled heat or by chemicals, and the modified toxin is called a **toxoid**.

In order to improve vaccines, the antigenic component is often coupled with additional chemical agents that reduce the solubility of the vaccine, ensuring that the release of the active agent is slower (a **depot injection**) and with agents to increase the immunological response, i.e. **adjuvants**. Alum is often used to fulfil both criteria. Complexing the antigen with specific molecules may also specifically fulfil both roles, and such complexes are known as **ISCOMs** (**immunostimulatory complexes**).

It is usual for more than one dose of a vaccine to be required, as the first dose has a priming effect, leading to the production mainly of IgM, while subsequent booster doses lead to the rapid and persistent production of IgG (Fig. 18.2). Booster injections are usually given at intervals to enhance antibody production. In between injections, antibody production is maintained by the persistence of antigen on follicular dendritic cells in lymph nodes, which provide a continuing source of antigen for restimulation of T and B cells.

Genetic engineering has been used specifically to produce vaccines. Large viruses such as *Vaccinia* can be used as vectors to carry DNA for antigens of other microbes, which will then be transcribed and translated in the host cells to produce the antigen of interest and engender an appropriate immune response. Similarly, genetically modified *Salmonella* has been used to target antigens to mucosal macrophages. There is also interest in using purified DNA directly as a vaccine, adsorbed onto gold particles. On injection into muscle, rather than being degraded as one would expect, this may actually lead to production of specific proteins, leading to an immune response against the proteins.

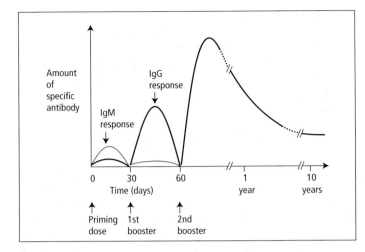

Figure 18.2 Immune response to immunization. The first dose primes the immune system and produces a response comprising mainly IgM. Subsequent doses produce high levels of IgG and retention of antigen within lymph nodes leading to long-term production of antibody through continued restimulation.

Immunization against infectious disease

There are many constraints on producing a successful vaccine against infectious disease. Effective vaccines will only be possible if there is a single strain of the virus or bacterium and there is no variation in the key antigens, or a single toxin. For example, there are over 80 strains of **Pneumococcus**, which can cause human disease, and developing a vaccine that can give complete protection is not possible. A compromise has to be accepted in vaccine production, such that the vaccine is targeted against the most common strains only, between 7 and 23 strains, depending on the vaccine. Likewise, **Influenza virus** changes its haemagglutinin (H) and neuraminidase (N) antigens each season in response to immunological selection pressure. Development of the annual vaccine is therefore based on predictions of the likely combinations of H and N antigens expected in the following winter, which may or may not be correct. In some cases, such as sleeping sickness (**trypanosomiasis**), the pathogen is capable of switching its coat proteins in direct response to the immune response, enabling it to escape from immune surveillance; this has made vaccine development impossible. The immune response must be protective rather than harmful and in some cases it has not proven possible to develop vaccines because the response produced is damaging. An example is

Table 18.2 Infectious diseases for which no satisfactory vaccines have yet been developed.

Human immunodeficiency virus (AIDS)
Human herpesvirus (EBV, CMV, HSV)
Rhinovirus (common cold)
Mycobacterium tuberculosis (TB)
Mycobacterium leprae (leprosy)
Vibrio cholerae (cholera)
All parasitic infections (malaria, trypanosomiasis, filariasis, schistosomiasis)

AIDS, acquired immunodeficiency virus; CMV, cytomegalovirus; EBV, Epstein–Barr virus; HSV, herpes simplex virus; TB, tuberculosis.

Neisseria meningitidis type B, where vaccines based on the type B polysaccharide induce autoimmunity in recipients because of similarities between polysaccharides of this meningococcal type and human cells. Some pathogens produce only poor immunity, such as **Mycobacterium tuberculosis**, and vaccine development is difficult. Table 18.2 identifies infectious diseases of worldwide importance for which no satisfactory vaccines have yet been developed.

One of the challenges to scientists in many diseases is that the key antigen against which protection is required is poorly immunogenic, i.e does not readily induce a suitable protective immune response. This is why the infection causes significant disease. The best example of this is the relatively poor response to polysaccharide antigens in children under the age of 2 years. This would normally be an IgG2 response. Organisims whose virulence factors include polysaccharide antigens, e.g. *Haemophilus influenzae* **type B (Hib)** and *Pneumococcus*, where there is a polysaccharide capsule, will thus readily cause disease in this age group and immunization with a pure polysaccharide does not lead to adequate protective immunity. Conjugation of the polysaccharide with a 'carrier' protein, e.g. tetanus toxoid or a diphtheria protein, increases the immunogenicity, and leads to the production of IgG1 antibodies against both the protein and polysaccharide. This is because such a conjugate facilitates the interaction of B cells and helper T cells (see p. 46 and Fig. 4.7). Thus, B cells that specifically bind the bacterial polysaccharides to their surface immunoglobulins will internalize and process the conjugated carrier protein, leading to the presentation of carrier peptides associated with HLA class II molecules on the surface of the B cells to elicit T cell help that stimulates the B cells to produce IgG1 antipolysaccharide antibodies. The introduction of conjugate vaccines for Hib has seen invasive Hib disease, epiglottitis and meningitis, disappear from the under 2-year-old population.

Successful immunization programmes are also dependent for their effect on the development of **herd immunity**, i.e. the development of immunity in the majority of a population at risk. The advantage of this is that it reduces or abolishes the circulation of the pathogen, as there are no susceptible hosts to maintain its life cycle. If the immunization levels can be maintained, then it is possible to eliminate a pathogen where humans are the sole host. The WHO sponsored programme of vaccination against **smallpox** led to the elimination of smallpox as a natural disease, although there remains concern about its potential use as a terrorist weapon now that the routine vaccination programmes have been halted. This success is not possible where there is a large animal reservoir for infection. Where immunization programmes are not kept up, then populations of susceptible individuals occur, and the disease can reappear. This

has been seen in the UK with whooping cough during the period of parental resistance to the vaccine, and after the collapse of communist Russia, where the decline in immunization against diphtheria has led to the reappearance of the disease.

Immunotherapy for cancer

There is great interest in the development of vaccines that will prevent or treat cancer. A major problem has been that the immune response to tumours is usually poor. Approaches have included vaccination against pathogens known to be implicated in tumorigenesis, such as **papillomaviruses** in cervical cancer, and the development, through genetic techniques, of vaccines against tumour-specific antigens, often coupled with genes for molecules such as IL-2, IL-6 and granulocyte–macrophage colony-stimulating factor (GM-CSF) which will stimulate the immune response.

Immunotherapy for allergy ('desensitization') and for autoimmune diseases

In diseases where tissue damage is caused by inappropriate immune responses to extrinsic or intrinsic antigens, i.e. the allergies and autoimmune diseases considered in Chapters 13 and 14, the aim of immunotherapy is to inhibit, rather than enhance, the immune response. This could involve attempting to re-establish lymphocyte nonresponsiveness (i.e. tolerance) to the stimulating allergens or autoantigens, boosting suppressive mechanisms (e.g. T_{Reg} cells; see p. 34), or diverting the immune response into less damaging pathways.

Allergic desensitization is a form of antigen-specific immunotherapy. Here purified allergen is injected subcutaneously on a weekly basis in increasing doses to patients with severe allergies. This leads to a reduction in clinical allergen reactivity that is specific for the allergen injected. The immunological mechanism for the reduction in reactivity is unknown, as allergen-specific IgE initially rises and then falls only slowly over 6–12 months. It is thought that IgG blocking antibodies, possibly of IgG4 class, may be involved although this remains controversial. Maintenance injections are usually continued at 4–6 weekly intervals for up to 3 years. This approach is used for severe allergic rhinoconjunctivitis caused by pollen, dust mite and animal exposure, and anaphylaxis to bee and wasp venom. Treatment of asthma is viewed as high risk (in the UK at least). Researchers are looking to develop safe vaccines for other causes of severe allergies such as peanut, shellfish and latex. Sublingual therapy is also being evaluated, although this appears to be slightly less effective and requires much higher antigen doses to achieve effects.

The goal for allergic immunotherapy is to develop allergy vaccines that are independent of the allergen, but this has not yet been achieved. The use of anti-IgE receptor monoclonal antibodies such as **omalizumab** may have potential in this respect and trials are under way.

Vaccination to modify autoimmune disease has been used in experimental animal systems and early clinical trials, e.g. in experimental autoimmune encephalomyelitis and multiple sclerosis, using either inactivated autoreactive T cells themselves as the vaccine or peptides derived from the T cell receptors of myelin basic protein-reactive T cells. Oral or parenteral administration of autoantigens has been performed in attempts to re-establish tolerance (eg. myelin basic protein in multiple sclerosis, collagen in rheumatoid arthritis and insulin in type 1 diabetes); however, despite encouraging results in animal models, trials in patients have given disappointing results.

Immunomodulatory therapy

In the previous chapter, a number of drugs were discussed for modulating the immune system in the context of transplantation. This is the sternest test of immunomodulation. The same drugs are also used, usually in lower doses, to modulate unwanted immune responses in the context of autoimmune disease. The mainstay of treatment of autoimmune disease is **corticosteroid** therapy, which has both immunomodulatory and anti-inflammatory properties.

Corticosteroids and other immunosuppressive drugs

Corticosteroids bind within the cell to high affinity glucocorticoid receptors and are transported to the nucleus where they have a direct effect on nuclear transcription through the production of IκBα, which inhibits the essential transcription factor NFκB. The effect is to prevent the production of essential cytokines and chemokines, reducing lymphocyte activation and proliferation. The effect is not antigen-specific. As well as the immunomodulatory effects on lymphocytes, corticosteroids also act on macrophages and neutrophils to reduce the inflammatory response, down-regulating the arachidonic acid and leukotriene pathways. At very high doses, corticosteroids are lymphocytotoxic. Corticosteroids have myriad side-effects, altering fat and glucose metabolism, suppressing adrenal function, causing osteoporosis and raising blood pressure. Other immunomodulatory drugs such as **methotrexate** (a folate antagonist which also inhibits the enzyme 5-aminoimidazole-4-carboxamide ribonucleotide transformylase), **azathioprine** (which interferes with nucleic acid synthesis), **ciclosporin** and **tacrolimus** (inhibitors of calcineurin) and **cyclophosphamide** (a lymphocytotoxic drug, which works by cross-linking DNA and preventing replication) are therefore combined with corticosteroids to reduce the dose of corticosteroid required.

Cytokines, interferons and colony-stimulating factors

Colony-stimulating factors (CSFs) have been used clinically for some time to treat the cytopenia associated with chemotherapy for malignant disease. In doses required to kill cancer cells, many drugs also lead to marked suppression of bone marrow, leading to severe neutropenia and consequent bacterial and fungal infection. The use of CSFs such as **GM-CSF** and granulocyte CSF (**G-CSF**) can abolish or reduce the neutropenia and have a beneficial effect in preventing secondary infection. They can also be used to treat rare primary immune deficiencies such as **cyclic neutropenia**, a disorder marked by cyclic drops in the neutrophil count every 21 ± 2 days.

α-Interferon (IFN-α) is used clinically as an antiviral agent as part of the treatment of **viral hepatitis**, particularly hepatitis C. Best results are obtained when it is used in combination with the antiviral drug ribavirin. IFN-α is also effective in treating the malignant B cells in patients with hairy cell leukaemia, although it has been superseded by even more effective drugs, such as **fludarabine**, which inhibit adenosine deaminase, and cause an iatrogenic ADA deficiency. It is also used in the treatment of Kaposi's sarcoma, a tumour caused by the herpesvirus **HHV-8**, in the context of HIV infection. **IFN-γ** is used as an adjunct to antibiotic therapy in the treatment of infections in **chronic granulomatous disease** (see p. 123). It is a potent immunostimulator, and can be used to increase the seroconversion rate to the hepatitis B virus vaccine in individuals who do not respond to the usual schedule of vaccination. It has also been used to improve immunity in patients with severe mycobacterial infection. **IFN-β** is used in the management of some cases of multiple sclerosis, although its full efficacy and its therapeutic mode of action are unclear.

In many instances, cytokines have been somewhat disappointing in clinical use. **IL-2** has been used as an adjunctive therapy in the treatment of renal tumours and melanoma, and it has also been used in HIV infection. However, in the latter case, the advent of combination chemotherapy, highly active antiretroviral therapy (**HAART**) has enabled virus production to be completely suppressed over long periods, which allows spontaneous immunological reconstitution to occur.

A new class of immunostimulatory drugs, which induce cytokine production and Th1-mediated responses, is represented by **imiquimod** which stimulates dendritic cells and macrophages by binding to toll-like receptor-7 (see p. 34). Imiquimod is licensed for the topical treatment of ano-genital warts caused by papillomavirus, and is proving effective against various types of skin cancer where its effects involve a combination of immunostimulation and direct induction of tumour cell apoptosis.

Monoclonal antibodies and soluble receptor molecules

Numerous mouse monoclonal antibodies that may have therapeutic effects in humans have been genetically modified to reduce the risk of a human antimouse antibody (**HAMA**) response in patients, without altering their antigenic specificities. **Chimaeric antibodies** are produced by linking the Fab regions of the mouse antibodies to a human immunoglobulin Fc region. In **humanized antibodies**, the hypervariable regions that form the antigen combining sites of the mouse antibodies (see p. 51 and Fig. 5.3) are grafted into human immunoglobulin heavy and light chain genes.

Inhibition of the effects of **TNF-α** using monoclonal antibodies (e.g. **infliximab**) has shown considerable promise as treatment for inflammatory bowel diseases such as **Crohn's disease** and also **rheumatoid arthritis**. It is also being used experimentally in other inflammatory autoimmune diseases. An alternative approach is to block the effects of TNF by using a **soluble TNF-receptor** fused to a human Fc fragment derived from IgG1 (**etanercept**). This has also been used in a similar range of diseases with positive benefit. Interestingly, the side-effects of this approach have been an increased risk of developing mycobacterial disease and also the production of autoantibodies. An **IL-1 receptor antagonist (anakinra)** has also been used in rheumatoid arthritis but, although of some benefit, the results have not been as exciting as had been hoped. The use of monoclonal antibody therapies against cytokines such as IL-4 in asthma has proven disappointing. It is likely that, because of immunological redundancy, combination biological therapy will be required to block the immune response.

Monoclonal antibodies have also been used in the management of malignant disease such as lymphoma (**rituximab**, an antibody against the B cell marker CD20) and breast cancer (**trastumab**, an antibody against the tumour antigen HER2), and have also been used in other fields of therapy.

Alemtuzumab (Campath-1H) is an antibody against the lymphocyte surface molecule CD52, and is used in the management of lymphoma, graft rejection, graft-versus-host disease and severe autoimmune disease. F(ab')$_2$ fragments of an antibody against digoxin, **digibind**, are used to treat acute digoxin toxicity, while **abciximab**, an antibody against the platelet glycoprotein receptor IIb/IIIa, is used in the management of unstable angina.

Experimental work is looking at the possibility of blocking the CD40–CD40L interaction (see p. 39) as a way of interfering with immune activation both in transplantation and in the treatment of autoimmune disease. CTLA4 has been produced as a soluble fusion protein that can be used to inhibit the CD28–B7 co-stimulatory interaction for T cell activation (see p. 34), but the therapeutic effects in humans have been disappointing. A humanized monoclonal antibody, **natalizumab**, specific for the α chain of the $α_4β_1$ integrin VLA-4 (see p. 101) blocks the interaction of lymphocytes and macrophages with vascular cell adhesion molecule-1 (VCAM-1) expressed by activated endothelium at sites of inflammation; this antibody reduces the formation of brain lesions in multiple sclerosis and causes clinical improvements in Crohn's disease.

Anti-inflammatory and antiallergic therapy

Corticosteroids are the most potent anti-inflammatory dugs but because of their side-effects other drugs are required to manage non-life-threatening inflammatory processes.

Non-steroidal anti-inflammatory drugs

Prostaglandins (PG) and leukotrienes are important inflammatory mediators. PGE_2 causes vasodilatation and bronchodilatation, while $PGF_{2α}$ cases bronchoconstriction. Leukotrienes have very similar effects to histamine, causing vasodilatation, increased vascular permeability and hypotension.

The non-steroidal anti-inflammatory drugs (NSAIDs) work by inhibition of the enzyme **cyclo-oxygenase** (COX) to prevent the production of prostaglandins from arachidonic acid (see p. 80 and Fig. 8.3). COX exists in two forms: COX-1, which is constitutively expressed in many tissues and is involved in the protection of the stomach; and the inducible COX-2, which is the enzyme found in macrophages. Older drugs such as **aspirin** are non-selective inhibitors, but newer drugs such as **celecoxib** are more selective inhibitors of COX-2, and work preferentially on inflammatory cells while leaving the gastric protective mechanism unaffected. These drugs are used, for example, in treating inflammatory autoimmune diseases of the joints such as rheumatoid arthritis.

Drugs that interfere with the inflammatory effects of leukotrienes include drugs that block their production by the inhibition of **lipo-oxygenase** (see p. 80 and Fig. 8.4), such as **zileuton**, and drugs that block the cysteinyl-leukotriene receptors, such as **monteleukast** and **zafirlukast**. These drugs are used as adjunctive therapy in the management of asthma and more recently in the management of urticaria, in combination with antihistamines.

Antiallergic drugs

The mainstay of antiallergic therapy is the use of antihistamines, which block the **H$_1$-histamine receptors** on blood vessels and smooth muscle. Older drugs such as **chlorphenamine** readily cross the blood–brain barrier and cause marked sedation, but have weak antihistaminic activity. Newer drugs such as **cetirizine** and **fexofenadine** do not readily cross the blood–brain barrier and therefore do not cause the same degree of sedation. They are more potent blocking agents and have long durations of action. H_2 receptors are found mainly in the stomach and are involved in control of gastric acid production, but play little part in allergic disease.

Drugs that interfere with histamine release from mast cells are also used; these include the **membrane stabilizers** such as **sodium cromoglicate**. These drugs tend not to be soluble and are therefore not adsorbed from the gut. They can only be used topically in the eye, nose and lung. Drugs that block cellular calcium channels, such as nifedipine or verapamil, will also block histamine release, although such drugs, which are mainly used for control of hypertension, are used only rarely in the therapy of allergic disease.

Key points

1 Passive immunotherapy can supply transient immunity, without producing long-term immunological memory. It is used in the long term to protect patients unable to make antibody of their own, or to replace missing factors such as C1-esterase inhibitor.

2 Active immunotherapy can produce long-lasting effects on the immune system and can be targeted to both T and B cells. It can be combined with passive immunotherapy to provide immediate protection.

3 Immunomodulation can be achieved using drugs such as corticosteroids, and cytotoxic drugs. Monoclonal antibodies, soluble receptors and fusion proteins can all be used to manipulate the immune system.

4 Anti-inflammatory drugs target the cyclo-oxygenase and lipo-oxygenase pathways.

5 Long-acting non-sedating antihistamines are the mainstay of allergy therapy.

Index

Page numbers in **bold** represent tables, those in *italics* represent figures.

abciximab 188
accessory cells *see* antigen-presenting cells
acid hydrolases 75
acquired immune deficiency syndrome *see* AIDS
activation *9*, 100
activation-induced cell death 35
active immunotherapy 182–6
acute lymphoblastic leukaemia 160
acute myeloblastic leukaemia 160–1
acute phase proteins **103**
acute phase response 102–3, *103*
adaptive immunity 5–6
  features of 6–7, *7*
Addison's disease 103, 133, **134**
addressins 43
adenosine deaminase 115
adhesion 84–5, 100
adhesion molecules *see* cell adhesion molecules
adjuvants 183
adrenal hyperplasia, congenital **153**
adult T-cell lymphoma/leukaemia 164
aetiological fraction 154
afferent lymphatics 41, *42*, 43
affinity 15, 52–3
affinity maturation 47
agglutination *61*
AIDS 3, 107–11
  clinical features 107
  epidemiology 107–8, **108**
  immunology 109–10
  management 110–11
  prevention 111
  virology 108–9, *109*
AIDS-related complex 107
AIRE (autoimmune regulator) gene 33, 117
alemtuzumab 188
allelic exclusion 58–9
allergens 131
allergic alveolitis **132**, *146*
allergic asthma 131, 145
  see also lung disease

allergic conjunctivitis 131
allergic rhinitis 131
allergy 12, 106, 131
  antiallergic drugs 188–9
  immunotherapy 185–6
alloantigens *172*
allotypes 53
alpha chain disease 167
alpha$_1$-acid glycoprotein 102
alpha$_1$-antichymotrypsin 102
alpha$_1$-antitrypsin 102
alpha$_1$-antitrypsin deficiency 182
alveolitis
  extrinsic (allergic) **132**, *146*
  intrinsic (cryptogenic) 147
Am system 53
amyloidosis **168**
anaemia
  autoimmune haemolytic 142
  pernicious 133, **134**, **153**
anakinra 187
anaphylaxis 131, 140–1
anaphylatoxins 65, 73, 77, 97
anaplastic large-cell lymphoma 163
anergy 30
angioimmunoblastic T-cell lymphoma 164
ankylosing spondylitis **153**
anti-GBM disease 133
anti-idiotype antibodies 52, 135
anti-inflammatory therapy 188–9
antiallergic drugs 188–9
antibodies **5**, 6
  anti-idiotype 52, 135
  autoanti-idiotype 177
  autoantibodies 135
  chimaeric 187
  humanized 176, 187
  idiotype 52, 135
  monoclonal 4, 61–2, 187–8
antibody diversity **58**
antibody-dependent cellular cytotoxicity 87, 145
antigens 6, 14
  autoantigens **130**, 133–8
  exposure to 14–15
  microbial 128–30, *129*, **130**
  nature of 14

non-microbial **130**, 131–3, **131**, **132**
  sequestered 137
  T-independent B-cell 135
  unidentified 138–9
antigen combining sites 15, 51–2, *52*
antigen determinants 15
antigen processing 19, 22–4, *22*, *23*, *24*
antigen receptors 15–17
antigen recognition 14–27
  B and T cells 17–19, *18*, *19*
antigen shedding 98
antigen-presenting cells 10, *18*, 19, 22–4, *22*, *23*, *24*, 144
antigenic determinant 51
antigenic variation/drift 98
antihistamines 188
antilymphocyte globulin 176
antimicrobial chemotherapy 105
antithymocyte globulin 176
antiviral state 11
APECED 117
apoptosis 29, 85, 87
appendix 41
arachidonic acid 78, 79
Arthus phenomenon 144
aspirin 188
associative recognition 19, 170
ataxia telangiectasia 117
atopic dermatitis 131
atopic disease 131, 150–2, **151**
atopic trait 131, 150
attachment inhibition 99
attenuation 183
atypical mononuclear cells 160
autoanti-idiotype antibodies 177
autoantibodies 135
autoantigens **130**, 133–8
autoimmune disease **134**
  immunotherapy 185–6
autoimmune haemolytic anaemia 142
autoimmunity 12, 106
  induction of 135–8, **135**, *136*
autologous transplantation 179–80
avidity 52–3

azathioprine 175
azurocidin 75
azurophilic lysosomal granules 71

B cells **5**, 6, 28
  activation and maturation
    30–1, *30*, *46*, *47*
  antigen receptors 15–17
  antigen recognition 17–19, *18*,
    19
  development 28–30, *29*
B cell deficiencies 118–20
  transient
    hypogammaglobulinaemia of
    infancy 120
  X-linked
    hypogammaglobulinaemia
    118–20
B cell hybridomas 61–2, *62*
B cell-specific tyrosine kinase 119
B lymphoblasts 164
B-1 cells 30–1
B-2 cells 31
B-ALL cells 160
Bacillus anthracis 99
bacteria **95**
bacterial lysis 9
bagassosis **132**
bare lymphocyte syndrome 115
basic cationic proteins 75
basophils **5**, 77–83
  triggering of 77–8, **78**
Bence Jones protein 165
Berger's disease 148
beta-glucuronidase *72*, 78, *79*, *82*
beta₂-microglobulin 20, 25, 98,
  168
biliary cirrhosis **134**
biological recognition systems
  7–8
biphasic reaction 140
bird fancier's lung **132**
blood transfusion effect 177
bone marrow 9
bone marrow transplantation
  178–80
  autologous 179–80
  graft-versus-host disease 178–9
  indications **179**
  laundering 179
  purging 179
bone pain 165
Bordetella pertussis 99
Brucella abortus 99
Bruton's disease 118–19
Burkitt's lymphoma 163
burns 127

C-reactive protein **5**, 102
C1 esterase inhibitor 65

C3 convertase 65–7, *66*, *67*
C3 receptor 65
C3 receptor deficiency 75
C4-binding protein 65
caeruloplasmin 103
calcium channels 78
calor 128
calreticulin 23
cancer immunotherapy 185
Candida albicans 99
carrier effect 135, *136*
catalase 74
cathepsins 24, 75
cationic proteins 82
CD proteins **21**
CD1 34
CD3 31, 115
CD4 21, 31
CD5 30
CD8 21, 31
CD45 115
CD94/NKG2A 86
cell adhesion molecules 100, 101
cell-reactive tissue damage 142–3
central tolerance 31
centroblasts 46
centrocytes 46
cetirizine 188
Chagas' disease 134
Charcot-Leyden crystals 82
Chédiak-Higashi syndrome 118,
  122, 123
cheese worker's lung **132**
chemokines **5**, 37, 73
chemotactic factors 78
chemotaxis 9, 72–3, 100
  inhibition of 99
chimaeric antibodies 187
chlorphenamine 188
chondroitin sulphate 79
chorea 129
chromium release assay 48–9
chromosomal translocations 159
chronic granulomatous disease
  75, 123–4, 187
chronic inflammatory diseases
  105
chronic lymphocytic leukaemia
  161, 163
chronic mucocutaneous
  candidiasis 117
chronic myeloid leukaemia 162
ciclosporin 175
class II expression 137
CLIP peptide 24
clonal deletion 133
clonal inhibition 133
clonal selection 17, *18*, 58–9
clone 17
Clostridium perfringens 99

coeliac disease 132, **153**
collectins **5**, 65, 73
common gamma chain 115
common variable
  immunodeficiency 119–20,
  182
complement **5**, 8, 9, 64–70, 156
  activation *65*
  activation inhibitors **68**
  alternative pathway 67–8, *68*
  classical pathway 64–7, *65–7*
  inactivation 99
  inadequate regulation of
    activation 69
  lectin pathway 64–7, *65–7*
  membrane attack pathway
    68–9, *69*
  polymorphisms and deficiencies
    70
complement deficiencies 124–6,
  125
  hereditary angio-oedema 69,
    124, 125–6
complement fixation *61*
complement receptors 9
complement resistance 98
complementarity-determining
  regions 51
congenital adrenal hyperplasia
  153
constant domains 16, 51
contact dermatitis 132
contact hypersensitivity 148
Coombs' test 143
corticosteroids 186
cowpox 4
CR1 73
CR3 73
CR4 73
Creutzfeldt-Jakob disease, variant
  182
Crohn's disease 138, 187
cross-presentation 24
cross-priming 24
cross-reaction 15, *16*
cryoglobulinaemia 167–8
  types of **167**
cryoglobulins 163, 164, 167
cryptogenic alveolitis 147
CTLA-4 35
cyclic neutropenia 187
cyclooxygenase 79, *80*, 188
cystic fibrosis 127
cytokines **5**, 10, 34, 37, 80, 97
  functions **38**
  immunotherapy 186–7
  inhibition of 99
  production by T-lymphocytes
    37–40, **38**, *39*, *40*
  T helper cell activation *45*

cytomegalovirus 98
cytotoxic T cells (Tc cells) **5**, 11,
    19, 33
    target cell recognition 84–5, *85*
    see also killer cells
cytotoxicity 98
cytotoxins **5**

defence 4–5, **5**, 10–11, *11*
    against infection 93–8, *94*,
        95–6
    immunological 10–11, *11*
defensins **5**, 71, 75
deficiency disorders 75
delayed type hypersensitivity
    144–5, 147
dendritic cells **5**, 10, 172
depot injection 183
dermatitis herpetiformis 132,
    147, *148*, **153**
dermatomyositis **134**
desensitization 185–6
diabetes mellitus **134**, **153**
differentiation markers 48
diffuse large B-cell lymphoma 163
DiGeorge syndrome 116
digestion 9
    resistance to 99
digibind 188
direct recognition 172
    HLA-dominant 173
    peptide-dominant 172–3
disguise 98
dolor 128
domains 16, 50–1, *52*
double diffusion 60
dual recognition *see* associative
    recognition
Duncan syndrome 118, 160

ECF 81
eczema 127
effector systems, triggering of
    55–6
efferent lymphatics 41, 44
eicosanoids **5**
elastase 75
ELISA *61*
endocytosis 23
endosomes 23
enhancement 4, 177
enteric fever 130
eosinophils **5**, 80–3
    Fc receptors **73**
    inflammatory products **83**
    products 81–3, *82*, **83**
    properties **80**
eosinophil cationic protein 97
eosinophil peroxidase 81
eosinophilia, pulmonary 138

epitopes 15, 51
Epstein-Barr virus 99, 160
equivalence 60
erythema nodosum 130
erythrocyte sedimentation rate
    103
etanercept 187
evasion *96*, 98–9, 105
exons 56
extended haplotype 154

Fab fragments 50
fabulation 98
factor H 65
factor I 65
farmer's lung **132**, 146
Fas 35, 87
Fas-ligand 35, 87
favism 132
Fc binding 98–9
Fc receptors 73, 77
fever 102
fexofenadine 188
fine needle aspiration biopsy
    174–5
flow cytometer 48
fluorescence-activated cell sorter
    48
follicles 41, *42*
follicular dendritic cells *42*, 46
follicular lymphoma 163
food allergy 131
frustrated phagocytosis 75
fungi **95**
fusagenic lipids 78

gastritis 130
genome nomenclature 155
genotype 154–6
germinal centres 41, *42*, *43*, 46
Ghon focus 147
glomerulonephritis 129
glucocorticoid release 103
Gm system 53
Goodpasture's syndrome **134**,
    142, *146*, 148, **153**
Good's syndrome 120
graft rejection 170–8
    acute 173
    afferent limb 171–3, *172*
    allograft response 174–5
    blood transfusion effect 177
    chronic 173
    efferent limb 173
    HLA typing and matching
        173–4
    hyperacute 173
    induction of *171*
    non-specific
        immunosuppression 175–6

recurrent and transferred
    disease 177–8
selection and preparation of
    recipient 174
source and preparation of graft
    174
specific immunosuppression
    176–7, *176*
graft-versus-host disease 115,
    178–9
granulocyte colony-stimulating
    factor 180
    immunotherapy 186–7
granulocytes 5
granzymes **5**, 87
Graves' disease **134**, **153**
gut-associated lymphoid tissue
    (GALT) *43*

HAART therapy 110–11, 187
haemolytic-uraemic syndrome
    69, 124
Haemophilus influenzae 98, 99,
    185
haplotype 154–6
haptoglobin 103
Hashimoto's thyroiditis **134**, **153**
Hassall's corpuscles 31
Heaf test 147
heavy chain disease 168
Helicobacter pylori 130, 163
helminths **95**
helper T cells *see* T helper cells (Th
    cells)
heparin 79
hepatitis 129, 187
herd immunity 185
hereditary angio-oedema 69, 124,
    125–6, 182
herpes simplex 99
herpesvirus 187
high endothelial cells 43
histamine **5**, 78
histocompatibility 170
HIV *see* AIDS
HLA 170
HLA expression 99
HLA matching 173–4
HLA system 19–26
    antigen processing and antigen-
        presenting cells 22–4, *22*, *23*,
        24
    HLA genes 25
    HLA molecules 19, 20–2, *20*, *21*
    polymorphism 25–6
HLA typing 173–4
HLA-A 173
HLA-B 173
HLA-DM 24
HLA-DR 173

HLA-G 87
HLA-related disease 152–6, **153**
  mechanisms of association
    155–6
  strength of associations 154
Hodgkin's disease 162
horror autotoxicus 133
host-pathogen interface 105–6,
    106
host-versus-graft disease 178
HTLV-1 164
human leucocyte antigen *see* HLA
humanized antibodies 176, 187
hydrogen peroxide 74
hydroxyl radical 74
hygiene hypothesis 151
hyper-IgE syndrome 123
hyper-IgM syndrome 117–18
hypercalcaemia 165
hypereosinophilic syndrome 83
hypersensitivity 12, 106
hypervariable regions 51
hyperviscosity 164
hyperviscosity syndrome 163
hypogammaglobulinaemias
    118–20
  Good's syndrome 120
  transient of infancy 120
  X-linked 118–20
hypohalite 74

idiopathic haemochromatosis
    153
idiopathic thrombocytopenic
    purpura 142
idiotype antibodies 52, 135
imiquimod 187
immature B cells 29
immediate hypersensitivity 146
immediate (type I)
    hypersensitivity 140–2
immobilization 9, 100
immune adherence 65, **69**, 73
immune complex disease 125,
    152
immune complex-mediated tissue
    damage 143–4
immune complexes 46, 60
  solubilization 68
immune reactions, types of 130
immune response 8–10
  regulation of 103
immune response genes 155
immunity 3
immunization 105, 184–5, **184**
immunodeficiency 12, 105
immunodeficiency disorders
    112–27, *113*
  B-cell deficiencies 118–20
  clues to 112

complement deficiencies
    124–6
  immunoglobulin deficiencies
    120–1
  investigation of 112, 114
  mediator defects 118
  natural killer cell defects 118
  phagocyte defects 121–4
  primary or secondary
    immunodeficiency 114
  secondary forms 126–7
  severe combined
    immunodeficiency **115**
  T-cell deficiencies 116–18
  thymic hypoplasia 116
immunodiffusion *60*
immunoelectrophoresis 61
immunofixation *166*
immunofluorescence *61*
immunogenicity 14–15
  exposure to antigen 14–15
  nature of antigen 14
  nature of recipient 15
  receptor-antigen interactions
    15
immunogens 14
immunoglobulins **5**, 6, 50–63
  affinity and avidity 52–3, *53*
  antigen combining site 51–2,
    52
  classes 17, 29, 53–4, *53*, *54*
  cleavage 98
  component deficiencies 121
  deficiencies 120–1
  exploiting properties of 59–62,
    60–2
  genes 56–9
  physical and biological
    characteristics **53**
  structure 50–3, *51*
  superfamily *16*, 51
  triggering of effector systems
    55–6
  variable and constant domains
    50–1, *52*
immunoglobulin alpha 30
immunoglobulin beta 30
immunoglobulin A 54–5
  cell/membrane-reactive tissue
    damage 142–3
  deficiency 121
  myeloma **165**
  nephropathy 148
immunoglobulin D 55
  myeloma **165**
immunoglobulin E 55
  myeloma **165**
immunoglobulin G 54
  cell/membrane-reactive tissue
    damage 142–3

deficiency 120–1
  myeloma **165**
immunoglobulin M 55
  cell/membrane-reactive tissue
    damage 142–3
  deficiency 121
  monoclonal 164
  myeloma **165**
immunological defence strategies
    10–11, *11*
immunological disease 140–9,
    141, *142–3*, **151**
  susceptibility to 150–7
  type I 140–2
  type II 142–3
  type III 143–4
  type IV 144–5
immunological synapse *34*, 35
immunological tolerance 4, 14,
    177
immunomodulation 186–8
immunopathology 12, 128
immunoregulation, impaired 137
immunoselection 167
immunostimulatory complexes
    (ISCOMs) 183
immunosuppression
  non-specific 175–6
  specific 176–7, *176*
immunotherapy 181–9
  active 182–6
  anti-inflammatory and
    antiallergic 188–9
  immunomodulation 186–8
  passive 181–2, *182*
infection
  defence against 93–8, *94*, **95–6**
  diagnosis of 103–4, **104**
  host-pathogen interface 105–6,
    106
  mechanisms of evasion 98–9
  non-immunological conditions
    predisposing to 126–7, **127**
  opportunistic 104–5, **105**
  systemic response to 101–2,
    102
  as trigger of autoimmunity
    133–4, **134**
  see also inflammatory response;
    and various diseases
infectious mononucleosis 160
inflammation 9, **69**, 128
inflammatory response 97,
    99–103
  acute phase response 102–3,
    103
  coordination of **102**
  fever 102
  glucocorticoid release 103
  leucocytosis 102

inflammatory response (cont'd)
  molecular basis 100–1, *101*
  regulation of 103
  systemic response to infection
    101–2, **102**
infliximab 187
Influenza 184
inheritance *155*
innate immunity 5–6
integrins 43, 44, 101, 122
intercellular adhesion molecule-1
    (ICAM-1) 84
interdigitating dendritic cells *42*
interference 97
interferons **5**, 11, **88**
  cooperation with killer cells
    88–9
  immunotherapy 186–7
interferon-alpha 187
interferon-beta 187
interferon-gamma 37, 187
interleukin receptor antagonists
    187
interleukins **5**, 37
  functions **38**
  immunotherapy 187
  see also cytokines
intermediate hypersensitivity 146
intracellular calcium 78
intraepithelial lymphocytes 41,
    43
introns 56
invariant chain protein 24
IPEX 137
isotype 53
isotype switching 59

J chains 54, 55
JAK-3 kinase 115
Jenner, Edward 3–4, 182–3
Job's syndrome 123

Kaposi's sarcoma 109
Kartagener's syndrome 127
keratoconjunctivitis sicca 133
kidney disease 148–9
killer cell immunoglobulin-like
    receptors 86
killer cells 84–9
  cooperation with interferons
    88–9
  cytotoxic T cells (Tc cells) **5**, 11,
    19, 33, 84
  membrane ligands 87–8
  natural killer cells **5**, 11, 25, 84
  secreted proteins 87
  target cell recognition 84–7, *85*,
    86
killing, resistance to 99
Km system 53

lactoferrin 75
lamina propria 41, *43*
Langerhans' cells 45, 144
large granular lymphocytes *see*
    natural killer cells
laudable pus 71
laundering 179
lectin pathway 64–7, *65–7*
left shift 102, 122
lens-induced uveitis 133
leprosy 129
lethal hit 85
leucocyte adhesion deficiency
    122–3
leucocytosis 102
leucotrienes **5**
leukaemias 160–2, **161**
leukotrienes 73, 79, *80*
light chain disease 165
linkage disequilibrium 154
lipoxygenase 79, 188
lung disease 145–7, *146*
  see also allergic asthma
lymph nodes 9, 41, *42*
lymphadenopathy 107, 158–9,
    159
lymphoblasts *29*, 30
lymphocyte transformation test
    48
lymphocytes
  activation 99
  isolation and identification 48
  recirculation and homing 43–5,
    44
  selection and maturation 45–8
  stimulation 48–9
  suppression 99
  see also B cells; T cells
lymphocytic choriomeningitis
    128, *129*
lymphocytic lymphoma 163
lymphocytosis 102, 158–9, *159*
lymphoid ablation 126–7
lymphoid stem cells 5
lymphoid system 41–3
lymphomas 162–4
lymphoproliferative disease 12,
    158–69
  amyloidosis **168**
  cryoglobulinaemia 167–8, *167*
  Epstein-Barr virus and
    infectious mononucleosis
    160
  leukaemias 160–2, **161**
  lymphocytosis and
    lymphadenopathy 158–9,
    159
  lymphomas 162–4
  monoclonal gammopathies
    164–7, **165**, **166**

viruses and oncogenes 159–60
lysis 9, *61*, 97
  bacterial 9
  osmotic 85, 87
  reactive 69
lysosomal digestion 97
lysozyme 75
lytic enzymes **5**

M cells 41
macroglobulinaemia 158, 164–5
macrophages **5**, *8*, 9, 71, *72*
  Fc receptors **73**
macropinocytosis 24
major basic protein 82
major histocompatibility complex
    19, 170
MALT *see* mucosa-associated
    lymphoid tissue
malt worker's disease **132**
maltoma 163
mannan-binding lectin **5**, 65
mannose-binding lectin 124
Mantoux test 147
mast cells **5**, 9, 77–80
  degranulation 77
  inflammatory products **83**
  properties **80**
  triggering of 77–8, **78**
mast cell mediators 78–80
  cytokines 80
  preformed 78–9
  secondary 79–80
measles 130
mediator defects 118
medulla 44
membrane attack complex 9, 68
membrane attack pathway 64,
    68–9, *69*
membrane ligands 87–8
membrane stabilizers 188
membrane-reactive tissue damage
    142–3
membranous glomerulonephritis
    149
membranous nephropathy 139,
    153
memory 6
memory lymphocytes 10
memory population 30
MHC *see* major histocompatibility
    complex
MHC class IB genes *25*
MICA 87
MICB 87
microbial antigens 128–30, *129*,
    130
microlymphocytotoxicity 153
minor histocompatibility antigens
    173

mitogens 30
mixed connective tissue disease **134**
mixed essential cryoglobulinaemia 168
mixed lymphocyte culture 171, *172*
molecular mimicry 136, 156
monoclonal antibodies 4, 61–2, 187–8
monoclonal gammopathy 164–7, **165**, **166**
　heavy chain disease 168
　macroglobulinaemia 158, 164–5
　myeloma 158, 164, 165–6, **165**, *166*
　of uncertain significance 166–7
monoclonal response 59
monocytes **5**
mononuclear cells 5
mononuclear phagocyte system 71
monteleukast 188
mucins 44, 101
mucosa-associated lymphoid tissue (MALT) 9, 28, 41, 43
multiple sclerosis **134**, **153**
mushroom worker's lung **132**
myasthenia gravis 133, **134**
Mycobacterium leprae **40**, 99, 129
Mycobacterium tuberculosis 99, 184
mycophenolate mofetil 176
mycosis fungoides 161, 163
myeloid stem cells 5, *159*, 161
myeloma 158, 164, 165–6, **165**, *166*
myeloma kidney 166
myeloperoxidase 74

naive helper T cells (Th0) 12
narcolepsy **153**
nasal polyps 138
natalizumab 188
natural killer cells **5**, 11, 25
　characteristics **85**
　defects 118
　target cell recognition 85–7, *86*
　see also killer cells
nef protein 110
Neisseria gonorrhoeae 98
Neisseria meningitidis 184
nephritic factor 69
neutrophil polymorphs 71
neutrophils **5**, 9, 71–2, *72*
　Fc receptors **73**
　properties **80**
nitric oxide 75
NOD2 protein 138
non-Hodgkin's lymphoma 162–4

non-microbial antigens **130**, 131–3, **131**, **132**
non-specific immunosuppression 175–6
non-steroidal anti-inflammatory drugs 188
Notch pathway 39

oligoclonal response 59
omalizumab 186
Omenn syndrome 115
oncogenes 159–60
opportunistic infection 104–5, **105**
opsonization 9, 68, 73, 97, 183
osmotic lysis 85, 87
oxidative killing 97

palivizumab 182
PAMPs see pathogen-associated molecular patterns
panning 48
papillomavirus 185
paracortex 41
paroxysmal cold haemoglobinuria 133
paroxysmal nocturnal haemoglobinuria 69
passenger leucocytes 172
passive immunotherapy 181–2, *182*
pathogen-associated molecular patterns (PAMPs) 6, **34**, 38
pathogens **95**, **96**
pattern recognition receptors 6
pemphigoid 133, **134**, 142, 147
pemphigus 133, **134**, 142, 147
pentraxins **5**, 73
perforins **5**, 87
periarteriolar lymphoid sheath 41
peripheral stem cell transfusion 179–80
pernicious anaemia 133, **134**, **153**
Peyer's patches 41, *43*
phagocytes 9, 71–6
　chemotaxis 72–3
　defects 121–4
　deficiency disorders 75
　ingestion *73*, *74*
　killing and degradation 74–5
　macrophages **5**, 8, 9, 71, *72*
　neutrophils **5**, 9, 71–2, *72*
　polymorphism 156
　target recognition 73–4, *73*
　toxicity 99
phagocytosis 183
　inhibition of 99
　see also phagocytes
phagolysosome 74

phagosome-lysosome fusion inhibition 99
phagosomes, escape from 99
phenotype 154–6
Philadelphia chromosome 160, 162
Pierrepont, Lady Mary 3
plasma cells 10, 30, 164
Plasmodium falciparum 98
platelet-activating factors 72, 80
pluripotent stem cells 28, *159*, 162
Pneumococcus 184, 185
Pneumocystis carinii 111
pneumonia 129
polyclonal B-cell stimulators 135
polyclonal response 59
polymorphism 20, 25–6
　complement 70
polymorphonuclear leucocytes 5
postcapillary venules *42*
pre-B cells 29
　receptors 29
prednisolone 175
premunition 98
primary lymphoid organs 9, 28
primary response 6, *7*
prions 182
privileged sites 171
professional antigen-presenting cells 23
prostaglandins **5**
proteinase G 75
protozoa **95**
PRRs see pattern recognition receptors
Pseudomonas aeruginosa 99
pulmonary eosinophilia 138
pulmonary tuberculosis 129, 147
purging 179
purine nucleoside phosphorylase deficiency 116

22q11 deletion syndromes 116

rabies 182
radial immunodiffusion 61
radioimmunoassay *61*
RAST test 131, 141
Raynaud's phenomenon 165
reactive lysis 69
receptor editing 30, 59
receptor interaction 156
receptor-antigen interactions 15
recognition 4–5, 5, 84–5, *85*, *86*
recombination activating genes (RAGs) 57, 115
Reed-Sternberg cells 162
regulatory T cells 34
Reiter's syndrome 130

rejection *see* graft rejection
relative risk 154
respiratory syncytial virus 130
reticular dysgenesis 115
rheumatic fever 129
rheumatoid arthritis 133, **134**, **153**, 187
rituximab 187
rofecoxib 188
rosetting 48, *49*
rubor 128

Samter's triad 138
sarcoidosis 138, 147
Schistosoma mansoni 98
Schulzberger-Chase phenomenon 15
Schwachman's syndrome **122**, 123
scleritis 130
second set reaction 173
secondary immunodeficiency **126**
secondary lymphoid organs 9, *10*, 28, 41
secondary response 6, *7*
secondary specific granules 72
secretory piece 54, 55
selectins 43, 100
self-discrimination *7*
self-ignorance 136
sequestration 98
serprocidins 71, 75
serum sickness 131, 144
severe combined immunodeficiency **115**
Sézary's syndrome 161, 163
sicca syndrome **153**
singlet oxygen 74
Sjögren's disease 133
skin disease 147-8, *148*
skin prick test 131
SLAM-associated protein 118, 160
slow reacting substance 72, 78, 79
smallpox 3-4, 185
sodium cromoglycate 78, 188
somatic mutation 46, 58
specific immunosuppression 176-7, *176*
specificity 6, 15
spleen 9, 41, *43*
standard quantitative precipitation test 59, *60*
Staphylococcus aureus 98, 99
Streptococcus pneumoniae 98, 99
subacute bacterial endocarditis 135
subcapsular sinus 41, *42*, 43
suberosis **132**
superoxide anion 74
superoxide dismutase 74

syphilis 129
systemic lupus erythematosus 133, **134**, 148, **153**
systemic sclerosis **134**

T cells 6, 28
  antigen receptors 15-17
  antigen recognition 17-19, *18*, *19*
  autoreactive 138
  cytokine production by 37-40, **38**, **39**, *40*
  development and education 31-3, *32*, *33*
  receptor for antigen *16*, 17
  receptor genes 59
  subpopulations 33-5, *34*
T cell deficiencies 116-18
  ataxia telangiectasia 117
  chronic mucocutaneous candidiasis 117
  hyper-IgM syndrome 117-18
  purine nucleoside phosphorylase deficiency 116
  Wiskott-Aldrich syndrome 116-17
T cell lymphoma 161
T helper cells (Th cells) **5**, 11, 19, 33, 37, **39**
T-ALL cells 160
T-independent B-cell antigens 135
T-suppressor cells 177
tapasin 25
target cells 19, 22, 84
  death 85
  recognition 84-7, *85*, *86*
Tc cells *see* cytotoxic T lymphocytes
TCR *see* T-cell receptor for antigen
tetanus 182
tetrahydrobiopterin 75
Th cells *see* T helper cells
Th0 cells *see* naive helper T cells
Th1 cells 12
Th2 cells 12, 37, **39**
thoracic duct *42*, *43*, 44
thymic hypoplasia 116
thymocytes 31
thymoma 120
thymus 9
thymus-dependent responses 30
thymus-independent responses 30
TI-1 antigens 30
TI-2 antigens 30
tickover C3 conversion 68
Tine test 147
tissue-specific antigens 32-3
titre 6
TNFR1 receptor 87

tolerogens 14
Toll-like receptors 34
tonsils 41
total allergy syndrome 133
toxic granulation 102
toxoids 183
Toxoplasma gondii 99
transforming growth factor-beta 39
transient hypogammaglobulinaemia of infancy 120, 181
transplantation 170-80
  bone marrow 178-80
  histocompatibility systems 170
  rejection 170-8
trastumab 187
Treponema pallidum 134
Trypanosoma cruzi 98, 99, 134, 136
trypanosomiasis 98, 184
tumor 128
tumour necrosis factors **5**, 37, 87, 187
two-dimensional immunoelectrophoresis 61
typhoid fever 130

ulcerative colitis 139
uveitis 133, 138

vaccination 3-4, 183
Vaccinia 183
valency 53
variable domains 16, 51
variolation 3-4, 183
vascular addressins 43
vascular permeability 9, 100
vasculitis 138, 144
vasodilatation 9, 100
V(D)J recombinase 57
ventilator pneumonitis **132**
viruses **95**, 159-60

Waldenström's macroglobulinaemia 163
Wiskott-Aldrich syndrome 116-17

X-linked agammaglobulinaemia 118-19, 182
X-linked lymphoproliferative syndrome 118, 160

Yersinia pestis 99

zafirlukast 188
ZAP-70 115
zileuton 188